Evidence-based practice
in speech pathology

Evidence-based practice in speech pathology

Edited by

SHEENA REILLY

Professor of Paediatric Speech Pathology,
School of Human Communication Sciences
La Trobe University
The Royal Children's Hospital
Murdoch Childrens Research Institute
Melbourne
Australia

JACINTA DOUGLAS

Senior Lecturer
School of Human Communication Sciences
La Trobe University
Melbourne
Australia

JENNI OATES

Associate Professor
School of Human Communication Sciences
La Trobe University
Melbourne
Australia

W
WHURR PUBLISHERS
LONDON AND PHILADELPHIA

First published 2004 by
Whurr Publishers Ltd
19b Compton Terrace, London N1 2UN

Reprinted 2004 and 2005

British Library Cataloguing in Publication Data

A catalogue record for this book is available from the British
Library.

ISBN 1 86156 320 5

Printed and bound in the UK by Athenaeum Press Limited,
Gateshead, Tyne & Wear.

Contents

Contributors

Stacey Baldac
School of Human Communication Sciences
La Trobe University
Melbourne
Australia

Sandy Barry
School of Human Communication Sciences
La Trobe University
Melbourne
Australia

Susan Block
School of Human Communication Sciences
La Trobe University
Melbourne
Australia

Louise Brown
School of Human Communication Sciences
La Trobe University
Melbourne
Australia

Jacinta Douglas
School of Human Communication Sciences
La Trobe University
Melbourne
Australia

Patricia Eadie
School of Human Communication Sciences
La Trobe University
Melbourne
Australia

Teresa Iacono
Centre for Developmental Disability Health
Monash University
Melbourne
Australia

Beverly Joffe
School of Human Communication Sciences
La Trobe University
Melbourne
Australia

Jenni Oates
School of Human Communication Sciences
La Trobe University
Melbourne
Australia

Sheena Reilly
School of Human Communication Sciences, La Trobe University
Royal Children's Hospital and Murdoch Childrens Research Institute
Melbourne
Australia

Miranda Rose
School of Human Communication Sciences
La Trobe University
Melbourne
Australia

Tanya Serry
School of Human Communication Sciences
La Trobe University
Melbourne
Australia

Foreword

You are asked to see a child with language delay or stuttering or to manage a stroke victim with aphasia. How often, at the end of such a consultation, are you left with unanswered questions for which you require more information? More often than not?

In order to practise efficiently and effectively, speech pathologists need to be armed with a battery of information or *evidence* to support their practice. This might include information about the frequency of a condition, its diagnosis, its treatment or its prognosis. Having identified a need for information, speech pathologists must set about finding the most up-to-date evidence available in the ever-increasing mass of scientific literature. They must evaluate and summarize the evidence from various sources. Then, speech pathologists must decide whether the information available will help in managing the patient at hand. They must make management decisions in consultation with patients and their families, and these decisions must be acceptable to patients. Furthermore, any such decisions made by speech pathologists must take into account the context and constraints, usually financial, of the health service setting.

The description above summarizes the process of evidence-based practice, which involves a number of steps:

- Evaluating the patient (history, examination, diagnostic tests).
- Identifying the need for information and structuring clinical questions to provide focus.
- Searching the literature for the current evidence.
- Critically appraising or evaluating the quality of the evidence.
- Assessing the applicability of the evidence to the patient and considering the restraints which might limit its implementation.
- Using the evidence in patient care and evaluating its effects – good and bad.

If we fail to follow these steps we risk compromising our patients' optimal care, wasting precious resources and potentially ending up ourselves in the hands of the lawyers!

Evidence-based Practice in Speech Pathology covers each of these steps as it introduces the concepts and the limitations of evidence-based practice. Through the use of clinical examples, this excellent book guides the reader towards making evidence-based decisions.

The term 'evidence-based medicine' (EBM) was coined at McMaster University in the early 1990s, but EBM was not incorporated into health sciences curricula until much later. Consequently, many speech pathologists may not have been taught the skills required for evidence-based practice. Although most people will be familiar with the randomized controlled trial, terms such as 'allocation concealment' or 'number needed to treat' may remain a mystery to those without training in critical appraisal. Lack of time to access and evaluate the literature is often cited by the busy clinician as a barrier to obtaining evidence. Some clinicians feel that they are drowning in information overload, whereas others need to develop the skills needed to master the challenges of information technology necessary to access available electronic databases.

Even with the necessary skills, a personal computer and sufficient time, speech pathologists cannot expect to fully search and summarize the literature for every question that arises in their practice. Fortunately, sources of summarized evidence are becoming more frequently available. For example, the Cochrane Library Database of Systematic Reviews contains reviews of the literature on specific interventions and these are regularly updated. Similarly, journals such as *Evidence-Based Medicine* and *ACP Journal Club* provide summaries of papers considered to use sound methodology and to be of immediate clinical relevance. These resources not only save the speech pathologist time but also provide a summary which has been subjected to peer review.

Evidence-based Practice in Speech Pathology provides a valuable source of summarized evidence for speech pathologists. Rather than trying to be all-inclusive, the authors have selected a range of conditions that might present at different ages to speech pathologists in a range of clinical settings. Topics range from the treatment of aphasia after stroke, to the treatment of stuttering, dysphagia, voice disorders, late talkers and paediatric motor speech disorders. This gives the book a wide appeal and broad relevance. For each topic addressed the relevant literature has been systematically traced, appraised and summarized, with an emphasis on management.

Speech pathology is a relatively new discipline, and there are major gaps in knowledge about the effectiveness of treatments that are used every day. The evidence presented in this book has been graded by use of standard criteria for assessing the strength of the method used to produce that evidence. For example, 'Level I' evidence represents a meta-analysis of a systematic review of all randomized controlled trials (which we are reminded will only be as good as the individual trials!), whereas 'Level IV' evidence represents 'opinion' alone. This process is useful in the context of this book because it highlights the lack of strong evidence to support many interventions used routinely in speech pathology. It also identifies areas where evidence is absent, where there is a need for high-quality research and where – for now at least – we and our patients must accept a degree of uncertainty.

The practice of evidence-based speech pathology requires the maintenance of clinical skills because best practice results only when clinical expertise is combined with application of the best available research evidence. In all areas of health care we must continue to question why we use a certain diagnostic test, why we use a particular treatment and whether what we are doing is with the approval and to the benefit of our patients. As we grapple with the need to acquire new skills and struggle to the surface of the ever-increasing mounds of literature, it important to remember that our patients are of prime importance and that, above all, evidence-based medicine is about solving clinical problems. None of us can ignore the need to acquire the necessary skills to ensure we are up to date in our area of practice.

Evidence-based Practice in Speech Pathology is one of the first texts to marry evidence-based practice with speech pathology, to discuss the available evidence and to highlight its shortcomings. I have no doubt that this important book will provide the stimulation and motivation needed to point speech pathologists in the direction of evidence-based practice and to encourage them to plan the research needed to make a difference to their patients.

Elizabeth Jane Elliott

(Elizabeth Elliott is Associate Professor in the Department of Paediatrics and Child Health at the University of Sydney and Consultant Paediatrician at The Children's Hospital at Westmead, NSW, Australia. She is Director of the Centre for Evidence Based Paediatrics, Gastroenterology and Nutrition and Senior Associate Editor of Evidence-based Pediatrics and Child Health *(Moyer VA, Elliott EJ, Davis RL, Gilbert R, Klassen T, Logan S, Mellis C, Williams K. Evidence-based paediatrics and child health. London: BMJ Books, 2000.)*

Preface

Evidence-based Practice in Speech Pathology is primarily directed at speech pathologists, but will be of interest to many other health professionals and researchers. The broad aims of this book are to:

- introduce speech pathologists to the concept of evidence-based practice
- discuss the advantages and disadvantages of evidence-based practice
- provide speech pathologists with information about how to become evidence-based practitioners
- provide an overview of the evidence for key areas of speech pathology practice
- address and summarize the challenges that speech pathologists face in ensuring that clinical practice and teaching are underpinned by best evidence.

This book is divided into three parts. Part One, 'Introducing Evidence-based Practice', addresses the first three broad aims outlined above. Part Two, 'Presenting the Evidence', created the greatest challenge both to us as editors and to the individual authors. It evolved after numerous discussions and much hard work. Our aim was to provide the profession with a summary of the evidence that underpins practice in some of the more common subspecialities in speech pathology. We also wished to do more than just provide an evidence level. Instead, we encouraged authors to discuss the reasons why certain levels of evidence exist (or do not exist) in their particular fields. Each chapter summarizes where future research is required in each area. Part Three, 'Examining Practice and Future Directions', contains two chapters: the first addresses how evidence is translated into practice, and the second looks at future directions for the speech pathology profession, summarizes where evidence is urgently required, and discusses the type of evidence that is most appropriate.

It was not our intention to review the evidence for every area of speech pathology practice. Nor did we set out to cover all aspects within any area. Some authors (for example, Douglas et al. in Chapter 3) reviewed the scope of practice in the whole area, whereas others (for example, Eadie in Chapter 9) focused on the evidence for intervention in one group. Some authors focused on adult populations (for example, Oates in Chapter 6) and others on children (for example, Eadie in Chapter 8). One chapter focuses on children only (Joffe and Reilly in Chapter 10) and one on both adults and children (Reilly, Chapter 7).

In Part Two, authors were provided with an outline and structure for their contributions. They were encouraged to undertake broad-based literature searches to ensure that they found all relevant information. Electronic databases were used to search for information and, understandably, these vary from chapter to chapter. It was the responsibility of each author to develop a set of search terms that were relevant to the disorder or condition that was being investigated. Search dates varied according to the database accessed and the information that was available. In the main, only English-language papers were considered. Electronic databases included the Cochrane Controlled Trials Register, the Cochrane Oral Health Group Specialized Register, MEDLINE (from 1996), MBASE (from 1980), CINAHL (from 1982), PsychInfo (from 1967) and AHMED (from 1985). In addition, hand searching was also carried out of journals specific to each area.

Broad inclusion criteria were used to ensure retrieval of any relevant information. General methods were used to identify studies that met inclusion criteria (that is, studies that contained data on patients). Each publication was examined in detail by the individual authors. The information obtained was generally organized into evidence tables and the information ranked according to an evidence hierarchy. We used the levels of evidence from the Joanna Briggs Institute for Evidence Based Nursing and Midwifery (www.joannabriggs.edu.au/) which were developed from the levels of evidence produced by Phillips R, Ball C, Sackett D, Haynes D, Straus S, McAlister F http://www.eboncall.co.uk/content/levels.html (1998) and displayed on the Centre for Evidence Based Medicine website (http://cebm.jr2.ox.ac.uk/). Each chapter in this book uses the evidence levels as a framework in which to describe quantitative data. The manner in which this has been done varies slightly from chapter to chapter, but in general contains information regarding the study methodology, design, subject characteristics, sample size, intervention and outcomes. Where possible, an evidence level has been attributed for each piece of information obtained.

The levels of evidence are as follows:

- Level I: evidence obtained from a systematic review of all relevant randomized controlled trials.
- Level II: evidence obtained from at least one properly designed randomized controlled trial.
- Level III.1: evidence obtained from well-designed controlled trials without randomization.
- Level III.2: evidence from a well-designed cohort or case-controlled analytic studies, preferably from more than one centre or research group.
- Level III.3: evidence obtained from multiple time series, with or without the intervention. Dramatic results in uncontrolled experiments.
- Level IV: opinions of respected authorities, based on clinical experience, descriptive studies or reports of expert committees.

In Part Two it becomes clear that there is variety in the types and levels of evidence in the various subspecialities in speech pathology. The type of methodology selected (qualitative and quantitative) also varies. For example, in the AAC literature (*see* Iacono, Chapter 12) the evidence is almost entirely at the single-case study level. In contrast, in aphasia (*see* Douglas et al., Chapter 3) a variety of types and levels of evidence, ranging from the systematic review to single-case studies, is available. In some specialties (*see again* Douglas et al., Chapter 3) there has been a marked shift from quantitative to qualitative methodologies.

The overall aim of this book has been to generate discussion within the speech pathology profession. Although some of the results may engender surprise, we hope that they will galvanize the profession into developing some clear research strategies for the future. Just as in other professions, there are many accepted practices in the field of speech pathology that are not evidence-based: many of these are addressed in Part Two. Our challenge for the future is to identify these areas, develop methodologically sound studies that address the problems that exist, and to translate the results from these studies into clinical practice.

Sheena Reilly, Jacinta Douglas and Jenni Oates
La Trobe University
July 2003

Acknowledgements

The editors wish to acknowledge the staff in the School of Human Communication Sciences, La Trobe University, many of whom contributed chapters to this book. In addition, thanks to our many colleagues who have patiently read drafts and through discussion and debate have contributed to and helped shape this book. We are grateful for administrative support we have received, in particular, from Lyndall Mulready, and to the Publications Committee at La Trobe University for their generous financial support.

We are indebted to copy-editor Charlotte Roseby for her editorial support and excellent advice and guidance.

Lastly, we would like to express our gratitude to our families for their patience, ongoing support and encouragement.

Part One
Introducing Evidence-based Practice

CHAPTER 1

The move to evidence-based practice within speech pathology

SHEENA REILLY

> The fact that an opinion has been widely held is no evidence whatever that it is not utterly absurd.
>
> Bertrand Russell (1872–1970)

Introduction: what is evidence-based practice?

The aim of this chapter is to define and discuss evidence-based practice and consider its relevance to the speech pathology profession. The most widely used definition of evidence-based medicine was developed by Sackett and colleagues (1997, p. 2): 'Evidence based medicine is the conscientious, explicit and judicious use of current best evidence in making decisions about the care of individual patients.' A few years later Guyatt and Rennie (2002) added that evidence-based medicine entailed solving clinical problems by using tools to assist clinicians to determine the benefits and the risks of different management strategies.

A number of similar definitions have since emerged that extend the application and principles of evidence-based medicine to all professionals involved in health care. In their book *Evidence Based Health Care: A practical guide for therapists*, Bury and Mead (1998) prefer to use the term 'evidence based health care', an all-encompassing definition that includes key strands such as evidence-based (EB) commissioning and purchasing, EB policy management, EB patient choice and EB practice.

We have adopted the use of the term 'evidence-based practice' throughout this book to encompass the varied work of the speech pathology profession.

What do we mean by 'evidence'? A broad dictionary definition is, 'ground for belief or disbelief; data on which to base proof or to establish truth or falsehood' (*Collins Modern English Dictionary*, 1988). Clinical practice would be much simpler if we could apply this definition directly to clinical practice, resulting in a straightforward process of establishing proof. However, proof comes in many forms; it may include both systematic and unsystematic observations of events and individuals, all of which constitute evidence. To enable clinicians to appraise and compare different types of evidence a hierarchy of evidence has been proposed. (In Chapter 2 the types and levels of evidence that form this hierarchy, both systematic and unsystematic, will be introduced and described.)

Is evidence-based practice the latest fad?

Many practitioners have asked if evidence-based practice is just the latest fad? Although some have argued strongly that it is, most believe it is here to stay. Throughout the 1990s evidence-based practice emerged as a fundamental element in Western-style clinical medicine and became an integral part of the clinical practitioner's method. The practice and its teaching have spread rapidly across Europe, Africa, eastern and south-eastern Asia, and Australasia.

Historically, evidence-based medicine is not a new concept. Although the use of the term evidence-based medicine first appeared in the literature as recently as the early 1990s, its origins may be traced back several centuries. Sackett et al. (1997) and others note that the philosophical origins of evidence-based medicine extend back to the middle of the nineteenth century in Paris. There is also evidence of the use of controlled trials in the eleventh, twelfth and early nineteenth centuries. (Readers may like to visit an interesting website (www.rcpe.ac.uk\controlled_trials), developed by the Royal College of Physicians in Edinburgh, which focuses on controlled trials throughout history.)

Evidence-based practice is not without its opponents and its introduction to clinical practice has not been without criticism. Interestingly, opponents tend to come from the ranks of the most experienced clinicians who believe that it is too prescriptive or menu-driven and therefore fear that their clinical practice risks becoming tyrannized. However, Sackett (1997) and others are quick to reassure that a critical component of evidence-based practice is the *integration* of individual clinical expertise with the best available external clinical evidence from systematic research.

Regardless of whether evidence-based practice is a modern or ancient concept, Bury and Mead (1998) argue that the challenge for all practitioners is to answer the question, 'How do you know that what you do works?' What is different about evidence-based practice is that it places a new emphasis on the use of scientific evidence to answer this question.

What does evidence-based practice mean to speech pathologists?

Evidence-based practice requires speech pathologists to integrate their individual clinical expertise with the best available evidence from systematic research, to demonstrate that what they do works! It means moving away from basing decisions on opinion, past practice and past teaching towards clinical decision-making that is guided by science and research – in other words, the evidence.

Because evidence-based practice is a lifelong process of self-directed learning it challenges not only clinicians but also educators, managers and academics. Without the evidence to underpin clinical practice, speech pathology is vulnerable. (Some sub-specialities may be more at risk.) Without access to and application of current best evidence our practice risks becoming rapidly out of date, to the detriment of our patients. Not only do speech pathologists require a mass of research and clinical knowledge to draw upon, they also need the critical appraisal skills necessary to evaluate this information or evidence. Although speech pathologists traditionally receive some training in research methodology, they have neither been trained to critically appraise the literature nor equipped with the fundamental skills required to adopt an evidence-based approach.

In 1995 Enderby and Emerson authored a very important book, *Does Speech and Language Therapy Work?* The book was essentially a review of the international literature, which aimed to 'establish the state of knowledge regarding the efficacy of speech and language therapy' (Enderby and Emerson, 1995 p.1). In the Introduction the authors pointed out that evidence about the efficacy of speech and language therapy is necessary in order to 'offer an improved quality of life to our client group, as effectively as possible, to the maximum number of people'. They stated that clinical practice must be based on research evidence and they pointed out that the National Health Service (NHS) research and development strategy objective is to 'ensure that the content and delivery of clinical care ... is based on high quality research relevant to improving the health of the nation' (NHS R&D, 1991). This objective remains paramount because research matters to clinical practitioners. Rutter (2000), discussing child language disorders, stated that research provides the means by which an audit is carried out in relation to planning of services, in the provision of individual treatment plans and in prevention strategies. Rutter (2000) went on to say that while research may affirm long-held beliefs and opinions, so might the results repudiate such beliefs and opinions.

In the last few decades in Australia, Europe and the USA one of the key concerns of policy-makers and governments has been health expenditure.

The allocation of limited health resources has been examined closely, resulting in policy-makers and managers wanting more and more information about the efficiency and effectiveness of current interventions. These decisions should be informed by evidence-based practice to ensure that interventions result in the best possible patient outcomes and are cost effective at the same time. Speech pathologists need to be proactive in initiating and leading these discussions about speech pathology services.

What if there is no evidence?

In many instances the evidence will alert clinicians to the most efficacious and cost-effective approach, but becoming an evidence-based practitioner does not provide all the answers. Clinicians will be surprised to find that in many instances there will be limited or no evidence to support a particular approach, thereby identifying future research directions for the profession. In situations where there is no or limited evidence of any benefit, clinicians need to ask: 'Should the service or treatment be offered at all?' Answering this question demands more than just an appraisal of the evidence (both systematic evidence and unsystematic observations); it requires an examination of whether the benefits of intervention are worth the costs involved (financial or other) as well as consideration of the values and preferences of the patient.

Where there is no direct evidence from basic or applied research, indirect evidence should be appraised for its applicability. This has occurred in the sub-specialities of dysarthria and dysphagia, where evidence from studies on the adult population with the same problem (being indirect evidence) has been applied to children with the same condition. The emphasis here should be on appraising the indirect evidence to ascertain if it is indeed transferable. In cases where there is limited evidence or low levels of evidence, priority setting and deciding on an appropriate division of resources will become necessary. (For a full discussion on levels of evidence see Chapter 2.)

Having reached this point, clinicians should not be discouraged by the growing realization that whereas some areas of speech pathology practice are strongly evidence-based, others may be based on no evidence, or on a limited and weak level of evidence. A number of surveys (see Sackett et al., 1991) of health professionals show that clinical decision-making is rarely based on the best evidence. In the early 1980s it was suggested that 10–20% of medical interventions were based on sound evidence (Williamson et al., 1979; Office of Technology Assessment of the Congress of the United States, 1983). Greenhalgh (2001) reported that these figures are disputed in recent evaluations, which classified 21% of health technologies as evidence-based and 60–90% of the clinical decisions (specialty dependent) as evidence-based (for example, Ellis et al., 1995; Gill et al., 1996; Howes et al., 1997).

Why should evidence-based practice make a difference to solving clinical problems?

Evidence-based practice is more than clinical problem-solving. Ultimately, EBP is about providing care 'that does more good than harm in terms of health gain and the patient experience' (Bury and Mead, 1998 p.1). In order to provide this care, clinical decision-making needs to become more explicit and accountable rather than being based on history and anecdote (Enderby and Emerson, 1995).

The components of evidence-based health care

Hicks (1997 p. 1) (www.jr2.ox.ac.uk/ bandolier/band39/b39-9.htm) used the term 'evidence-based health care' and defined this as care that 'takes place when decisions that affect the care of patients are taken with due weight according to all valid, relevant information'. Hicks (1997) defined each component of this definition and provided supporting statements to assist with the interpretation as follows.

'Decisions that affect the care of patients' are taken regularly, not only by allied health clinicians such as speech pathologists, but by managers and policy-makers as well as doctors. Furthermore, patients (or their carer(s)) will also be involved in the decision-making process. Evidence-based practice is therefore relevant to all involved with patient care. Taken further, educators and trainers have an indirect but important role to play in ensuring that they produce evidence-based practitioners and that their teaching is evidence-based.

'Due weight' acknowledges that there are many factors that contribute to decisions about the care of patients. There are many factors, other than simply the results of clinical trials, that may affect clinical decision-making (for example, patient preferences and resources). Although the result of a clinical trial might indicate a good outcome, it may not be one valued by individual patients. For example, survival from major illness is without doubt a positive outcome after intervention. However, many individuals will want to understand the cost of that intervention because if the resulting quality of life is poor they may choose a different or no treatment option. Therefore, clinicians should evaluate and discuss all evidence in light of the main outcome measures and their relevance to individual patients. This definition does not assume that any one sort of evidence should necessarily be the determining factor in a decision.

'All' implies that there should be a broad search for all valid, relevant information.

'Valid, relevant' implies that the information found should be critically appraised before it is used in a clinical decision. That is, clinicians should evaluate the accuracy of the information and its applicability to the clinical decision in question and the individual to which it pertains.

'Information' remains deliberately unspecified. Information is evidence of which there are many types that may be valid and relevant to particular circumstances. There is no need to exclude any particular type of information, as long as clinicians make an appraisal of the validity and relevance of the information and the information is given due weight. (Levels of evidence are discussed in more detail in Chapter 2, as are the critical appraisal skills required to make informed decisions about the validity and strength of the evidence.)

Why should speech pathologists bother with evidence-based practice?

Numerous writers, including Sackett et al. (1997), have proposed reasons why all clinicians should bother with evidence-based practice. These apply equally to speech pathologists.

The amount of evidence available is increasing

Mulrow (1994) estimated that approximately two million articles are published annually on medical issues. The diversity of the professional activities of many speech pathologists means that there is no 'speech pathology literature' as such. Research by speech pathologists is published in an enormous variety of journals in areas such as linguistics, psychology, education, medicine (and all its specialties), surgery, paediatrics, behavioural and neuro-science and engineering.

There is no doubt that the trend in medicine for an increase in the number of papers being published also exists in speech pathology (Reilly and Perry, 2001). This phenomenon raises a number of challenging questions for clinicians, educators and academics:

- How do we filter all this information?
- How do we tell the good from the bad and the strong from the weak evidence?
- How do busy clinicians access the evidence in a timely manner?
- How does evidence-based practice help?

What do you do when you are handed a long list of references to read or you have retrieved far too many items following a MEDLINE search? How do you make sense of the many different types of articles, judge the quality of each and its relevance to your patients? What conclusion do you draw when, 'for every bit of research that comes to any specific conclusion, there is at least one research report that disagrees' (Light and Pillemer, 1984; Sommers et al., 1992)? As Guyatt and Rennie (2002) emphasized, evidence-based practice helps by equipping clinicians with the necessary skills in critical appraisal to evaluate the benefits and risks associated with particular treatments in the context of an individual patient's experiences and values. Evidence-based practice provides a framework or hierarchy so that individual clinicians can appraise and classify the information according to the strength of the evidence. (These concepts will be expanded and levels of evidence will be defined and fully explained in Chapter 2.)

We need, but fail to access, new evidence

Sackett et al. (1997) demonstrated that in order to keep abreast of the literature a general physician would have to read, on average, 19 articles a day, 365 days of the year. Sackett et al. (1998) polled medical grand round audiences about their average reading times. He found that up to 75% of junior doctors (house officers) had not read anything about the problems presented by their patients in the last week. What was more, they were being taught by senior consultants, 40% of whom had not read anything either. Are speech pathologists any different? Brener et al. (2002) polled 53 speech pathologists attending a master class in paediatric dysphagia at a Speech Pathology Australia conference regarding their reading habits in the preceding week. Just over half said they did no reading; 15% had spent up to 30 minutes reading in the preceding week, 11% spent between 30 and 60 minutes and just nine per cent spent more than one hour reading about their patients (Brener et al., 2002). Lack of access to technology was not solely to blame for this situation as 52% of respondents had access to a computerized database for literature searching (for example MEDLINE, CINAHL) but stated that they did not access it regularly (50% accessed technology on a monthly basis).

New evidence creates changes in patient care

There are numerous, excellent examples of the ways new evidence creates changes in patient care. (Some of the best examples are available from one of the many evidence-based discussion groups (www.hsc.usf.edu/~bdjulbeg/oncology/RCT-practice-change.htm), which provides a list of randomized controlled trials that have changed medical practice.) Examples are available from cardiology, gastroenterology, nephrology, oncology, obstetrics and gynaecology, ophthalmology and neurology. One of the oldest examples, published in 1948 in the *British Medical Journal*, is reported as the first, truly randomized controlled trial. The trial compared streptomycin, as a treatment for pulmonary tuberculosis, with bed rest (standard treatment at the time). As expected the trial established the superiority of streptomycin.

An excellent speech pathology example of new evidence creating changes in patient care may be found in the management of adults with Parkinson's disease. Smith et al. (1995) compared the effectiveness of two treatment types to increase vocal loudness in Parkinson's disease. The study found that Lee Silverman Voice Treatment (LSVT) resulted in marked improvements, whereas the alternative, aimed at increasing respiratory effort only, did not. Later studies showed that the treatment effects were long term (Ramig, 1997) and individuals with Parkinson's disease reported a significant reduction of the impact of their disease on their communication after treatment (Berger et al., 1981). These studies are of interest for two reasons: first, because they demonstrate the effectiveness of one treatment over another; and second, because they challenge influential statements in the literature such as the following: 'Voice treatment for disorders that are degenerative is controversial since there is no expectation for recovery of function, or that any improvements secondary to ... speech pathology ... will be maintained in the long term' (Hillman et al., 1990, p. 308).

There are major unanswered questions about treatment efficacy in speech pathology

Enderby and Emerson (1995) highlighted that approximately 70% of speech and language therapy resources in the UK were spent on children with speech and language difficulties, yet the amount (and perhaps the quality) of research in the area was woeful. How then do we make decisions about the allocation of resources in the area? Should primary prevention versus secondary prevention versus management programmes receive equal resources? If not, how should resources be split between these programmes? Given that the instruments used to define early child language delay are not sufficiently sensitive (currently a high percentage of false positives is obtained; that is, many children with early language delay resolve spontaneously over time) we would run a grave risk of unnecessary and costly therapy, and possibly poor compliance, if resources were weighted towards primary or universal prevention (Wake and Reilly, 2001). Because we are some way from understanding which children in the at-risk groups require early therapy or early diversion into special services as opposed to those suitable for 'watchful waiting', the argument for early screening and the instigation of primary prevention programmes is not strong. Despite this lack of evidence, significant resources are being spent on primary prevention programmes (for example, the Sure Start programme in the UK (Sure Start Unit, 1999)) even though the benefits of these programmes have not been strongly demonstrated. Similarly, some often costly management programmes (such as FastForward) have been promoted without their efficacy being established (Windsor, 2001).

There is disparity between clinical practice and research evidence for effective interventions

Disparity between clinical practice and the research evidence for effective interventions is one of the main arguments for adopting evidence-based practice. Do such disparities exist in speech pathology? To date, little has been written on the subject. However, a recent publication concerning fluency programmes for young children addressed the disparity between the research evidence and clinical practice as well as discussing some of the reasons why this might have occurred (Rousseau et al., 2001).

Rousseau et al. (2001) investigated the use of the Lidcombe programme (a well-known intervention programme for young stutterers that incorporates operant methods) by speech pathologists in Australia. Specifically, the authors set out to ascertain the extent to which the programme was used, to determine the level of satisfaction among users and to uncover barriers to its application. A questionnaire was sent to 400 speech pathologists across Australia and achieved a 75% response rate. The majority of respondents had heard of and reported use of the programme or parts of it. Interestingly, only about half the respondents reported that they used the Lidcombe programme as recommended. The reasons for this were largely related to workplace restrictions and included:

- The workplace was not set up to see clients weekly.
- The demands of the Lidcombe programme exceeded the time allocated per case.
- The way in which the service was structured meant that only parts of the Lidcombe programme were used.

Rousseau et al. (2001) clearly illustrated that despite research teams' best efforts to get evidence into clinical practice (via research publications and education) not all clinicians used the Lidcombe programme or used it in the manner in which it was recommended. Instead they adopted the 'bits' that suited the mode of service delivery (about 50%). Those not using the programme were almost certainly using interventions for which there was poorer or perhaps even no evidence.

Many specialist areas in speech pathology have developed from a clinical base and lack academic underpinning

The fact that many specialist areas in speech pathology lack academic underpinning is not surprising for a relatively young profession. The first clinic in Australia was opened just over 70 years ago. In many situations, clinical priorities override the necessity for scientific underpinning because of the urgent need to address the presenting clinical problem. Unfortunately, in some areas these priorities resulted in a lack of scientifically rigorous tools and treatment protocols and an interesting debate as to whether speech pathology 'constitutes an art or a science' (Enderby and Emmerson, 1995, p. 166).

Williams and Mellis (2000) wrote that they did not expect 100% of paediatric medical practice to be evidence-based as there will always be 'art' in the practice of medicine. They went on to define areas often considered as art, such as communication with families, history-taking, examination and teaching. Although few would disagree that there is an art to communicating (for example, some individuals are simply more skilled than others and this may facilitate their history-taking), this should not be an excuse for failing to understand or develop an evidence base. Williams and Mellis (2000) pointed out that clinical care should never be compromised just because we do not understand the evidence base.

Is there a role for evidence-based practice in education and research?

Although the focus of this chapter has been on clinical practice, clearly, evidence-based practice extends to research and education. Finding no or limited evidence should result in the development of research questions and drive research direction. Often, tensions exist between clinicians who fear that research will become the sole driver of clinical practice and academics who value basic science over clinically relevant research. Although both views are important, it is vital to acknowledge that the relationship between clinical work and research is a cyclic and symbiotic one (Figure 1.1).

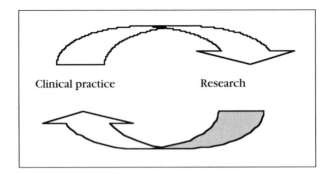

Clinical practice   Research

Figure 1.1 The cyclical and symbiotic relationship between clinical work and research.

As part of postgraduate and continuing education, speech pathologists are required to attend a certain number of events each year. In addition, many individuals will also attend special interest groups and regard these as a way of staying in touch and keeping up to date. Many of these events will involve talks from local or visiting experts and subsequently raise a number of questions. First, is the presentation evidence-based or is it the expert's opinion? The clinician must decide between what is the expert's opinion and what is expert opinion based on scientific evidence. Relying solely on the expert's opinion means abdicating responsibility for undertaking a review and adopting the words of others. Sackett et al. (1991) described this as the 'Seduction' method. Second, let us suppose the presentation is evidence-based; is this an effective way of keeping up to date? Third, is there any carryover from continuing education events to clinical practice? Strong evidence has emerged to suggest that despite clinicians' best attempts to keep up to date, traditional methods (as described above) do not necessarily result in improved learning outcomes (Thompson et al., 1998). Davis et al. (1995) used the randomized controlled trial to test the efficacy of continuing education programmes for doctors. These authors discovered that traditional methods in common use failed to modify clinical performance, although there is no doubt that traditional methods substantially increased the knowledge level of participants (Davis et al., 1995). There was minimal carryover into patient care and clinical decision-making. The researchers concluded that traditional methods of clinical education were judged ineffective in improving the health outcomes of the patients concerned and did not address the problem of declining clinical competence.

Where should speech pathologists begin?

Speech pathologists should begin by acknowledging that there are numerous reasons for adopting an evidence-based approach to patient care (including the six reasons proposed earlier in this chapter) and therefore making a commitment to become an evidence-based practitioner. Sackett et al. (1997), Moyer and Elliot (2000) and others have described some excellent strategies and steps towards becoming an evidence-based practitioner. In the first instance, speech pathologists have to learn how to become evidence-based practitioners. One of the best ways to do so is to complete a course on evidence-based practice. Alternatively, there are numerous online tutorials available (for example, www.nelh.nhs.uk and www.clinicians.vic.gov.au/) that help educate clinicians about the principles of evidence-based practice. Library training (specifically, in how to conduct literature searches efficiently) may also be necessary (see Chapter 2). Most crucially though, speech pathologists will increasingly be required to demonstrate that what they do works, by using the best scientific evidence to answer the question. Speech pathology clinical practice requires the development and adoption of evidence-based practice clinical protocols that are reviewed regularly and used to audit clinical practice (Brener et al., 2002).

Conclusions: what are the challenges for speech pathologists in becoming evidence-based practitioners?

Much of the information available on evidence-based practice stems from the medical and nursing professions. Although evidence-based practice appears to have been adopted by these professions, and by some professions allied to medicine, speech pathologists appear to have been largely unaffected by these changes: to date there are few publications on evidence-based practice and speech pathology. There are a few exceptions, including *Does Speech and Language Therapy Work?* (Enderby and Emerson, 1995) and, more recently, *Evidence-based Practice in Voice* (Carding, 2000). Numerous evidence-based practice health care initiatives have arisen from other professions (for example, the Centre for Evidence-based Medicine, Nursing and Mental Health and the Joanna Briggs Institute for Evidence-based Nursing and Midwifery). However, until recently there was no such development for the speech pathology profession.

Although many of the challenges in the evidence-based practice area are not particular to any one discipline, could speech pathologists' lack of involvement suggest that profession-specific barriers exist that prevent us from embracing the principles of evidence-based practice? Clearly, there is a need to explore this further. It has been suggested in several reports that research is necessary to investigate potential barriers and to examine the effectiveness of evidence-based clinical pathways in allied health professions such as speech pathology (Thomas et al., 2000). However, to date these have not been explored (either nationally or internationally) in the profession.

There are numerous challenges ahead for the speech pathology profession. Like our medical and allied health colleagues, we must all strive to ensure that results from research find their way into clinical practice to improve patient outcomes. Evidence-based practice also challenges educationalists to ensure that future speech pathologists are graduates in evidence-based practice and that they are lifelong learners, equipped with the skills necessary to appraise the literature critically and apply their findings to their future patients. A priority, therefore, is to underpin undergraduate and postgraduate training with the principles of evidence-based practice. Teachers need to understand thoroughly the evidence for and against different approaches and to be able to impart this knowledge to their students. Educational content, therefore, must be current and presented within an evidence-based framework.

Box 1.1

Five steps towards becoming an evidence-based practitioner

Sackett and colleagues (1997) outlined five steps towards becoming an evidence-based practitioner. In this book we focus primarily on steps 2 and 3.

1   Convert a clinical need into an answerable question. This may be about diagnosis or prognosis as well as therapeutic intervention. In a broader sense it could include almost any clinical or health care issue.
2   Search for and find the best evidence to answer the question. (Chapter 2 addresses sources of evidence and finding the evidence.)
3   Critically evaluate the evidence you find for its validity, strength and applicability (usefulness) to the individual patient.
4   Apply the results of the search and appraisal to your clinical practice.
5   Evaluate or audit your performance.

It is important to realize that in speech pathology types and levels of evidence vary enormously in the various sub-specialties, as does the type of methodology selected (qualitative and quantitative). For example, in the augmentative and alternative communication literature (see Chapter 13) the evidence is almost entirely at the single-case study level. In contrast, in aphasia (see Chapter 3) a variety of types and levels of evidence ranging from the systematic review to single-case studies is available. In some specialties (for example, aphasia, see Chapter 3) there has been a shift from quantitative to qualitative methodologies.

In 1999 the NHS R&D Centre for Evidence-based Medicine in Oxford (www.jr2.ox.ac.uk/cebm) identified several areas requiring further development. These include:

- The need to better understand how clinicians seek information and the factors that influence and limit the application of knowledge, once found, to changing practice.
- The need to continue to develop innovative (going beyond paper to CD, websites, video clips and so on) evidence-based patient care guides for frontline health professionals in all disciplines.

- The need to promote ways to integrate evidence into information systems that can support the decisions of patients and practitioners.
- The need to better understand how health professionals, patients and managers understand, value and use evidence in decisions.
- The need for researchers who are interested in studying these problems.

These areas all have direct relevance to the speech pathology profession and information obtained from research within the profession is of vital importance. In addition, speech pathologists need to take a long, hard look at clinical practice, education and research priorities if they are to meet the challenges facing them.

References

Berger M, Bobbit RA, Carter WB, Gilson BS. Sickness impact profile: development and final version of a health status measure. Medical Care 1981; 19: 787–805.

Brener L, Vallino-Napoli L, Reid J, Reilly S. Accessing the evidence to treat the dysphagic patient: can we get it? Is there time? Asia Pacific Journal of Speech, Language and Hearing 2002 8(1): 36–43.

Bury T and Mead J. Evidence Based Health Care: A practical guide for therapists. Oxford: Butterworth Heinemann, 1998.

Carding P. Measuring the Effectiveness of Voice Therapy. London: Whurr Publishers, 2000.

Collins Modern English Dictionary. Glasgow: William Collins & Sons Co. Ltd, 1998.

Davis DA, Thomson MA, Oxman AD, Haynes RB. Changing physician performance: a systematic review of the effect of continuing medical education strategies. Journal of the American Medical Association 1995; 274: 700–5.

Ellis J, Mulligan I, Rowe J, Sackett DL. Inpatient general medicine is evidence based. Lancet 1995; 346: 407–10.

Enderby P, Emerson J. Does Speech and Language Therapy Work? London: Whurr Publishers, 1995.

Gill P, Dowell AC, Neal RD, Smith N, Heywood P, Wilson AE. Evidence based general practice: a retrospective study of interventions in one training practice. British Medical Journal 1996; 312: 819–21.

Greenhalgh T. How to Read a Paper: The basics of evidence based medicine (second edition). London: BMJ Books, 2001.

Guyatt G, Rennie D. The Users' Guide to the Medical Literature: A manual for evidence based clinical practice. Chicago, IL: American Medical Association Press, 2002.

Hicks N. Evidence-based health care. Bandolier 1997; 39(5) May.

Hillman R, Gress C, Hargrave J, Walsh M, Bunting G. The efficacy of speech and language pathology intervention: voice disorders. Seminars in Speech and Language 1990; 11: 297–309.

Howes N, Chagla L, Thorpe M, McCullough P. Surgical practice is evidence based. British Journal of Surgery 1997; 84: 1220–23.

Light RJ, Pillemer DB. Summing up: the science of reviewing research 1984. Cambridge, MA: Harvard University Press, 3–4.

Moyer VA, Elliott EJ, Davis RL, Gilbert R, Klassen T Logan S, Mellis C, Williams K. Evidence Based Paediatrics and Child Health. London: BMJ Books, 2000.

Mulrow CD. Rationale for systematic reviews. British Medical Journal 1994; 309: 597–9.

NHS R&D. Research for Health. 1991.

Office of Technology Assessment of the Congress of the United States. The Impact of Randomized Clinical Trials on Health Policy and Medical Practise. Washington DC: US Government Printing Office, 1983.

Ramig LO. How effective is the Lee–Silverman Voice Treatment? ASHA 1997; 39: 34–5.

Reilly S, Perry A. Is there an evidence base to the management of paediatric dysphagia? Asia Pacific Journal of Speech, Language and Hearing 2001; 6: 1–8.

Rousseau I, Onslow M, Packman A, Robinson R. The Lidcombe program in Australia. In: M Onslow, A Packman, E Harrison (eds). The Lidcombe Program of Early Stuttering Interventions: A clinicians guide. Austin, TX: Pro-Ed, 2001.

Rutter M. Research into practice: future prospects. In: Bishop DVM, Leonard LB (eds) Speech and Language Impairments in Children: Causes, characteristics, intervention and outcome. London: Taylor & Francis, 2000.

Sackett DL. Surveys of self-reported reading times of consultants in Oxford, Birmingham, Milton-Keynes, Bristol, Leicester and Glasgow. In: DL Sackett, WS Richardson, WMC Rosenberg, RB Haynes (eds). Evidence Based Medicine. London: Churchill Livingstone. 1997.

Sackett DL, Haynes RB, Guyatt GH, Tugwell P. Clinical Epidemiology – A Basic Science for Clinical Medicine. London: Little Brown, 1991.

Sackett DL, Richardson WS, Rosenberg WMC (eds). Evidence Based Medicine. London: Churchill Livingstone, 1997.

Sackett DL, Richardson WS, Rosenberg WMC, Haynes RB (eds). Evidence Based Medicine: How to Practise and teach EBM. London: Churchill Livingstone, 1998.

Smith M, Ramig L, Dromey C, Perez K, Samandari R. Video laryngoscopy in Parkinson's disease following intensive voice treatment. Journal of Voice 1995; 9: 453–9.

Sommers RK, Logsdon BS, Wright JM. A review and critical analysis of treatment research related to articulation and phonological disorders. Journal of Communication Disorders 1992; 25: 3–22.

Sure Start Unit. Sure Start 'Trailblazer' Edition: A guide to EBP. London: Sure Start Unit, 1999 (www.surestart.gov.uk/).

Thomas L, Cullum N, McColl E, Rousseau N, Soutter J, Steen N. Guidelines in Professions Allied to Medicine. Cochrane Effective Practice and Organisation of Care Group (EPOC), 2000.

Thomson MA, Oxman AD, Davis D. Outreach visits to improve health care, professional practice and health care outcomes. In: L Berow, R Grilli, J Grimshaw, A Oxman (eds). Cochrane Collaboration on Effective Professional Practice module of the Cochrane Database of Systematic Reviews (updated 1 December 1997). Oxford: Update Software, The Cochrane Collaboration, Issue 1, 1998.

Wake M, Reilly S. Now we're talking ... but who are we talking about? Journal of Paediatric and Child Health 2001; 37: 421–2.

Windsor J. Editorial. American Journal of Speech Language Pathology 2001; 10: 194.

Willams K, Mellis C. Putting evidence into practice. In: VA Moyer, EJ Elliott, RL Davis, R Gilbert, T Klassen, S Logan, C Mellis, K Williams (eds). Evidence Based Paediatrics and Child Health. London: BMJ Books, 2000.

Williamson JW, Goldschmidt PJ, Jillson IA. Medical Practise Information Demonstration Project: Final report. Baltimore, MD: Policy Research, 1979.

CHAPTER 2

What constitutes evidence?

SHEENA REILLY

Introduction: what is evidence?

Speech pathology is a relatively new discipline. The profession was founded about 70 years ago and focused initially on the treatment of head-injured soldiers returning from war. Speech pathology developed initially as a caring profession in response to clinical needs and concern for individuals with communication disorders. It is not surprising, therefore, that anecdote has played a role in the development and direction of the profession. Although the response to clinical needs is admirable, it has meant that in some areas of practice there is a lack of scientific underpinning, with an urgent need for scientifically rigorous tools and empirically derived treatment protocols. Evidence-based practice has emerged at a crucial time for the profession.

Numerous definitions of evidence-based practice have been proposed to date. The majority emphasize that the clinical decision-making process should integrate best evidence with clinical expertise and patients' rights and wishes.

Evidence may originate from numerous and diverse sources, including both systematic (for example, scientific studies) and unsystematic observations (for example, a clinical observation). Evidence is also proof obtained from experimental approaches about the efficacy of a treatment, diagnostic technique, prognosis or economic analysis. Evidence comes in numerous forms and some types are considered stronger than others. In this chapter we will define and explain different types of evidence and their relevance to speech pathology.

How do we tell good from bad evidence?

How do we tell good from bad evidence and differentiate strong from weak evidence? The answer to this question lies in accurate and critical appraisal.

The question implies that all sources of evidence are not equal. A filtering process is required to rank or order evidence according to its value or level, from high to low. High-level or strong evidence means that there has been a systematic scientific evaluation of the problem or question, whereas low-level or weak evidence implies there has been no or poor scientific evaluation. For example, the existing evidence may originate from clinical observations and experience and therefore be supported only by unsystematic observations. It is worthwhile exploring further what constitutes low or weak levels of evidence.

What is *not* evidence-based practice?

Greenhalgh (2001) outlined four decision-making approaches that could not be regarded as evidence-based practice. They included decision-making by:

- Anecdote.
- Press-cutting.
- Expert opinion.
- Cost minimization.

Examples of almost all of these may be found in speech pathology as well as medicine and other areas of allied health or nursing practice.

Decision-making by press-cutting

An excellent example of decision-making by press-cutting occurred in Australia in 2000. The following headline appeared in the *Medical Observer*, a magazine-style newspaper for general practitioners, 'Speech therapy may be wasted on pre-schoolers' (27 October 2000). The opening paragraph of the article read: 'Doubt has been cast over the benefits of speech therapy for pre-school children after the release of new British research showing that it is no better than a "wait-and-see" approach' (p. 30).

The article appeared in response to a randomized controlled trial of community-based speech pathology in pre-school children published by Glogowska et al. (2000) in the *British Medical Journal*. The study was carried out in 16 community clinics in south-west England (specifically, the Bristol area). The results showed that there was little difference between language-delayed children who were given low levels of speech pathology intervention when compared to those whose difficulties were simply monitored.

Conti-Ramsden and Law (2000), in an accompanying editorial in the same journal, stated: 'At first glance the picture painted by Glogowska et al. in this issue of the BMJ (p. 923) is gloomy.' These authors went on to say: 'there are some features of the study that should be interpreted cautiously. On average the children spent just six hours with their speech and language therapist in 12 months' (Conti-Ramsden and Law, 2000, p. 908). The study conducted by Glogowska and colleagues reflected what was happening in a National Health Service (NHS) community setting. The service was almost certainly stretched very thinly as it was providing an average of just six hours of therapy per year to each child.

Conti-Ramsden and Law (2000) highlighted that there was evidence that improvements could be achieved with intensive intervention and that the major implication of this study was the way in which services to such children were structured and resourced. Commenting on the study, Parsons (Chair of the Royal College of Speech and Language Therapists (RCSLT) at the time) was quoted as saying: 'If a patient needs ten tablets and you give them only one, it is not surprising if the medication does not work. The challenge for the profession is to produce guidance about minimum levels of effective treatment' (RCSLT press release (www.rcslt.org.uk)).

Reilly and Eadie (2000) wrote to the *Medical Observer* highlighting that this study did not prove or disprove the efficacy of speech pathology for pre-school children. Most importantly, the study demonstrated that children with specific speech and language disorder do not get better spontaneously (in other words, 'watchful waiting' is not an option) and that the provision of limited amounts of therapy (for example, six hours in 12 months) is not a tenable solution.

It would have been interesting to conduct a survey of general practitioners and paediatricians to ascertain how many of them actually accessed the original article and how many relied on the press-cutting for their information. The dangers of decision-making by press-cutting are clear. Equally disturbing was the view that emanated from some speech pathology quarters (albeit largely uninformed groups) that the authors should not have published the paper. Why? Because they feared the interpretation that speech pathology does not work. This is an excellent example of what Greenhalgh (2001) refers to as 'decision-making by press cutting'.

Decision-making by expert opinion

Decision-making by expert opinion also occurs in speech pathology. As in other professions, the traditional approach for novices wanting to know about an unfamiliar area of practice was to send them off to find a good review article or chapter in a book. However, as Mulrow and Oxman (1997), and Oxman and Guyatt (1993), ably demonstrated, there was no guarantee that a review or chapter of a book would contain the latest information, would be unbiased and – most importantly – result from a critical appraisal of all the existing literature. In fact, more often than not such sources contained writer or expert bias. Critical information may be ignored because it does not support the writer's theoretical stance; the review therefore may not be considered scientific and at best could be construed as decision-making by expert opinion or 'eminence-based medicine', as labelled by Greenhalgh (2001, p. 7). The lack of objectivity in such reviews led to the systematic review, which is essentially an overview and summary of a series of studies. (The systematic review will be further defined and discussed later in this chapter.)

Decision-making by cost minimization

There are examples of decision-making by cost minimization in speech pathology – although they are less dramatic than some from medicine, they are important nonetheless. Two examples include the use of group rather than individual therapy and the use of volunteers or aides to deliver therapy. Although both have a place in the delivery of speech pathology services, there have been occasions when such strategies have been used to prop up services, to plug gaps and to reduce attention from growing waiting lists. It is in these instances that concern arises about cost minimization.

Recently, a senior mentor was heard advising a junior colleague (who had just commenced a new job in an area previously unserviced by speech pathology) to think about running therapy groups to reduce the waiting list for therapy. What is the evidence that group therapy is more effective, and for whom? Perhaps a more useful strategy might have been a more politically aware approach, involving regular reporting to management and the government about the success of the service, highlighting previously unidentified and unmet needs that have been uncovered since beginning this service. In addition, in the campaign for better services, the engagement and support of parents of children on the waiting list might have been useful.

For many years there has been debate about the use of aides and volunteers in speech pathology to deliver some aspects of therapy. There is no doubt that provided they receive training, there is such a role. Some countries now have recognized training programmes for speech pathology aides. However, there have also been numerous attempts to use untrained and even unpaid volunteers to maintain inadequately funded and under-resourced speech pathology services.

Where is the evidence?

As alluded to earlier, evidence is found in numerous formats. So, how do we decide the worth of the evidence and if it should be considered or included in the decision-making process? Judgements about evidence are made according to study design, the quality of methodology used in the design, the degree of certainty about the treatment and the treatment effect. It is through this process that evidence hierarchies have been formed. But first we have to find the evidence.

Given the information explosion, it is vital that clinicians become skilled and resourceful users of the literature. The only way to do this is to keep abreast of library searching techniques and to attend regular tutorials. There has been a move towards the use of journal articles, rather than textbooks, as the best way to access evidence. There are good reasons for this. First, new research appears in health care journals and is almost always peer-reviewed. This means that before being published, an article will have been appraised for its scientific validity, originality and importance. Second, journal articles generally contain adequate description of the methodology of a study to enable clinicians to replicate the work. The information provided will enable the reader to critically appraise the validity and applicability of the information to patients and practice. Third, the large electronic databases (for example, MEDLINE – the world's largest and the most popular medical database), now accessible from most desktop computers, contain the majority of the literature on health care. Lastly, online text versions of the very latest journal articles, which can be instantly downloaded and printed from personal computers, are now a reality.

As in other professions, speech pathology evidence is found on office and home computers that are linked to libraries. The libraries contain the latest electronic versions of relevant databases, such as MEDLINE, CINAHL, EMBASE and the Cochrane Library. Having defined a clinical question and devised a search strategy, clinicians conduct an electronic search of the databases. This may result in just a few, hundreds or even thousands of articles. The next skill clinicians need is deciding the relevance of the articles, which may originate from a wide variety of journals including discipline-specific journals (for example, *International Journal of Communication Disorders*), journals that focus on specific disorder or disease groups (for example, *Dysphagia*, *Aphasiology*) or specialist journals grouped by subject (for example, *Archives of Diseases in Childhood*, *Journal of Clinical Epidemiology*).

Finding the evidence is dependent on a number of steps, beginning with the composition of a focused and clearly defined clinical question. The question is followed by the identification and selection of information sources (for example, databases) and the development of a search strategy.

Search strategies

Many excellent articles and book chapters have been written on developing answerable questions and developing search strategies. Here is a selection of resources.

- *Finding the evidence*: Booth A, Madge B. In: Bury T, Mead J. *Evidence Based Healthcare: A practical guide for therapists*, 1998.
- Searching the literature: Greenhalgh T. In: Greenhalgh T. *'How to Read a Paper: The basics of evidence based medicine*, 2001.
- *Searching for the best evidence*: Sackett et al. In: Sackett et al. *Evidence Based Medicine: How to practise and teach EBM*, 1998.
- *Finding the evidence*: McKibbon et al. In: Guyatt R, Rennie D (eds). *The Users' Guide to the Medical Literature: A manual for evidence based clinical practice*, 2002.
- Framing questions: Logan S, Gilbert R. In: Moyer AA et al. *Evidence Based Paediatrics and Child Health*, 2000.
- *Finding the evidence*: Hunt et al. In: Moyer AA et al. *Evidence Based Paediatrics and Child Health*, 2002.

How do we appraise and interpret the evidence?

There is no doubt that most clinicians feel confident reading the abstract and the beginning of a journal article, followed by the discussion and conclusion sections. However, many clinicians are least confident with the middle, the most important section, that deals with results and statistics.

Confidence with methodology and procedures might also falter, depending on the level of training clinicians have had in research methodology. One of the best ways for the uninitiated to learn critical appraisal skills is to attend a workshop or to participate in an online tutorial such as that offered by the Critical Appraisal Skills Programme (CASP) (www.ihs.ox.ac.uk/casp/ and www.shef.ac.uk/~scharr/ir/netting/) in the UK. There are many similar programmes in the USA and Canada (http://hiru.mcmaster.ca/ebm.htm) and Australia (www.clinicians.vic.gov. au/links.htm). For those who prefer paper versions there is the excellent series of articles, the 'Users' Guide to the Medical Literature' by Guyatt and Rennie (1993), Guyatt et al. (1995) and Oxman et al. (1993, 1994).

Critical appraisal skills are also essential to develop new areas of practice and discard areas of practice that have been shown to be ineffective. A series of tools or checklists have been devised by various authors to assist with their deveolopment. These exist for studies concerning diagnostic tests, clinical interventions, prognosis and clinical guidelines. Greenhalgh (2001) lists 12 checklists (see Box 2.1) for finding, appraising and implementing evidence. These checklists help clinicians to decide if a study is valid and to determine whether the results are applicable to particular patients and practice contexts.

Box 2.1

Checklist for finding, appraising and implementing evidence

1 Checklist for individual clinical encounters.
2 Checklist for searching MEDLINE or the Cochrane Library.
3 Checklist to determine what a paper is about.
4 Checklist for the method section of a paper.
5 Checklist for the statistical aspects of a paper.
6 Checklist for material provided by a pharmaceutical company representative.
7 Checklist for a paper that claims to validate a diagnostic or screening test.
8 Checklist for a systematic review of meta-analyses.
9 Checklist for a set of clinical guidelines.
10 Checklist for an economic analysis.
11 Checklist for a qualitative research paper.
12 Checklist for healthcare organizations working towards an evidence-based culture for clinical and purchasing decisions.

(Source: Greenhalgh, 2001, pp 200–9)

What is an evidence hierarchy?

An 'evidence hierarchy' is a framework for ranking the strength of the available evidence, from strong to weak. There are numerous published examples available in the literature for evaluating the strength of the evidence for treatment studies. Some of the more well-known evidence hierarchies for evaluating treatment are listed below:

- The National Health and Medical Research Council (www.health.gov.au/nhmrc/index.htm).
- The Centre for Evidence Based Medicine – levels of evidence and grades of recommendation (http://cebm.jr2.ox.ac.uk).
- The Joanna Briggs Institute for Evidence Based Nursing and Midwifery – levels of evidence (www.joannabriggs.edu.au)
- Guyatt et al. (1995).

In addition, evidence hierarchies are also available for assessing the level of evidence for non-treatment studies; for example, evidence about prognosis, diagnosis, and economic and decision analyses. For a comprehensive summary, readers are directed to the Centre for Evidence Based Medicine website (http://cebm.jr2.ox.ac.uk). The levels of evidence on this website are updated periodically and list levels of evidence from one to four, where one is the strongest level of evidence (systematic review of randomized controlled trials) and four the weakest level of evidence, expert opinion without explicit critical appraisal. A summary of the information available from this source is given in Figure 2.1. Within each of the four levels of evidence there are further grades of recommendation. Within levels I and II there are three grades, and in level III there are two grades. Full explanations for these may be obtained from the website.

As outlined in the Preface, we have adopted levels of evidence from the Joanna Briggs Institute for Evidence Based Nursing and Midwifery (www.joannabriggs.edu.au), which are reproduced in Figure 2.2.

The Levels of Evidence from the Joanna Briggs Institute for Evidence-based Nursing and Midwifery for the evaluation of treatment follow the traditional evidence hierarchy. That is, Level I evidence (evidence from a systematic review) is considered the strongest evidence, whereas Level IV (the opinion of respected authorities) is considered weak.

Although there are many similarities across the evidence hierarchies, the Joanna Briggs Institute for Evidence-based Nursing and Midwifery Levels of Evidence was chosen for the following reasons. First, the levels of evidence are relatively straightforward, uncomplicated and easy to apply. Second, Level IV (opinion of respected authorities, clinical experience and reports of expert committees) is still included in the evidence hierarchy, whereas it has been omitted from some other published evidence hierarchies. Although this is at the weakest end of the evidence hierarchy (and some would argue that it

Type of study	Therapy/ Prevention/ Aetiology/ Harm	Prognosis	Diagnosis	Differential diagnosis/ symptom prevalence study	Economic decision analysis
Level					
I	Systematic review		(RCT)		Strong
II					
III					
IV	Expert opinion				Weak

Figure 2.1 Levels and grades of evidence available from the Centre for Evidence Based Medicine (http://cebm.jr2.ox.ac.uk). These levels are updated periodically and readers are advised to check the website for the latest guidelines.

Level I	Evidence obtained from a systematic review of all relevant randomized controlled trials.
Level II	Evidence obtained from at least one properly designed randomized controlled trial.
Level III	
1	Evidence obtained from well-designed controlled trials without randomization.
2	Evidence obtained from well-designed cohort or case control analytic studies, preferably from more than one centre or research group
3	Evidence obtained from multiple time series, with or without the intervention. Dramatic results in uncontrolled experiments.
Level IV	Opinion of respected authorities, based on clinical experience, descriptive studies, or reports of expert committees.

Figure 2.2 The Joanna Briggs Institute for Evidence Based Nursing and Midwifery – levels of evidence.

does not constitute evidence at all) it is an important category to include for the speech pathology profession, where either the gathering of evidence, in some areas, is at a very early stage or, in other areas, where longstanding practices have developed from a non-existent evidence base.

How do we rank evidence to create an hierarchy?

To understand evidence hierarchies fully it is necessary to understand some basic information about research methodology. This is essential because literature searches reveal a range of research methodologies. Research methods are often dichotomized into *qualitative* and *quantitative* methodologies. These methods are complementary, and in treatment studies in particular, serve to answer two important questions: 'Does it work?' and 'Is it acceptable?' (Bury and Jerosch-Herold, 1998, p. 145). The traditional evidence hierarchy reproduced in Figure 2.1 and the Joanna Briggs levels of evidence (Figure 2.2) regarding treatment evaluate only quantitative evidence in intervention studies. Although medicine has been slow to accept the role of qualitative research (traditionally the domain of the social scientists) the situation is changing; as Greenhalgh (2001, p. 167) points out, qualitative research is becoming mainstream.

Definitions of the main quantitative research methodologies are provided in Table 2.1 to enable the reader to understand and interpret the data contained in the remainder of the book. It is well beyond the scope of this chapter to do so in a comprehensive fashion. Examples of studies have been

Table 2.1 Levels of evidence, definitions and examples from speech pathology

Evidence level	Evidence obtained from	Definitions and study types	Examples from speech pathology
I	A systematic review of all relevant randomized controlled trials*	A *systematic review* is a summary of all published randomized controlled trials on the topic of interest	Greener, Enderby, Whurr. Speech and language therapy for aphasia following stroke (Cochrane review). In: The Cochrane Library 1999; Oxford: Update Software.
		A *systematic review* of all published primary studies on the topic of interest	Law, Boyle, Harris, Harkeness, Nye. Screening for speech and language delay: a systematic review of the literature. Health Technology Assessment 1998; 2: 1–184.
II	At least one properly designed randomized controlled trial	A *randomized controlled trial* is used to compare one or more interventions or to compare an intervention(s) against no treatment. Participants are randomly assigned to the group(s) and the results of previously defined outcomes are evaluated in treated and non-treated groups	MacKenzie, Millar, Wilson, Sellars, Dreary. Is voice therapy an effective treatment for dysphonia? A randomised controlled trial. British Medical Journal 2001; 323: 658–61.
III.1	Well-designed controlled trials without randomization	Occasionally randomization is not possible for ethical or practical reasons and in these circumstances a controlled trial is undertaken – identical in all respects apart from participants being randomized to treatment groups. This category should be used if randomization procedures are not adequately described	Pamplona, Ysunza, Espinosa. A comparative trial of two modalities of speech intervention for compensatory articulation in cleft palate children, phonologic approach verses articulatory approach. International Journal of Pediatric Otorhinolaryngology 1999; 49: 21–6.

(contd)

Table 2.1 (contd)

Evidence level	Evidence obtained from	Definitions and study types	Examples from speech pathology
III.2	Well-designed cohort or case-controlled analytic studies preferably from more than one centre or research group	In a *cohort* study a group of people, the cohort, are followed over time. The cohort may be studied to examine sub-sets within the cohort (for example, those exposed or not exposed to an intervention or item of interest) or to study the natural history of disease/disorder (for example, speech and language development)	Rescorla and Schwartz. Outcome of toddlers with expressive language delay. Applied Psycholinguistics 1990; 11: 393–407. Hawdon, Beauregard, Slattery, Kennedy. Identification of neonates at risk of developing feeding problems in infancy. Developmental medicine and Child Neurology 2000; 42(4): 235–9.
		Case-controlled studies involve the comparison of an intervention versus comparison group. They differ from the controlled trials without randomization because they are often retrospective and rely on the identification of a group of people with an outcome or disorder of interest being compared retrospectively with a control group who do not have the outcome or disorder. Case-controlled trials are almost always the design used in rare conditions	Reilly and Skuse. Characteristics and management of feeding problems in young children with cerebral palsy. Developmental Medicine and Child Neurology 1992; 34: 379–88.

III.3	Multiple time series with or without the intervention. Dramatic results obtained from uncontrolled experiments	Guyatt et al. (1990) relabelled what psychologists and many allied health researchers term 'multiple baseline', 'single-case' or 'single-subject' research the 'n of 1 trial'. This involves a single participant and an experiment designed to determine the effect of an intervention	Blood. Efficacy of a computer-assisted voice treatment protocol. American Journal of Speech-Language Pathology 1994; 3: 57–66.
IV	Opinions of respected authorities based on clinical experience, descriptive studies or reports of expert committees	A case report is usually a preliminary report that describes an aspect of an individual (it may be an unusual presentation, diagnosis or response to treatment). Sometimes a number of cases are reported together and this is known as a *case series*	Gibbon, Stewart, Hardcastle, Crampin. Widening access to electropalatography for children with persistent sound system disorders. American Journal of Speech-Language Pathology 1999; 8: 319–34. Thomas-Stonell, Leeper, Young. Evaluation of a computer-based program for training speech rate with children and adolescents with dysarthria. Journal of Medical Speech-Language Pathology 2001;9(I): 17–29.

* Systematic reviews sometimes include primary studies if few or no RCTs are available. Two examples are provided – the review by Law et al. (1998) included all primary studies, whereas the review by Greener et al. (1999) was of RCT's only.

provided from the speech pathology literature to illustrate the types of studies that would be included in each level of evidence.

Do evidence hierarchies help or hinder?

Evidence hierarchies are based on the validity (or accuracy) of the quantitative scientific methodology used in a particular study. Each study is appraised (see 'How do we interpret the evidence?' in this chapter) and then ranked according to the strength of the evidence obtained. Established hierarchies are based on high-quality studies within each level of evidence. However, this does not mean that they are set in stone. For example, there are situations where a Level I or Level II study will not outrank a Level III study. A poorly constructed randomized controlled trial will not outrank Level III.1 or Level III.2 evidence obtained from a controlled trial without randomization or a well-designed cohort study.

As highlighted in Figure 2.1, evidence hierarchies differ according to the type of study being appraised (for example, intervention versus diagnosis). Just as quantitative methodologies are appraised and the evidence ranked according to its strength, so is qualitative research, although as Greenhalgh (1997, p. 743) pointed out, the critical appraisal of qualitative research is a relatively underdeveloped science. Malterud (2001) and Greenhalgh (2001) have, however, provided some helpful guidelines and checklists for authors and reviewers of qualitative studies.

A randomized controlled trial (see Table 2.1) is a prospective study (that is, the data are collected after the study is designed) and usually involves the evaluation of a single variable (for example, thickening of liquids versus thin liquids) in a defined patient group (for example, children with dysphagia and spastic quadriplegia). Its greatest strength lies in the fact that it removes bias and usually seeks to disprove the proposed hypothesis. Randomized controlled trials are considered 'gold standards' in health care, but only to answer specific clinical questions concerned with the evaluation of therapy and/or prevention. As stated previously, the research methodology applied depends entirely on the clinical question being asked. That is, a randomized controlled trial would not be used to answer a question about the natural history of a disorder (for example, language disorders), instead a longitudinal cohort study design would be more appropriate (Guyatt et al., 1990). Similarly, in low prevalence or rare disorders (for example, Rett syndrome) a multiple baseline or 'n of 1' trial, or a case-controlled trial (without randomization) would be more appropriate. Similarly, if information is sought about patients' attitudes and views concerning a particular intervention a qualitative approach will be best adopted.

Even though the randomized controlled trial may well provide strong evidence in support of the intervention, patients' views about the procedure may well outweigh the benefits demonstrated through the trial (for example, 'It's too painful', 'The side-effects are not tolerable' or 'The quality of life outcomes are unacceptable'). In addition, there are occasions where randomization is not possible for ethical reasons (such as where there is dramatic evidence from previous research supporting the superiority of the treatment) and in some areas (for example, early intervention for disability) individual or parental choice may prevent the conduct of such a trial.

In speech pathology there has been lively debate about methodological approaches. One extreme view expressed is that randomized controlled trials are 'the gold standard for medical research' and 'wholly appropriate for use in drug trials', however they are 'totally inappropriate in speech and language therapy' (Mobley, 2000, p. 7). The reasons given to support this view include the fact that speech pathologists deal with 'behaviours rather than pathology' and that the 'verbal behaviours of patients ... vary widely' (Mobley, 2000, p. 7). The author went on to ask in a randomized controlled trial 'can we control for factors such as motivation and previous language experience and use?' (Mobley, 2000, p. 7).

The objections raised by Mobley (2000) concentrate mainly on the heterogeneity of the population and the complexity of measuring multiple aspects of therapy in populations of people with communication disorders. However, heterogeneity does not preclude the conduct of randomized controlled trials, as Glogowska et al. (2001) have suggested. When conducted properly, both randomization and stratification (that is, allocation to groups based on known or suspected prognostic factors) balance the groups and ensure that any differences are due to chance and not bias. Glogowska et al. (2001) pointed out that the children in the treatment and control groups with speech and language disorders were well balanced on factors known to affect speech and language development (for example, maternal education) as well as variables thought to affect progress, about which far less is known.

Perhaps a greater challenge in speech pathology is the issue of complexity. In many areas of speech pathology this involves moving the measurement of outcomes beyond changes in the level or severity of the impairment, to include consideration of the consequences of the impairment and how this disadvantages individuals' participation in society. In a thought-provoking editorial, McConachie (2002, p. 196) questioned whether in some complex conditions (such as autistic spectrum disorders) a discrete treatment can be defined and 'one or a small number of effects measured after a short space of time'. McConachie stated that because autistic spectrum disorders are life-long conditions and these complex children require multifactorial approaches over long periods of time, alternative models for evaluation are required. She argued that even if the management of complex conditions such as autism could be answered satisfactorily in well-designed, multi-centred early intervention studies, randomization of such children shortly after diagnosis to one treatment group or another would be extremely difficult given current estimates of five or six per 1000 pre-school children. McConachie (2000, p. 196) went on to ask if it may be more appropriate (and perhaps more cost-effective) to use other experimental models of evaluation but highlighted that that this would require among other things 'family needs assessment, individual goal setting for children'. This would clearly demand the development of much broader outcome measures and a complex study design involving more than one methodology.

It is perhaps not surprising, therefore, that there is a strong assertion by many in the profession that a randomized controlled trial will not show 'the changes that therapy brings about' (Glogowska et al., 2001, p. 7). However, it is vital to ensure that the outcomes of interest cover the relevant areas (that is, not just change in impairment levels) and that the measures chosen are capable of demonstrating the change clinicians believe will occur regardless of the study design.

What is the future of evidence-based practice in speech pathology?

The most powerful evidence in speech pathology will come from matching the question to the appropriate research design and recognition that the use of a combination of methodologies (for example, survey and in-depth qualitative research within the framework of a randomized controlled trial) will best meet the needs of a profession working with populations of people in whom cures will often not be possible. As emphasized by Enderby (1997), outcome measurement needs to be broader than that traditionally measured and must include, among other things, the ability to participate in society.

There is no doubt that limiting the application of one type of evidence or one hierarchy will not meet the needs of the speech pathology profession. In Chapters 13 and 14 some of these issues will be revisited and explored further.

References

Blood GW. Efficacy of a computer-assisted voice treatment protocol. American Journal of Speech. Language Pathology 1994; 3: 57–66.

Booth A, Madge B. Finding the evidence. In: Bury T, Mead J. Evidence Based Healthcare: A practical guide for therapists. Oxford: Butterworth Heinemann, 1998.

Bury T, Jerosch-Herold C. Reading and critical appraisal of the literature. In: Bury T, Mead J. Evidence Based Healthcare: A practical guide for therapists. Oxford, Butterworth Heinemann, 1998.

Bury T, Mead J. Evidence Based Healthcare: A practical guide for therapists. Oxford, Butterworth Heinemann, 1998.

Conti-Ramsden G, Law J. Treating children with speech and language impairments. British Medical Journal 2000; 321: 908-9.

Enderby P. Therapy Outcome Measures (Speech and Language Therapy). London: Singular Publishing, 1997.

Gibbon F, Stewart F, Hardcastle WJ, Crampin L. Widening access to electropalatography for children with persistent sound system disorders. American Journal of Speech-Language Pathology 1999; 8: 319-34.

Glogowska M, Roulstone S, Enderby P, Peters TJ. RCTS: myths, misconceptions and mastery. RCSLT Bulletin 2001; March: 6-7.

Glogowska M, Roulstone S, Enderby P, Peters TJ. Randomised controlled trial of community based speech and language therapy in preschool children. British Medical Journal 2000; 321: 1-5.

Greener J, Enderby P, Whurr R. Speech and language therapy for aphasia following stroke (Cochrane review). The Cochrane Library, Issue 4, Oxford: Update Software, 1999.

Greenhalgh T. How to read a paper: papers that go beyond numbers (qualitative research). British Medical Journal 1997; 315: 740-3.

Greenhalgh T. How to Read a Paper: The basics of evidence based medicine. London: BMJ Books, December 2001.

Guyatt GH, Rennie D. Users' guides to the medical literature. Journal of the American Medical Association 1993; 270: 2096-7.

Guyatt G, Rennie D (eds). The Users' Guide to the Medical Literature: A manual for evidence based clinical practice. Chicago, IL: American Medical Association Press, 2002.

Guyatt GH, Keller JL, Jaeschke R, Rosenbloom D, Adachi JD, Newhouse MT. The n-of-1 randomized controlled trial: clinical usefulness. Our three-year experience. Annals of Internal Medicine 1990; 112: 293-9.

Guyatt GH, Sackett DL, Sinclair JC, Heywood R, Cook DJ, Cook RJ. User's guide to the medical literature. IX. A method for grading health care recommendations. Journal of the American Medical Association 1995; 274: 1800-4.

Hawdon JM, Beauregard N, Slattery J, Kennedy G. Identification of neonates at risk of developing feeding problems in infancy. Developmental Medicine and Child Neurology 2000; 42: 235-9.

Hunt D, McKibbon K, Moyer V. Finding the evidence. In: Moyer AA, Elliott E, David R, Gilbert R, Klassen T, Logan S, Mellis C, Williams K. Evidence Based Paediatrics and Child Health. London: BMJ Books, 2002.

Law J, Boyle J, Harris F, Harkeness A, Nye C. Screening for speech and language delay: a systematic review of the literature. Health Technology Assessment 1998; 2: 1-184.

Logan S, Gilbert R. Framing questions. In: Moyer AA, Elliott E, David R, Gilbert R, Klassen T, Logan S, Mellis C, Williams K. Evidence Based Paediatrics and Child Health. London: BMJ Books, 2000.

MacKenzie K, Millar A, Wilson JA, Sellars C, Dreary IJ. Is voice therapy an effective treatment for dysphonia? A randomised controlled trial. British Medical Journal 2001; 323: 658-61.

Malterud K. Qualitative research: standards, challenges, and guidelines. Lancet 2001; 358: 483-8.

McConachie H. Appropriate research design in evaluating interventions for children with disabilities. Child: Care, Health and Development 2002; 28: 195-7.

McKibbon K, Hunt D, Scott Richardson W, Hayward R, Wilson M, Jaeschke R, Haynes B, Wyer P, Craig J, Guyatt G. Finding the evidence. In: Guyatt R, Rennie D (eds). Users' Guide to the Medical Literature: A manual for evidence based practice. Chicago, IL: American Medical Association Press, 2002.

Mobley P. Research renaissance. RCSLT Bulletin 2000; April: 7.

Mulrow CD, Oxman AD (eds). Critical Appraisal of Studies. Cochrane Collaboration Handbook. The Cochrane Collaboration. Oxford: Update Software: issue 4, 1997.

Oxman AD, Guyatt GH. The science of reviewing research. Annals of the New York Academy of Science 1993; 703: 125-33, discussion 133-4.

Oxman AD, Sackett DL, Guyatt GH for the Evidence-based Medicine Working Group. Users' guides to the medical literature, I: How to get started. Journal of the American Medical Assocation 1993; 270: 2093-5.

Oxman AD, Cook DJ, Guyatt GH for the Evidence-based Medicine Working Group. Users' guides to the medical literature. VI. How to use an overview. Journal of the American Medical Association 1994; 272: 1367-71.

Pamplona M, Ysunza Espinosa J. A comparative trial of two modalities of speech intervention for compensatory articulation in cleft palate children, phonologic approach verses articulatory approach. International Journal of Pediatric Otorhinolaryngology 1999; 49: 21-6.

Reilly S, Eadie P. Speech therapy has its place (letter). Medical Observer, 2000; 8 December: 24.

Reilly S, Skuse D.Characteristics and management of feeding problems in young children with cerebral palsy. Developmental Medicine and Child Neurology 1992; 34: 379-88.

Rescorla L, Schwartz E. Outcome of toddlers with expressive language delay. Applied Psycholinguistics 1990; 11: 393-407.

Royal College of Speech and Language Therapists. Press release (www.rcslt.org.uk).

Sackett D, Richardson W, Rosenberg W, Haynes, RB. Evidence Based Medicine: How to practice and teach EBM. London: Churchill Livingstone, 1998.

Thomas-Stonell N, Leeper HA, Young P. Evaluation of a computer-based program for training speech rate with children and adolescents with dysarthria. Journal of Medical Speech Language Pathology 2001; 9: 17-29.

Part Two
Presenting the Evidence

CHAPTER 3

The evidence base for the treatment of aphasia after stroke

JACINTA DOUGLAS, LOUISE BROWN AND SANDRA BARRY

Introduction: defining aphasia

Although the definitions of aphasia are many and varied, all encompass or imply four principal defining features of the disorder:

- It results from damage to the brain.
- It is acquired.
- It is a disorder of language processing that can affect all modalities.
- It excludes primary sensory or intellectual impairment.

These inclusionary features not only describe the nature of the disorder but also provide the basis for extreme heterogeneity in its clinical presentation.

Aphasia is most commonly caused by stroke associated with haemorrhagic or ischaemic cerebrovascular disease. The incidence of stroke is between one and two people per 1000 population per year (Kurtzke, 1980) with half this number dying as a result of the stroke (Bonita, 1992). Overall, stroke accounts for 10–12% of all deaths and is the third most common cause of death after heart disease and cancer (Bonita, 1992). The incidence of stroke increases as a function of age with rates being less than one per 1000 for people under the age of 50 but approaching 10 per 1000 at age 70 and 20 per 1000 at age 80 (Kurtzke, 1980; Mlcoch and Metter, 2001). Prevalence estimates are between four and six per 1000 population (Kurtzke, 1980). Stroke is responsible for 25% of chronic adult disability, including paralysis, sensory loss, cognitive changes and speech and language disturbances (National Stroke Foundation, 2000).

Data about the incidence of aphasia as a result of stroke vary as a function of sampling conditions. In their report on aphasia after stroke, Wade and colleagues (1986) noted that 25% of conscious stroke survivors presented with aphasia within seven days of stroke onset. A larger proportion of 40% was reported by Pedersen et al. (1995) who evaluated patients within the first three days of stroke onset. When stroke site is limited to the left hemisphere, not surprisingly, the proportion rises yet again. For example, Scarpa and colleagues (1987) found that 55% of patients with left hemisphere stroke had aphasia when examined 15–30 days after stroke onset. Enderby and Davies (1989) estimated that 30% of patients who have a first or recurrent stroke have aphasia and that the prevalence of persisting speech and language disorders in the stroke population approximates 50%. As the incidence of stroke increases dramatically with age, so too does the incidence of aphasia. Thus, with a ten-fold increase in the incidence of stroke for 50–70-year-old individuals, the vast majority of the aphasic population is elderly.

Communication is a dynamic and complex process; it is the medium through which we establish and maintain our social self at home, at work, in our local community and in society generally. Language is fundamental to our ability to communicate. As a consequence, the onset of aphasia can trigger disturbance in many aspects of personal, family and societal functioning. People with aphasia, their families and friends face many adjustment hurdles as they live with their acquired language impairment in a society in which their participation may be limited by frequent attitudinal and environmental barriers. Over many years, the far-reaching ramifications of aphasia have created the impetus for clinicians to develop treatments that promote beneficial change in the communication ability of people with aphasia.

Aphasia therapy in the context of evidence-based practice

The first reference, albeit indirect, to a treatment for aphasia was made as early as 1700 BC:

> Now when thou findest that man speechless, his relief shall be sitting; soften his head with grease – gazelle fat, and the grease of the serpent, the crocodile, and the hippopotamus – and pour milk into both his ears.
> (Breasted, 1930, p. 286)

No evidence for the efficacy of this treatment remains and to our knowledge neither does the treatment. What does remain, however, is the quest for effective aphasia treatment; that is, treatment for which effectiveness has been established through the collection and synthesis of evidence. This quest has given rise to many and varied treatment techniques with equally varied degrees of supporting evidence. Indeed, Joseph Wepman's comment in 1953 that there were as many methods of treating aphasia as there were people with aphasia applies as readily to speech pathology practice today as it did nearly 50 years ago. Given the individual experience of aphasia and the heterogeneous nature of its presentation, such a multiplicity of treatment methods is neither surprising nor counterproductive. It provides clinicians with a rich resource from which treatments can be selected logically with the outcomes for individual clients being observed and measured.

For each person with aphasia, the process of treatment selection requires the speech pathologist to answer the clinical questions posed by Wepman in 1968: '*Who* should do the therapy; of *what* should therapy consist or *how* should it be done; *when* should it be instituted, *when* discontinued?' (Wepman, 1972, p. 436). These clinical decisions made about the care of patients with aphasia fit well into the definition of evidence-based health care provided by Hicks (1997, p. 8): 'Evidence-based health care takes place when decisions about the care of patients are taken with due weight accorded to all valid, relevant information' (see Chapter 1).

In his description of this definition, Hicks (1997) made several important points that bear repetition in the context of evidence-based aphasia therapy. In particular, the phrase 'due weight accorded to all valid, relevant information' requires speech pathologists to search actively for and consider valid, relevant evidence alongside all relevant factors and information that may apply in the particular circumstances. Hicks' phrase acknowledges that there are many factors (for example, resources, patient and or family preference, presence of comorbidities) beyond just the results of randomized controlled trials that may and should contribute significantly to our clinical decisions. This definition does not imply that any one sort of evidence should necessarily be the determining factor in a decision. Indeed, the limitations of randomized controlled trials for examining the effectiveness of aphasia therapy have been well documented and much discussed among aphasiologists (for example, Howard, 1986; Pring, 1986; Robey et el., 1999; Code, 2000). Further, the hallmark heterogeneity of aphasia and the resulting individual treatment techniques certainly support the use of single-case methodology to establish an evidence base for aphasia therapy.

Hicks' (1997) use of the adjectives *valid* and *relevant* serves to highlight another important characteristic of aphasia therapy practice within an evidence-based health care framework. These terms suggest that before information or evidence is used in a decision about the care of a person with aphasia, it must be appraised. We must assess the accuracy of information and ascertain the applicability of the evidence to the decision and the case in question. In many instances, although evidence of systematic reviews and randomized controlled trials may well support the efficacy of a particular aphasia treatment, appraisal of the evidence clearly identifies its lack of suitability for a specific patient. On the other hand, careful appraisal of a comprehensively documented single-case investigation may well provide adequate evidence for the applicability of the evaluated treatment procedure to that patient.

The preceding discussion goes some way to underscoring the very active, evaluative nature of evidence-based aphasia therapy. It is a process which requires the aphasia therapist to use a broad range of skills and knowledge. It is the process that most aphasia therapists practise every time they work with a person with aphasia. It is a process that is clearly evident in the writings of aphasiologists throughout the twentieth century (for example, Head, 1920; Goldstein, 1948; Wepman, 1953 Schuell et al., 1964; Luria, 1970; Sarno et al., 1970; Darley, 1982). Within this process, however, there are new variables and much new information that bring with them opportunities to help speech pathologists improve the therapy received by people with aphasia.

Evidence for treatment efficacy and clinical effectiveness

In the field of aphasia therapy, we now have more and better information upon which to base treatment decisions and develop practice guidelines. In 1995, Enderby and Emerson commented: 'There have been more studies into the efficacy of speech and language therapy for dysphasia, published over the past two decades, than for any other client group' (p. 13). At that time, these authors added that it was 'still difficult to answer categorically the question of whether speech and language therapy works' (p. 15). The past five years have seen further considerable growth in information relevant to this question, and the noteworthy appearance of systematic reviews, some of which have used meta-analytic techniques. As its name implies, a 'systematic review' is a review in which all the primary studies have been systematically identified, appraised and summarized by use of a transparent methodology (MacDonald, 2000). An advantage of systematic reviews is the possibility of applying meta-analytic techniques to estimate the magnitude of the effect of intervention. Meta-analytic techniques are the quantitative procedures that statistically synthesize the results from a collection of studies and, hence, are a means of determining the weight of scientific evidence bearing on a particular research hypothesis (Hall et al., 1994).

Well-conducted and clearly reported systematic reviews allow clinicians to draw their own conclusions about the validity and relevance of the findings to the care of a particular person with aphasia. In order for clinicians to decide on the clinical relevance of a review to a case, the reviewers must have clearly stated their objectives and have included a detailed description of their methodology. For example, the Cochrane Library requires systematic reviews to address specified decision points in their primary research protocol before they are approved for publication (Moher et al., 1996).

(Typical decision points in a primary research protocol for a systematic review are shown in Table 3.1. Aphasia-specific examples for each decision point are also included.) The most widely accepted means for evaluating

Table 3.1 Typical decision points with examples in a primary research protocol for a systematic review

Decision point	Examples
Objective(s)	To assess the effects of language therapy for people with aphasia following stroke To calculate estimates of statistical power based on the effect sizes obtained from the meta-analysis
Criteria for considering studies	Studies concerned with language therapy for aphasia
Types of studies	Prospective randomized controlled trials, prospective cohort studies, retrospective case-control studies, clinical series with controls, studies with appropriate single-subject methodology
Types of participants	Adults with all types of acquired aphasia after stroke
Types of intervention	Language therapy delivered in a formal speech pathology setting
Types of outcome measures	Pre- and post-test scores for communication Rating scales, including satisfaction Measures of disability or quality of life
Search strategy	Electronic databases Speech pathology journals (general) Specific aphasia and stroke journals Aphasia texts Scanning reference lists of papers Personal contact with aphasia experts (academic and research institutions) Requests on internet discussion lists
Methods	Independent reviewers or assessors
Selection of studies	Application of inclusionary and exclusionary criteria (for example, effect size able to be calculated)
Assessment of methodological quality	Protection from sources of bias (for example, selection or exclusion bias, presence of co-interventions)
Data management	Coding (for example, amount and type of treatment)
Data synthesis	Specify method for dealing with incomplete data Specify analysis methods for dichotomous and continuous data Specify criteria for meta-analysis

treatment efficacy are randomized controlled trials that compare the intervention in question with a no-treatment control condition or another treatment condition. In clinical practice, however, these conditions may be difficult or impossible to establish. Although single-case controlled studies of clinical effectiveness are less useful for initially establishing the general effectiveness of intervention, they provide an excellent means of determining whether a particular treatment offers specific benefits, compared with an alternative intervention. Optimally, the clinical effectiveness of a specific intervention should be established by a comparative evaluation of its benefits with the best available treatment with known effectiveness. For this reason, single-subject research designs or controlled multiple baseline designs across subjects and interventions provide a sound model for the evaluation of aphasia treatment effectiveness.

A search of relevant electronic databases (for example, MEDLINE, EMBASE, ERIC, CINAHL, Psychlit, Dissertation Abstracts) and journal sources (for example, *Aphasiology, Brain and Language, Clinical Aphasiology, Journal of Speech, Hearing and Language Research* (formerly *Journal of Speech and Hearing Research, Journal of Speech and Hearing Disorders*), *International Journal of Disorders of Communication* (formerly *European Journal of Disorders of Communication, British Journal of Disorders of Communication*), *Stroke, Archives of Physical Medicine and Rehabilitation*) reveals more than 500 articles with potential relevance to the evaluation of the clinical effectiveness of treatments for aphasia. Not surprisingly, such a large resource has spawned several systematic reviews. These reviews provide aphasiologists with revealing summaries of the research conducted into the efficacy of aphasia therapy.

Published overviews of the evidence base for the treatment of aphasia

At the time of writing, ten published overviews with clearly stated objectives were identified (Pedro-Cuesta et al., 1992; Whurr et al., 1992; Robey, 1994, 1998; Enderby and Emerson, 1995; Pearson, 1995; Holland et al., 1996; Greener et al., 1999; Robey et al., 1999; Cicerone et al., 2000). Three of these reviews (Pedro-Cuesta et al., 1992; Enderby and Emerson, 1995; Pearson, 1995) are narrative reviews and the remaining seven are listed chronologically in Table 3.2. Four of the overviews met all the essential criteria outlined in Table 3.1 for classification as systematic reviews (Robey, 1994, 1998; Greener et al., 1999; Cicerone et al., 2000). Robey et al. (1999) set out to complete a meta-analysis of single-subject aphasia treatment research. However, too few of those studies that provided quantifiable outcomes were sufficiently similar to warrant statistical averaging. As a result, their report examined the experimental design issues necessary for the results of single-subject research to be meta-analysed. Although Whurr et al. (1992) and Holland and colleagues (1996) completed extensive overviews, they did not specify the search strategies they used. With the exception of Greener et al. (1999), the reviewers did not limit primary studies for inclusion to randomized controlled trials. Across the evidence base, outcome measures were confined generally to measures of impairment or deficit. In five of these six studies, the authors intended to use meta-analytic techniques. Following identification of primary studies, meta-analysis was completed in three of the reviews. Within the confines of their stated objectives, these studies provide informative overviews of the current evidence base for aphasia therapy. (The objectives and conclusions drawn from each of the overviews are outlined in Table 3.3.)

Overall, the weight of the evidence accumulated over the years and

Table 3.2 Overviews of the evidence base for the treatment of aphasia

Study	Year	Objective(s) stated	Search strategy defined	Studies included (identified)	Meta-analysis
Whurr et al.	1992	+	−	45	+
Robey	1994	+	+	21 (48)	+
Holland et al.	1996	+	−	9 (58)	−
Robey	1998	+	+	55 (479)	+
Greener et al.	1999	+	+	12 (60)	−
Robey et al.	1999	+	+	63 (479)	−
Cicerone et al.	2000	+	+	41 (655)	−

synthesized in these systematic reviews supports the broad conclusion that, on average, aphasia therapy is effective. Further, some of the long-held clinical notions that have guided the decision-making of aphasiologists have some support within the evidence base. Clearly, the magnitude of the effect sizes reported by Robey (1998) supports the clinical belief that treatment early in the recovery process provides maximum positive effect. The positive relationship between treatment intensity and outcome assumed by many clinicians is also supported by the weight of evidence. Intensive treatment (defined as two or more hours per week) was associated with outcomes more than twice as great as no-treatment outcomes, in Robey's second review. In addition, the effects of post-acute (3–12 months post-onset (MPO)) and even chronic stage (on or after 12 MPO) treatment when evaluated against a no-treatment effect are supported objectively to be effective by statistical analyses. This latter finding directly challenges the notion that later

Table 3.3 Objectives and conclusions of overviews conducted in the area of aphasia therapy

Study	Objective(s)	Findings
Whurr et al. (1992)	To examine empirical evidence for the efficacy of speech and language therapy for adults with aphasia by completing a meta-analysis of language intervention studies from 1946 to 1988	Mean effect size for treated individuals compared to untreated individuals matched for age and sex was 0.592 (d > medium-sized effect criterion).
Robey (1994)	To conduct a valid synthesis of research findings on the treatment of aphasic people in order to evaluate the efficacy of treatment offered by speech and language pathologists To calculate estimates of statistical power based on the effect sizes obtained from a meta-analysis	The effect of treatment commenced in the acute stage of recovery is nearly twice as large as the effect of spontaneous recovery alone Treatment initiated after the acute stage of recovery achieves a smaller but appreciable effect The difference between treated and untreated populations approaches the criterion for a large-sized effect when treatment is begun in the acute stage of recovery In the chronic stage of recovery, the difference between treated and untreated populations corresponds to a small-to medium-sized effect
Holland et al (1996)	To provide a summary of available literature on the efficacy of treatment for aphasia To present available programme evaluation data	Generally treatment for aphasia is efficacious Treated patients make more gains than untreated patients or than could be attributed to spontaneous recovery Improvement is maximized when treatment is frequent (more than two hours per week) and is of long duration (five to six months) Treatment can be effective long after onset of aphasia
Robey (1998)	To analyse a large set of primary studies in order to determine the replicability of Robey's (1994) findings	Outcomes for treated individuals are superior to those for untreated individuals in all stages of recovery (acute < 3 months post-onset (MPO), post-acute 3–12 MPO, chronic

Table 3.3 (contd)

Study	Objective(s)	Findings
		> 12 MPO). Outcomes are greatest when treatment is begun in the acute stage of recovery. The average effect sizes for treated individuals compared to untreated individuals in each stage of recovery were: *acute*: 1.83 times greater ($d = 1.15$; > medium-sized effect criterion); post-acute: 1.68 times greater ($d = 0.57$; > small-sized effect criterion)
	To conduct focused analyses focusing on each of four clinical dimensions of aphasia treatment: (1) amount of treatment; (2) type of treatment; (3) severity of aphasia; (4) type of aphasia	Clinical dimensions: (1) Treatment length in excess of two hours per week was associated with greater gains than those gains that result from shorter duration treatment; (2) The most frequently reported form of treatment was that coded as 'non-specified', presumably individualized, with an average effect size of 0.81 (small). The most frequently reported named treatment was Schuell–Wepman–Darley multimodality treatment with an average effect size of 1.39 (small); (3) Large gains are achieved by people with moderately severe and severe aphasia when they are treated by speech and language pathologists. No study included in the systematic review was specifically designed to assess the effect of treatment on mildly aphasic people; (4) There were too few studies for examining differential effects of treatments for differing aphasia types
Greener et al. (1999)	To assess the effects of formal speech-language therapy and non-professional support from untrained providers for people with aphasia after stroke: (1) speech and language therapy compared to no	None of the 12 randomized controlled trials judged to be eligible for this Cochrane Review contained sufficient detail to allow complete description and analysis to be carried out

(contd)

Table 3.3 (contd)

Study	Objective(s)	Findings
	support of any kind; (2) therapy from trained speech and language therapist compared to informal support from volunteer, trained or untrained; (3) untrained support from volunteer compared to no support of any kind; (4) formal therapy from trained therapist compared to supportive counselling from trained therapist; (5) different types of treatment	Owing to the quality of the trials identified, it was concluded that speech and language therapy treatment had not been shown to be clearly effective or clearly ineffective within a randomized clinical trial. Decisions about the management of people with aphasia need to be based on forms of evidence, other than randomized controlled trials
Robey et al. (1999)	To assess the state of single-subject aphasia treatment experimentation. To assess available effect sizes thus, constituting an elementary meta-analysis	The large majority of aphasia-treatment single-subject quasi experiments are hypothesis-driven and well-controlled. The available evidence suggests that effect sizes for treatment of aphasia, as indexed by single-subject research, are remarkably large. Only 19% of the single-subject studies included in the review presented quantifiable outcomes. Without quantifiable outcomes it is not possible to use meta-analysis to synthesize findings statistically across studies
Cicerone et al (2000)	To establish evidence-based recommendations for the clinical practice of cognitive rehabilitation (including remediation of language), derived from a methodical review of the scientific literature concerning the effectiveness of cognitive rehabilitation for persons with traumatic brain injury or stroke.	Good evidence exists to support the effectiveness of cognitive–linguistic therapies beyond the period of spontaneous recovery for the treatment of people with language deficits as a result of left hemisphere stroke. Language therapy was recommended as a practice standard during acute and post-acute rehabilitation for people with language deficits secondary to left hemisphere stroke

stage treatment is ineffective and, as a consequence, provides support for provision of treatment funds across the recovery continuum. Although it is heartening for clinicians to see that several of the general conclusions drawn from these systematic reviews support their clinical assumptions, it is imperative that speech pathologists explore this evidence base further in order to judge the strength of these conclusions.

Exploring the evidence

There are four important issues that need to be taken into account when the synthesized evidence for aphasia therapy is explored. These issues relate directly to the quality or the strength of the evidence base and include:

- The type and quality of primary studies included in the overview.
- The form in which treatment results are reported across primary studies.
- Consideration of threats to validity within the meta-analysis or overview.
- The extent to which outcome-related variables have been accounted for within the evidence base.

Primary studies

The specifications for inclusion of primary studies varied considerably across the reviews considered here. For example, by virtue of the Cochrane Review requirements, Greener and colleagues (1999) included only randomized controlled trials and only 12 trials were identified as eligible for review. In direct contrast, the Robey et al. (1999) study was specifically concerned with evaluating the contribution of single-subject research, studies that are normally excluded from systematic reviews and meta-analyses. Sixty-three primary studies were included in this review. Between these two extremes, Cicerone and colleagues (2001) included three classes of studies in their review. Class I studies were defined as prospective randomized controlled trials; Class II studies were defined as prospective cohort studies, retrospective case-control studies or clinical series with well-designed controls; and Class III studies were defined as clinical series without concurrent controls or studies with appropriate single-subject methodology. A total of 41 primary studies contributed to this review in the area of remediation of language and communication deficits; eight were categorized as Class I studies, seven were Class II studies and 26 were Class III studies.

Holland et al. (1996) used the categorization of evidence developed by the Therapeutics and Technology Assessment Subcommittee of the American Academy of Neurology (1994). In this classification, Class I evidence is provided by well-designed randomized controlled trials; Class II evidence is provided by well-designed randomized clinical studies, such as case-control or cohort studies; and Class III evidence includes expert opinion, non-randomized historical controls and case reports. Holland et al. (1996) further categorized their evaluation of studies according to the size and focus of the study. They reviewed nine large group studies ($n > 60$) that addressed the general question of efficacy of aphasia treatment. Of these, three were identified as Class I, two were considered Class II and five Class III. They also listed a further 21 well-designed and controlled small group or single-subject Class III studies that addressed specific treatment approaches. Robey (1998) included a total of 55 quasi-experiment group studies where, unlike true experiments, group membership is determined by subject attributes rather than random assignment. Thus, across these reviews several levels of evidence have been sampled and an interesting trend has emerged. Rather than an increase in the number of randomized controlled trials conducted since the 1980s, there appears to have been a significant decrease in their numbers with only one of the 12 included by Greener et al. (1999) being reported within the 1990s.

The shift away from randomized controlled trials in aphasia therapy research was not simply a random occurrence. As Code (2000) noted, this reduction in the number of randomized controlled trials was associated with a concomitant shift towards studies employing single-subject methodology. This move towards single-case design in aphasia research reflects general acknowledgment of its superiority over group design for the evaluation of the effectiveness of specific treatments for people with disorders associated with brain damage (Shapiro, 1966; Shapiro et al., 1973; Shallice, 1979; 1988, Howard, 1986; Pring, 1986; 1987). The superiority of single-case methodology lies in its ability to account for and even capitalize on the hallmark heterogeneity associated with the aphasia population. In fact, the findings of well-controlled, multiple-baseline single-case studies can be more readily applicable to clinical practice than are generalized findings across a heterogeneous sample. Further, multiple baseline studies are well suited to comparative evaluation of effectiveness across treatments.

Treatment results

Whether considering studies that use group design or those that employ single-subject methodology, research outcomes bearing on treatment-related hypotheses may be synthesized objectively by use of meta-analytic techniques to estimate an average effect size from the available evidence. The type of research (single-subject versus group design) dictates the mathematical techniques used in meta-analysis and the two types of design cannot be combined in the same analysis. However, regardless of study type, studies must produce quantifiable results if they are to contribute to a synthesized conclusion drawn from converging evidence. To date, lack of quantifiable results in primary studies is clearly a severe limitation for the body of evidence that has used single-subject methodology. Of the 63 studies included in the review by Robey et al. (1999) of single-subject clinical outcome research, only 12 (19%) studies presented quantifiable outcomes. This finding alone led Robey and colleagues (1999, p. 468) to conclude: 'the capacity for single-subject designs to produce standard evidence regarding the effectiveness of a treatment for an individual is largely unrealized.'

Unfortunately, the picture with respect to reporting quantitative data is not particularly healthier with group clinical outcome studies. Indeed, 46% of all group clinical outcome studies of the treatment of aphasia were considered inadequate with respect to provision of quantitative information necessary for the application of meta-analytic techniques (Robey, 1998). Similarly, Greener et al. (1999) stated that the most striking finding from their review of randomized controlled trials was not only the small number and the advanced age of randomized controlled trials that had been carried out but also how many methodological short-comings they had. Based on this finding, Greener et al. (1999, p. 16) concluded that there was justification 'for large scale, good quality randomised controlled trials of speech and language therapy for people who have aphasia following stroke'. These authors recommended a no-treatment versus formal speech and language therapy trial, although acknowledging the inherent ethical dilemma of treatment refusal in such a design. In contrast, Robey (1998) concluded that further studies to reinforce the general conclusion that outcomes for treated individuals are superior to those of untreated individuals would waste resources better spent on more focused investigations. Robey (1998) based this conclusion on the magnitude of the averaged effect size across 12 group studies without randomization that had investigated treatment versus no-treatment or control outcomes.

Threats to validity

It seems then that methodological shortcomings abound in the studies comprising the evidence base for the efficacy of aphasia therapy. Consequently, the conclusion from this literature cannot go beyond support for the broad hypothesis that, generally considered, aphasia therapy is effective. Indeed, practitioners using strict appraisal guidelines (for example, Sackett et al., 1997) may well consider that even this broad conclusion is not valid because it is not based on good quality, randomized controlled trials.

As well as the quality of primary studies, there is a further threat to the validity of systematic reviews that needs consideration. This threat relates to the degree of representativeness of the sample of primary studies synthesized or the sampling bias within the pool of primary studies. A non-representative sample of primary studies may arise for two reasons. First, the search strategy employed by the reviewers may have missed eligible primary studies. In order for the results to be valid all methods for identifying primary studies need to be implemented. Minimally, it is important that coverage of all relevant databases, and hand-searching of relevant journals not already searched, are demonstrated. Second, a general bias may exist in the literature which reflects a tendency not to publish or even submit primary studies that report negative findings. Such a bias is referred to as 'publication bias', and it is difficult to detect even when reviewers have used search strategies that included contacting academic institutions and individual researchers to identify unpublished material. Presence of publication bias means that an overview of published studies is likely to overestimate treatment efficacy.

The four systematic reviews (Robey, 1994, 1998; Greener et al., 1999; Cicerone et al., 2000) implemented comprehensive search strategies. In addition, Greener et al. (1999) reported approaching colleagues and authors of randomized trials to identify other relevant published and unpublished studies. Robey (1998) employed two statistical techniques to detect the possibility of publication bias. The first involved plotting sample size over effect size for each of the primary studies included in the review. Publication bias is unlikely to be present if the plot takes the form of an inverted funnel or a triangle resting on its base. The desired funnel profile was apparent for the plot of studies used to evaluate the within-effect, that is, pre-treatment versus post-treatment effect. A similar funnel configuration, although from fewer studies, was apparent for the between effect (treatment versus no treatment) plot. The second statistical technique used by Robey (1998) to examine the validity of his review involved calculating the number of null findings (that is, findings showing 0.0 effect size) that would be required to reduce the average treatment effect to a level less than or equal to the untreated effect. Across the hypotheses tested in the meta-analysis, the number of null findings required to produce such an outcome ranged from 6 to 66. These statistical analyses further support the validity of the results of the review.

Outcome-related variables

Given that synthesis of the current evidence base provides general support for the notion that people with aphasia who receive treatment by speech pathologists achieve superior clinical outcomes than those who do not, it is important to consider the evidence further with respect to individual-specific variables (for example, sex, age, language, handedness), aphasia-related variables (for example, severity, aetiology, type) and treatment variables (for example, type, amount, provider). For the most part, efforts to synthesize clinical outcomes around these variables have not been fruitful. Notable exceptions are the findings concerning the variables of aphasia severity and treatment intensity reported by Robey (1998). A total of 34 effects in the pool of pre–post-treatment effects were available to assess treatment outcomes in relation to aphasia severity. None of these addressed the effect of treatment on mildly aphasic individuals. Nine were coded as moderate severity, six as severe and the remaining 19 as heterogeneous (mixed severity in the primary study). These effects were further divided into the reference period in which treatment commenced (that is, acute, post-acute and chronic). The average effect size for moderately severe (d = 1.87) and severely (d = 2.76) aphasic people who began treatment in the acute period of recovery exceeded the criterion for a medium- and a large-sized effect, respectively. Only two effects were calculable for treatment commenced during the chronic phase. Both these effects were derived for people with moderately severe aphasia and their average size (d = 1.39) further supports the contention that treatment can promote large change even when begun in the chronic stage of recovery. It is important to acknowledge here that this large chronic stage treatment effect was derived from two studies (Doyle and Bourgeois, 1986; Helm-Estabrooks and Ramsberger, 1986) both of which evaluated the same treatment programme: *Helm's Elicited Language Training Program for Syntax Stimulation* (HELPSS) (Helm-Estabrooks, 1981). Thus, this effect may represent a treatment-specific effect that is further specific to patients with Broca's aphasia. As indicated by Robey (1998) in his discussion of the relatively large effect sizes obtained for moderately severe and severe aphasia, such a finding is not surprising given that people with severe deficits certainly have large scope for positive change in their performance. The potential for people with aphasia to achieve positive outcomes late in the recovery process is also supported by many single-subject experiments in the literature (for example, Nickels and Best, 1996; Robson et al., 1998; Rose et al., 2002) as well as the randomized controlled trial conducted by Elman and Bernstein-Ellis (1999).

Decision-making with respect to amount of treatment is by no means straightforward. A simple time estimate may reflect treatment regimes which vary significantly with respect to scheduling and duration factors (for example, distribution of treatment time throughout the day or the week, number and duration of treatments per week). Such time-related factors are generally acknowledged as important treatment planning variables and a 'more is better' flavour has underpinned much of the treatment literature in aphasia. From his analysis of amount of treatment, Robey (1998, p. 184) concluded: 'Treatment length in excess of two hours per week brings about gains exceeding those that result from shorter durations. Two hours of treatment per week should constitute a minimum length for patients who can withstand the rigours of receiving treatment.' His conclusion is based on the trend revealed in the 12 of the 60 pre–post-treatment effects that could be coded for amount of treatment. The average across three effects for high intensity treatment in the acute stage was better than twice the corresponding value for untreated recovery. In addition, effect size across the 12 pre–post-treatment comparisons was positively and moderately correlated with duration of treatment in weeks ($r = +0.76$, $p = 0.004$) and the total number of treatment hours at discharge ($r = +0.64$, $p = 0.026$). These findings together provide preliminary evidence for the clinical tenet that high intensity treatment effects greater performance change. However, due to the small number of effects available for analysis, the results are general and not specific to periods within the time post-onset continuum.

Although reviewers have set out to synthesize research findings around some of the other variables that potentially shape treatment outcomes, attempts have been thwarted by the limitations of the evidence base. For example, Greener et al. (1999) addressed the issue of treatment provider when they included as one of their five objectives an assessment of whether formal speech and language therapy from trained speech and language therapists was more effective than non-professional support from volunteers, trained or untrained, in improving expressive and receptive language disorders after stroke. They identified four trials relevant to this objective that met their inclusion criteria (Meikle et al., 1979; David et al., 1982; Wertz et al., 1986; Leal et al., 1993). Only outcome data in the form of drop-out rates were available for all four trials and odds ratio analysis found no statistically significant difference in the number of drop-outs from treatment whether treated by therapists or volunteers. Their conclusion regarding this objective stated: 'There was little evidence to judge whether informal support from a trained or untrained volunteer was any more or less effective as treatment from a trained speech and language therapist' (Greener et al., 1999, p. 15). They acknowledged that in small trials, like the ones conducted by David et al. (1982) and Meikle et al. (1979), the presence of variability due to individual participants and the effect of spontaneous recovery tends to favour acceptance of the null hypothesis or reduce the likelihood of a clear difference being demonstrated.

Clearly, the preceding brief exploration of the evidence base for aphasia therapy has revealed limitations. At present, the causes for this somewhat limited evidence base may be summarized effectively by a single word: *heterogeneity*. There is the marked heterogeneity of the aphasic patient population with which speech pathologists are so familiar. Added to that inherent population heterogeneity is the large amount of heterogeneity that exists within the primary studies that comprise the database used to evaluate treatment effectiveness. Variables underlying this heterogeneity include study design, treatment type, hypotheses tested, outcome measures and the quality of published reports. The heterogeneity within the pool of studies reporting clinical outcomes limits reliable and valid combination of data and provides significant challenges for the future development of aphasia therapy research.

Meeting the challenge

Perhaps the first and easiest challenge to address is the variable and often low quality of research reports. *Quality* here relates to the inclusion of scientific detail, that is, the detail that is necessary in order to be able to interpret and combine findings across aphasia treatment studies reliably. Almost 20 years ago, Kertesz (1984) and more recently Whurr et al. (1992) identified many important dimensions necessary for the interpretation of outcomes reported in aphasia therapy studies. In all the overviews included in this chapter, the authors acknowledged or discussed the issue of lack of essential detail in the pool of studies they reviewed. Greener et al. (1999) reported that there were missing and poorly reported data in many of the trials they included. Similarly, when Robey (1998) attempted to code reports for sex, language, neurologic history and side of lesion, only one of the 55 reports analysed had included each of the codified dimensions. He further pointed out that description of the treatment protocol being investigated was largely ambiguous or absent. In fact, the most frequently reported form of treatment was that coded as 'not specified'. Like Robey (1998), we may well presume that these treatments were appropriately designed to meet individual patient needs; however, we will continue to lose future potential benefits for our patients if clear, replicable descriptions of successful and unsuccessful treatment protocols are the exception rather than the rule of research reports.

As already indicated, the validity of the current evidence base is constrained by methodological shortcomings. Clearly, if 46% of all group clinical outcome studies of the treatment of aphasia are inadequate with respect to provision of quantitative information and if only 19% of published single-subject design studies present quantifiable outcomes, there is much room for improvement. Many suggestions have been made for improving the quality of quantitative information reported in treatment outcome studies (for example, Ware et al., 1986; Moher et al., 1994; Robey, 1994, 1998; Robey and Schulz, 1998; Robey et al., 1999; Slinger and Moher, 2000). Specific suggestions include reporting a priori statistical power analysis to determine appropriate sample size, a variety of descriptive statistics (for example, means, standard deviations, correlation coefficients, exact test statistics (t value), exact rather than < probability (p) values and effect size (d) values). Recommendations specific to single-subject research include insuring a sufficient number of baseline observations, combining visual analysis with statistical analysis and the use of statistical analysis procedures that are sensitive to the presence of autocorrelation in the data (for example, Matyas and Greenwood, 1990; Crosbie, 1993, 1995). Adoption of these suggestions will allow for synthesis of results across efficacy studies that address related questions. Consequently, the informative value of our research base will be enhanced.

Robey, who has conducted the majority of systematic reviews in this area, is clearly of the view that the basic issue of aphasia therapy effectiveness has been settled positively. In his discussion of the 'next era of clinical outcome research' (Robey, 1998, p. 183), he recommended that resources be dedicated to testing focused hypotheses programmatically. Focused hypotheses will provide evidence on which to base those thorny decisions such as treatment selection and termination that we make every day in clinical practice. Programmatic research is important because much of our current outcome evidence is composed of unitary independent studies without systematic replication. Systematic replication provides further support for clinical decisions, such as those that relate to the optimal amount and the stage of treatment provision, and differential effects relating to severity and level of language processing breakdown. Robey (1998) also recommended that programmatic research should combine single-subject experimental research testing focused hypotheses with group clinical trials testing similarly focused hypotheses. In this way, the field reaps the best of both worlds of outcome research, and the body of evidence for the effectiveness of aphasia treatment protocols will advance optimally. Whether single-subject or multiple-subject designs are employed, it is important that long-term maintenance of communication improvements produced by aphasia therapy is evaluated. Currently, short-term follow-up information is relatively scarce and long-term follow-up information is lacking.

Unlike medical treatments, which attempt to reverse pathology, aphasia therapy is primarily concerned with reducing levels of disability and increasing participation. Much of the clinical outcome research to date has evaluated treatment effectiveness by measuring change in the level of impairment. In fact, the outcome measures employed in efficacy research to date have dealt exclusively with diminution of impairment, measuring only a small component of outcome. Even when positive change in language impairment can be attributed to aphasia therapy, the relationship between this change and functional everyday improvement may, at best, be unclear or, at worst, be non-existent because of lack of generalization to everyday activities in home and community situations. This emphasis on change in impairment as the sole measure of outcome is clearly inappropriate when use of adaptive or compensatory strategies is the goal of a particular aphasia treatment. With compensatory treatments, real benefits are not likely to be apparent on impairment measures that do not provide the opportunity to mobilize adaptive strategies. Further, similar to the domains of disability and participation, patient and family satisfaction, and well-being are outcome domains in which aphasia therapy efficacy has rarely, if ever, been evaluated. It is important that outcome measures employed in future efficacy studies, are tailored to the specific, expected effects of the intervention. Ideally, outcome measures should reflect change in functional ability, such as performance of valued everyday activities at home and in the broader community, quality of life and subjective well-being. Recent developments of tools to measure change in these outcome domains (for example, *Therapy Outcome Measures*; Enderby, 1997) make it possible to diversify the dimensions upon which efficacy is evaluated. Promising, too, is the recent increase in qualitative research which has brought to the field the added richness of personal and sociological viewpoints in the constructivist paradigm (for example, Simmons-Mackie and Damico, 1999). Such research provides an additional means of evaluating treatment efficacy within the lived experience and culture of the person with aphasia. In addition, qualitative data presents its own challenge with respect to synthesis of findings across studies investigating related questions. This challenge is already being addressed and meta-syntheses of qualitative data have been attempted in other disciplines and fields (for example, Jensen and Allen, 1996; Noblit and Hare, 1988; Sandelowski et al., 1997; Suri, 1999).

At the beginning of the twenty-first century, there is not only much new information and new challenges for speech pathologists but also many tools that bring with them opportunities to help us evaluate and consequently improve the therapy received by people with aphasia.

References

Bonita R. Epidemiology of stroke. Lancet 1992; 339: 342–4.

Breasted JH. The Edwin Smith Surgical Papyrus. Chicargo: Chicago University Press, 1930.

Cicerone K, Dahlberg C, Kalmar K, Langenbahn D, Malec J, Bergquist T, Felicetti T, Giacino J, Harley P, Harrington D, Herzog J, Kneipp S, Laastch L, Morse P. Evidence-based cognitive rehabilitation: recommendations for clinical practice. Archives of Physical Medicine and Rehabilitation 2000; 81: 1596–1615.

Code C. The problem with RCTs. RCSLT Bulletin 2000; March: 14–15.

Crosbie J. Interrupted time-series analysis with brief single-subject data. Journal of Consulting and Clinical Psychology 1993; 61: 966–74.

Crosbie J. Interrupted time-series analysis with short series: why is it problematic? How can it be improved? In: Gottman JM (Ed.). The Analysis of Change. Mahwah, NJ: Lawrence Erlbaum, 1995.

Darley FL. Aphasia. Philadelphia, PA: WB Saunders Co., 1982.

David R, Enderby P, Bainton D. Treatment of acquired aphasia: speech therapists and volunteers compared. Journal of Neurology, Neurosurgery and Psychiatry 1982; 45: 957–61.

Doyle P, Bourgeois M. The effects of syntax training on 'adequacy' of communication in Broca's aphasia: a social validation study. In: Brookshire RH (Ed.). Clinical Aphasiology (Vol. 16). Minneapolis, MN: BRK Publishers, 1986.

Elman R, Bernstein-Ellis E. The efficacy of group communication treatment in adults with chronic aphasia. Journal of Speech, Language, and Hearing Research 1999; 42: 411-19.

Enderby P. Therapy Outcome Measures. San Diego, CA: Singular Publishing Group, 1997.

Enderby P, Davies P. Communication disorders: planning a service to meet the needs. British Journal of Disorders of Communication 1989; 24: 151-65.

Enderby P, Emerson J. Does Speech and Language Therapy Work? A Review of the Literature. London: Whurr Publishers, 1995.

Goldstein K. Language and Language Disturbances. New York, NY: Grune & Stratton, 1948.

Greener J, Enderby P, Whurr R. Speech and language therapy for aphasia following stroke (Cochrane Review). In: The Cochrane Library, Issue 4, Oxford: BMJ Books/Update Software, 1999.

Hall J, Rosenthal R, Tickle-Degnen L, Mosteller F. Hypotheses and problems in research synthesis. In: Cooper H, Hedges L (eds). The Handbook of Research Synthesis. New York, NY: Russell Sage Foundation, 1994.

Head H. Aphasia and kindred disorders of speech. Brain 1920; 43: 87-165.

Helm-Estabrooks N. Helm's Elicited Language Program for Syntax Stimulation. Austin, TX: Exceptional Resources Incorporated, 1981.

Helm-Estabrooks N, Ramsberger G. Treatment of agrammatism in long-term Broca's aphasia. British Journal of Disorders of Communication 1986; 21: 39-45.

Hicks N. Evidence-based health care. Bandolier 1997; 5: 8.

Holland A, Fromm D, DeRuyter F, Stein M. Treatment efficacy: aphasia. Journal of Speech, Language, and Hearing Research 1996; 39: S27-S36.

Howard D. Beyond randomised controlled trials: the case for effective case studies of the effects of treatment of aphasia. British Journal of Disorders of Communication 1986; 21: 89-102.

Jensen L, Allen M. Meta-synthesis of qualitative findings. Qualitative Health Research 1996; 6: 553-60.

Kertesz A. Neurobiological aspects of recovery from aphasia in stroke. International Journal of Rehabilitation Medicine 1984; 6: 122-7.

Kurtzke J. Epidemiology of cerebrovascular disease. In: Cerebrovascular Survey Report for Joint Council Subcommittee on Cerebrovascular Disease. Bethesda, MD: NINCDS, 1980.

Leal M, Farrajota L, Fonseca J, Guerriero M, Castro-Caldas A. The influence of speech therapy on the evolution of stroke aphasia. Journal of Clinical and Experimental Neuropsychology 1993; 5: 399.

Luria AR. Traumatic Aphasia: Its syndromes, psychology and treatment. The Hague: Mouton, 1970.

MacDonald G. Assessing systematic reviews and clinical guidelines. In: Moyer V (Ed.). Evidence Based Paediatrics and Child Health. London: BMJ Books, 2000.

Matyas T, Greenwood K. Visual analysis of single-case time series: effects of variability, serial dependence and magnitude of intervention effects. Journal of Applied Behaviour Analysis 1990; 2: 341-51.

Meikle M, Wechsler E, Tupper A, Benenson M, Butler J, Mulhall D, Stern G. Comparative trial of volunteers and professional treatments of dysphasia after stroke. British Medical Journal 1979; 2: 87-9.

Mlcoch A, Metter EJ. Medical aspects of stroke rehabilitation. In: Chapey R (Ed.). Language Intervention Strategies in Aphasia and Related Neurogenic Communication Disorders. New York, NY: Lippincott Williams & Wilkins, 2001.

Moher D, Dulberg C, Wells G. Statistical power, sample size and their reporting in randomized controlled trials. Journal of the American Medical Association 1994; 272: 122-4.

Moher D, Jadad A, Tugwell P. Assessing the quality of randomised control trials: current issues and future directions. International Journal of Technological Assessment and Health Care 1996; 12: 195-208.

National Stroke Foundation. Introducing the National Stroke Foundation and National Stroke Research Institute. Australia: National Stroke Foundation, 2000.

Nickels L, Best W. Therapy for naming disorders (Part II): specifics, surprises and suggestions. Aphasiology 1996; 10: 109-136.

Noblit G, Hare R. Meta-ethnography: Synthesising Qualitative Studies. Newbury Park, CA: Sage Publications, 1988.

Pearson V. Speech and language therapy: is it effective? Public Health 1995; 109: 143-53.

Pedersen P, Jorgensen H, Nakayama H, Raashou H, Olsen T. Aphasia in acute stroke: Incidence, determinants, and recovery. Annals of Neurology 1995; 38: 659-66.

Pedro-Cuesta J, Widen-Holmquist L, Bach-y-Rita P. Evaluation of stroke rehabilitation by randomised controlled studies: a review. Acta Neurologica Scandinavia 1992; 86: 433-9.

Pring T. Evaluating the effects of speech therapy for aphasics: developing the single case methodology. British Journal of Disorders of Communication 1986; 21: 103-15.

Robey R. The efficacy of treatment for aphasic persons: a meta-analysis. Brain and Language 1994; 47: 582-608.

Robey R. A meta-analysis of clinical outcomes in the treatment of aphasia. Journal of Speech, Language and Hearing Research 1998; 41: 172-87.

Robey R, Schultz M. A model for conducting clinical outcome research: an adaptation of the standard protocol for use in aphasiology. Aphasiology 1998; 12: 787-810.

Robey R, Schultz M, Crawford A, Sinner C. Single-subject clinical outcome research: design, data, effect sizes and analyses. Aphasiology 1999; 13: 445-73.

Robson J, Marshall J, Pring T, Chiat S. Phonological naming therapy in jargon aphasia: positive but paradoxical effects. Journal of the International Neuropsychological Society 1998; 4: 675-86.

Rose M, Douglas J, Matyas T. The comparative effectiveness of gestural and verbal treatments for a specific phonological naming impairment. Aphasiology 2002; 10: 1001-30.

Sackett D, Richardson W, Rosenberg W, Haynes R. Evidence-based Medicine: How to practice and teach EBM. New York, NY: Churchill Livingstone, 1997.

Sandelowski M, Docherty S, Emden C. Focus on qualitative methods. Qualitative meta-synthesis: issues and techniques. Research in Nursing and Health 1997; 20: 365-71.

Sarno M, Silverman M, Sands E. Speech therapy and language recovery in aphasia. Journal of Speech and Hearing Research 1970; 13: 607-23.

Scarpa M, Colombo P, Sorgato P, DeRenzi E. The incidence of aphasia and global aphasia in left brain-damaged patients. Cortex 1987; 23: 331-6.

Schuell H, Jenkins J, Jimenez-Pabon E. Aphasia in Adults: Diagnosis, prognosis and treatment. New York, NY: Harper & Row, 1964.

Shallice T. Case-study approach in neuropsychology. Journal of Clinical Neuropsychology 1979; 1: 183-211.

Shallice T. From Neuropsychology to Mental Structure. Cambridge: Cambridge University Press, 1988.

Shapiro MB. The single case in clinical psychological research. Journal of General Psychology 1966; 74: 3-23.

Shapiro MB, Litman GK, Nias DK, Hendry ER. A clinician's approach to experimental research. Journal of Clinical Psychology 1973; 29: 165-9.

Simmons-Mackie N, Damico J. Qualitative methods in aphasia research: ethnography. Aphasiology 1999; 13: 681-7.

Slinger R, Moher D. Assessing therapy. In: Moyer V (Ed.). Evidence Based Paediatrics and Child Health. London: BMJ Books, 2000.

Suri H. The Process of Synthesizing Qualitative Research: A Case Study. Paper presented at the annual conference of the Association for Qualitative Research, Melbourne, July, 1999.

Wade D, Langton-Hewer R, David R, Enderby P. Aphasia after stroke: natural history and associated deficits. Journal of Neurology, Neurosurgery and Psychiatry 1986; 49: 6-11.

Ware J, Mosteller F, Inglefinger J. P values. In: Bailar J, Mosteller F (eds). Medical Uses of Statistics. Waltham: NEJM Books, 1986.

Wepman J. A conceptual model for the processes involved in recovery from aphasia. Journal of Speech and Hearing Disorders 1953; 18: 4-13.

Wepman J. Aphasia therapy: some relative comments and some purely personal prejudices. In: Taylor Sarno M (Ed.). Aphasia: Selected Readings. New York, NY: Appleton-Century-Crofts, 1972.

Wertz R, Weiss D, Aten J, Brookshire R, Garcia-Bunuel L, Holland A, Kurtzke J, LaPointe L, Milianti F, Brannegan R, Greenbaum H, Marshall R, Vogel D, Carter J, Barnes N, Goodman R. Comparison of clinic, home, and deferred language treatment for aphasia: a Veterans Affairs cooperative study. Archives of Neurology 1986; 43: 653-8.

Whurr R, Lorch M, Nye C. A meta-analysis carried out between 1946 and 1988 concerned with efficacy of speech and language therapy treatment for aphasic patients. European Journal for Disorders of Communication 1992; 27: 1-18.

CHAPTER 4

The evidence base for the treatment of cognitive-communicative disorders after traumatic brain injury in adults

JACINTA DOUGLAS

Introduction: traumatic brain injury in context

In 1998 the National Institutes of Health (NIH) Consensus Development Panel on Rehabilitation of Persons with Traumatic Brain Injury concluded that traumatic brain injury, broadly defined as 'brain injury due to externally inflicted trauma', is a heterogeneous disorder of major public health significance. The significance of the disorder is based not only on the incidence of traumatic brain injury but also on the resultant life-long impairment of survivors' physical, cognitive and psychosocial functioning. The economic costs of traumatic brain injury are enormous with estimates for average lifetime costs of care for people with severe traumatic brain injury in the USA ranging from US$ 600,000 to US$ 1,875,000 (NIH, 1998). As the Consensus Development Panel pointed out, these figures may grossly underestimate the economic burden to families and to society because they do not include costs to state-funded social service systems, lost earnings for injured individuals and the value of time and lost earnings of family members who care for injured relatives.

Epidemiology

Current incidence estimates of traumatic brain injury in Australia, the UK and the USA are similar and reflect annual rates of approximately 100–160 per 100,000 people (NIH, 1998; Tate et al., 1998; Guerrero et al., 2000; Lovasik et al., 2001). These estimates are based mainly on information about patients admitted to hospital and those who die before hospitalization. Thus, there is a tendency for these figures to suffer from ascertainment bias, whereby people with mild injuries who are treated in a medical clinic rather than a hospital setting or who are only seen through the emergency departments of hospitals and not admitted are not counted by this method. Consequently, there is likely to be a significant underestimation of the overall incidence of traumatic brain injury, in particular for mild injuries. Until reliable data that are based on more than patients admitted to hospital become available, our understanding of the full spectrum of the disorder will continue to be incomplete.

Several trends, potentially significant from the perspective of prevention and rehabilitation, are evident across epidemiologic studies (Kraus et al., 1984; Tate et al., 1998; Guerrero et al., 2000). Males are more than twice as likely as females to sustain traumatic brain injury. The population distribution is bimodal with the highest incidence among adolescents and young adults, aged 15-24 years, and the elderly, aged 75 years and older. There is a lower peak in incidence in young children and toddlers five years of age and younger. Figures indicate that alcohol, either in the person causing the injury or in the person with the injury, is associated with as many as half of all injuries. Road traffic accidents, including motor vehicle, bicycle and pedestrian–vehicle incidents, are the most common cause – accounting for 50% of injuries and even more in the 18-25-year age group. Over the past 20 years there has been a gradual decline in the number of deaths and injuries related to road traffic accidents. This trend may be attributed to changes in road and automobile safety standards, including the increased use of restraints and airbags as well as reduced speed limits and improved road design and traffic control.

Falls are the second most common cause of traumatic brain injury among the very young and the elderly. Alcohol, medication and osteoporosis are risk factors for the elderly. About one-fifth of all injuries are caused by violence-related incidents, in particular in the 15–24-year age group but also in the very young. Domestic violence affects children and adults of both sexes, and although unintentional injury accounts for 75% of paediatric injuries, child abuse (for example, shaken baby syndrome) is a significant causal issue. Domestic violence-related brain injuries are also reported in the elderly. Sports and recreation-related traumatic brain injury is most common in the 5-24-year age group and responsible for approximately three per cent of admissions to hospital. Because of the mild nature of these injuries, they are thought to be under-reported and subsequently underestimated in incidence figures.

In addition to the overall trends described here, causal variations that reflect geographic or cultural variations have been noted. Examples include increased incidence of brain injury due to firearm and non-firearm assaults in the Bronx (Cooper et al., 1983), skiing accidents in Colorado (Hunter, 1999), bicycle accidents in China (Wang et al., 1986) and golf-related injuries in children in Scotland (McGuffie et al., 1998).

Pathophysiology

Acceleration or deceleration forces causing differential tissue movements within the skull are regarded as the major mechanism by which primary brain damage occurs following traumatic brain injury (Levin et al., 1982; Pang, 1985; Richardson, 1990; Katz, 1992). Differential tissue movements cause diffuse axonal injury as well as focal contusions. Regardless of the point of impact, the anterior and inferior surfaces of the frontal and temporal lobes are particularly vulnerable to such injury due to their proximity to the bony shelves of the skull. Diffuse axonal shearing also occurs particularly in the corpus callosum, the internal capsule, deep grey matter and in various tracts of the brain stem. Traumatic brain injury may either be closed (the skull and dura remain intact) or open (the skull is fractured and the cerebrum is penetrated). In addition to diffuse axonal injury and contusions associated with primary brain injury, intracranial and extracranial complications can cause secondary brain injury, either as a result of cerebral ischaemia or distortion and compression of the brain. Secondary complications include intracranial haematoma, oedema, raised intracranial pressure, infection, widespread hypoxia due to changes in cerebral blood flow or chest and airway injuries, and metabolic changes (Levin et al., 1982; Pang, 1985).

The complex nature of the pathophysiology of traumatic brain injury leads to marked heterogeneity of injury across individuals. Traumatic brain injury usually results in immediate loss or impairment of consciousness, followed by a period of confusion known as 'post-traumatic amnesia'. Severity may be indexed by the depth and length of coma and the length of post-traumatic amnesia. The duration of recovery is lengthy and the rate of recovery varies over time. Recovery may incorporate substages that have unique pathophysiology, and regional and functional differences in recovery may be exhibited over time. The neurobiological mechanisms responsible for functional recovery and their relative contribution to recovery at different stages after traumatic brain injury remain unclear and continue to be investigated (NIH, 1998).

The consequences of traumatic brain injury

Rarely are the consequences limited to one set of symptoms, clearly delineated impairments, or a disability that affects only one part of a person's life. Rather, the consequences of TBI often influence human functions along a continuum from altered physiological functions of cells through neurological and psychological impairments, to medical problems and disabilities that affect the individual with

TBI, as well as family, friends, community, and society in general. (NIH, 1998, p. 11)

The cognitive, behavioural and emotional sequelae of traumatic brain injury form part of the complex picture of its overall consequences, so clearly represented in the above quote from the NIH Consensus Statement (NIH, 1998). Much research has been dedicated to describing the consequences of injury for individuals (for example, Livingston et al., 1985; Tate et al., 1989; Hinkeldey and Corrigan, 1990; Ponsford et al., 1995; Corrigan et al., 1998; Douglas and Spellacy, 2000) and their families (for example, Brooks, 1991; Allen et al., 1994; Kreutzer et al., 1994; Douglas and Spellacy, 1996). In most cases, it is the cognitive, behavioural and emotional changes that prove to be the most disruptive and disabling chronic problems. The most persistent cognitive problems include: memory impairment; difficulties in attention and concentration; and impaired executive skills, such as problem-solving, abstract reasoning, insight, judgement, planning, information-processing and organization. Common behavioural deficits include: decreased ability to initiate responses; verbal and physical aggression; agitation; difficulties in learning; egocentricity; lack of self-awareness; altered sexual functioning; impulsivity; and social disinhibition. Depression, anxiety, altered emotional control and personality changes are also prevalent. These consequences occur in differing combinations, are variable in terms of their effects on individuals and can change in severity and presentation over time. They have a significant effect on an individual's capacity to participate in society and their social consequences are many and serious, including chronic unemployment, divorce, family breakdown, increased risk of suicide and substance abuse.

Cognitive-communicative impairment after traumatic brain injury

Communication is a complex interpersonal phenomenon dependent upon cognitive, linguistic and behavioural skills. Given the prevalence of cognitive and behavioural deficits following traumatic brain injury, it is not surprising that a large range of communication difficulties are described in the traumatic brain injury literature. The persistent communication difficulties associated with the diffuse damage of traumatic brain injury are rarely those associated with focal damage and aphasia (Heilman et al., 1971). They have been variously described as 'subclinical aphasia' (Sarno, 1980), 'non-aphasic language disturbances' (Prigatano et al., 1985), 'cognitive-language disorder' (Hagen, 1984) and 'cognitive-communicative impairment' (ASHA, 1988). Essentially, cognitive-communicative impairments associated with traumatic brain injury are a reflection of the underlying pathophysiology of the disorder. Indeed, the most common communication symptoms following traumatic brain injury are associated with damage to the frontal lobes, limbic structures and the connections between these structures (Ylvisaker et al., 2001). Ylvisaker et al. (2001, p. 755) list the following impairments as those most frequently associated with frontolimbic damage:

- Disorganized, poorly controlled discourse or paucity of discourse (spoken and written).
- Inefficient comprehension of language related to increasing amounts of information to be processed (spoken or written) and to rate of speech.
- Imprecise language and word retrieval problems.
- Difficulty understanding and expressing abstract and indirect language.
- Difficulty reading social cues, interpreting speaker intent and flexibly adjusting interactive styles to meet situational demands in varied social contexts.
- Awkward or inappropriate communication in stressful social contexts.
- Impaired verbal learning.

Clearly, these deficits reflect the interplay of cognitive and communicative functions. Consequently, rehabilitation of cognitive-communicative impairment after traumatic brain injury has developed within the broad context of cognitive rehabilitation.

Cognitive rehabilitation after traumatic brain injury

There is a large body of literature which describes various approaches to cognitive rehabilitation and outlines particular programmes (for example, Prigatano, 1986; Wood, 1987; Sohlberg and Mateer, 1989; Kreutzer and Wehman, 1991; Ponsford et al., 1995; Gillis, 1996; Ylvisker and Feeney, 1998). In addition, there are several contributions dedicated specifically to rehabilitation of cognitive-communicative disorders following traumatic brain injury (for example, Hagen, 1981; Hartley, 1995; Gillis, 1996; Snow and Ponsford, 1995; Snow and Douglas, 1999; Ylvisaker et al., 2001). Although there is no standard definition of cognitive rehabilitation, it generally involves 'a systematic, functionally oriented service of therapeutic activities that is based on assessment and understanding of the patient's brain–behavioural deficits' (Cicerone et al., 2000, p. 1596). Assessment and treatment planning are undertaken collaboratively by the rehabilitation team; the speech pathologist being primarily responsible for all aspects of communication. The person with the brain injury and his or her family are important members of the collaborative team and play a particularly active role in goal-setting. Whether interventions are described in traditional terms as 'restorative', 'compensatory', or indeed both, their essential purpose is to reduce the activity limitations experienced by people with traumatic brain injury and to increase optimally their participation in society. Just as communication deficits after traumatic brain injury reflect the interplay between cognitive and communicative impairments so, too, do the interventions used to address these deficits. Thus, it is not surprising to find that the current evidence base for the treatment of cognitive-communicative disorders after traumatic brain injury is contained within the evidence base for cognitive rehabilitation in general.

The practice of cognitive rehabilitation has not been without controversy over the years, and active debate concerning the theoretical foundations of various approaches to cognitive rehabilitation continues. Ylvisaker and colleagues (2002) reflect current debate in their recent reconsideration of theoretical paradigms in cognitive rehabilitation. Their statement emerged from the collaboration between the Joint Committee on Interprofessional Relationships for the American Speech, Language and Hearing Association (ASHA) and Division 40 (Neuropsychology) of the American Psychological Association (APA) and encompassed three purposes:

1 Exploration of the historical and conceptual foundations of cognitive rehabilitation.
2 Description of alternative paradigms for service delivery.
3 Promotion of studies by use of novel and theoretically sound paradigms to examine efficacy of cognitive rehabilitation.

The traditional approach to cognitive rehabilitation is outlined and compared with an alternative contextualized approach. In the context of their discussion, Ylvisaker et al. (2002) emphasize that, to date, most published studies of the effectiveness of cognitive rehabilitation have evaluated interventions from the traditional approach. Thus, the evidence base reviewed in this chapter must be considered within this constraint. Clearly, future research efforts need to be directed towards producing empirical evidence to support the comparative effectiveness of traditional and alternative approaches to cognitive rehabilitation.

Reviewing the evidence

Practitioners from the multiple disciplines involved in providing services for people with traumatic brain injury have acknowledged the need to establish empirically based recommendations for the practice of cognitive rehabilitation since the early 1980s. Indeed, health professional organizations and multidisciplinary panels have played a significant role in evaluating the existing literature on the effectiveness of cognitive rehabilitation. At the time of writing, the three most recent reviews of the cognitive rehabilitation literature arose from initiatives of the Consensus Statement, *Rehabilitation of Persons with Traumatic Brain Injury*, (NIH, 1998); the Agency for Health Care Policy and Research (AHCPR) (Carney et al., 1999; Chestnut et al., 1999); and the Brain Injury-Interdisciplinary Special Interest Group of the American Congress of Rehabilitation Medicine (BI-ISIG) (Cicerone et al., 2000). In 1996, ASHA also included a paper on cognitive-communicative disorders resulting from traumatic brain injury (Coelho et al., 1996) in the special supplement on treatment efficacy published in the *Journal of Speech and Hearing Research*. Together, these publications provide practitioners with an overview of the current state of available evidence to support the effectiveness of cognitive rehabilitation for people with traumatic brain injury. The objectives outlined by the authors of each review are listed in Table 4.1. Three of the reviews (NIH, 1998; Carney et al., 1999; Cicerone et al., 2000) included the intention to make evidence-based practice recommendations in the objectives, whereas the objective of the fourth review (Coelho et al., 1996) was limited to summarizing the evidence.

Although Coelho and colleagues (1996) specified the target of their review as cognitive-language disorders, like other recent reviews they addressed the broad spectrum of cognitive rehabilitation. Findings from samplings of two types of studies were presented: first, those focusing on the effects of general traumatic brain injury rehabilitation programmes; and second, specific interventions for discrete deficits. Treatments for attention, memory, executive function and social skill deficits were examined in the second category. The summary of treatment efficacy of general rehabilitation programmes referred to five studies (Prigatano et al., 1985; Harrington and Levandowski, 1987; Ruff et al., 1989; Ruff and Niemann, 1990; Mills et al., 1992), all of which were presented as providing support for treatment efficacy. Three broad descriptive categories of 'sample size', 'treatment focus' and 'improvements or findings reported' were used to summarize 38 treatment efficacy studies addressing specific deficits. With only one clear exception (Fussey and Tyerman, 1985), all the studies were described as reporting findings consistent with treatment-related improvement. The majority of studies (31) had a sample size of fewer than 10 participants; 17 of these were single-case studies.

Within their review, Coelho et al. (1996) also reported programme evaluation data for patients receiving speech and language pathology services from five inpatient rehabilitation services in the USA. Results were summarized by use of two variables: 'amount improvement' and 'number of

Table 4.1 Objectives and scope of reviews of the evidence base for cognitive rehabilitation

Review	Stated objectives	Scope of review
Coelho et al. (1996)	To summarize the evidence pertaining to treatment efficacy for cognitive-communicative disorders secondary to traumatic brain injury	Not specified
NIH Consensus Statement (1998)	To provide state of the art information and recommendations regarding effective rehabilitation measures for people who have suffered a traumatic brain injury	MEDLINE (1988–1998) Articles identified by experts
Carney et al. (1999)	To articulate the evidence for the effectiveness of cognitive rehabilitation, using methods and standards with demonstrated utility in other areas of medical research To illustrate controversies about the use of such standards in evaluating traumatic brain injury rehabilitation, particularly when applied to cognitive rehabilitation To compose reasonable recommendations for practice and for future research	MEDLINE (1976–1977) HealthSTAR (1995–1997) CINAHL (1982–1997) PsycINFO (1984–1997) Cochrane Library Reference lists of identified articles Peer recommendations
Cicerone et al. (2000)	To establish evidence-based recommendations for the clinical practice of cognitive rehabilitation, derived from a methodical review of the scientific literature concerning the effectiveness of cognitive rehabilitation for persons with traumatic brain injury or stroke	MEDLINE Articles identified by experts Reference lists from identified articles

patients improved', both reported as a percentage. Although outcomes were evaluated on a variety of functional status measures (for example, functional assessment measure, (FAM); functional independence measure, (FIM)) all employed a seven-point rating scale, and admission and discharge measures were taken. The average amount of improvement for the six treatment areas of receptive language, expressive language, speech production, reading, writing and cognition ranged from a low of 9.7% for speech production to a high of 26.1% for cognition. The average number of patients improving in these areas ranged from 69.4% for receptive language to 88% for reading. As the authors stated, these trends 'support the notion that a period of intensive inpatient rehabilitation is beneficial for cognitive-communicative deficits secondary to traumatic brain injury' (Coelho et al., 1996, p. S13). Clearly, beyond this general conclusion lay many specific patient- and treatment-related variables that need further investigation.

The summary of studies provided by Coelho et al. (1996) leaves the reader with a clear sense that the efficacy of treatments for cognitive-communicative disorders is supported by empirical evidence in the literature. However, critical appraisal of this review from an evidence-based practice perspective reveals several shortcomings that undermine the validity of the findings to some degree. As already indicated in Chapters 2 and 3, the validity of the results of a subject review or summary is measured by the transparency of the methods used to identify and evaluate the primary studies that are included. Consequently, it is disappointing to note that a clear methodology for the review was not included in the publication. Without clear explication of the search strategy, the criteria for considering studies, the types of studies and the types of participants, it is not possible to evaluate whether relevant studies were likely to be missed by the search strategy, whether those primary studies that were included were valid and whether they were selected without bias. Notwithstanding these limitations, the broad conclusion that 'there are a number of treatment techniques that have been successfully applied to deficits of attention, memory, and executive functions in various traumatic brain injury patients/clients' (Coelho et al., 1996, p. S13) has been reiterated in subsequent reviews, which have formed the basis of current practice recommendations.

Establishing evidence-based practice recommendations for cognitive rehabilitation of people with traumatic brain injury

In rehabilitation, as in other areas of healthcare, a desire for evidence-based guidance has led to increased use of systematic reviews as a basis for establishing practice recommendations, clinical guidelines or practice guidelines. Practice guidelines are statements that have been systematically developed to direct clinician and client decision-making in particular clinical circumstances. The NIH Consensus Panel, Carney et al. (1999) and Cicerone et al. (2000) all included practice recommendations in their reports. When setting out to develop practice recommendations, the development group needs to include all key stakeholders, including service users. It is also important that there be multidisciplinary representation, in order to avoid biased evaluation of evidence by groups with vested interests (MacDonald, 2000). The evidence upon which recommendations are based is crucial to their validity. Consequently, practice recommendations are frequently graded according to the quality of the supporting evidence upon which they are based. Of the reviews discussed here, only that conducted by Cicerone et al. (2000) graded recommendations. These authors did so by use of three levels from 'practice standards' (highest level of supporting evidence), through 'practice guidelines' to 'practice options' (lowest level of supporting evidence). (The recommendations from all three overviews and the evidence upon which they are based are discussed in the following sections.)

NIH Consensus Statements

The NIH Consensus Statements result from consensus development conferences that are convened to evaluate available scientific information and resolve safety and efficacy issues in health. These statements are prepared by non-advocate, non-federal panels of experts, based on three sources of information:

- First, presentations of investigators working in areas relevant to the consensus questions.
- Second, questions and statements from conference attendees during public discussion sessions.
- Third, closed deliberations by the panel.

The final independent report is intended to advance understanding of the issue in question and to be of benefit to health professionals and members of the public in general. A 16-member panel representing the fields of neuropsychology, neurology, psychiatry, behavioural medicine, family medicine, paediatrics, physical medicine and rehabilitation, speech and hearing, occupational therapy, nursing, epidemiology, biostatistics and the public prepared the consensus report for this issue, emphasizing the multidisciplinary nature of rehabilitation for people with traumatic brain injury. A further 23 experts from these same disciplines presented information to the panel and an audience of 883 people. Like the review completed by Coelho et al. (1996), the published consensus report does not have the same transparency of methodology characteristically required of systematic reviews. Thus, although there was a clear declaration of the intent and the source of information of the review, variables including the criteria for considering studies, the types of studies included, types of participants, types of outcome measures used and the methods of the review were not uniformly made explicit.

Evidence used to inform consensus development was derived from a review of the literature for cognitive rehabilitation identified via a search through MEDLINE from January 1988 to August 1998. The panel addressed five key questions concerning epidemiology, consequences, recovery, therapeutic interventions and models of rehabilitation. Two of these key questions specifically evaluated evidence-based issues in management: 'What are the common therapeutic interventions for the cognitive and behaviour sequelae of traumatic brain injury, what is their scientific basis, and how effective are they?' and 'What are common modes of comprehensive, coordinated, multidisciplinary rehabilitation for people with traumatic brain injury, what is their scientific basis, and what is known about their short-term and long-term outcomes?' (NIH, 1998, p. 7). Based on the answers to these questions, 15 recommendations regarding rehabilitation practices for people with traumatic brain injury were made and a further 30 research needs within the field were identified. (Recommendations made by the panel are summarized in Table 4.2.)

Perhaps one of the most telling findings of this review was that the research needs the panel identified clearly outnumbered the recommendations. Further, several of the recommendations concerning rehabilitation programmes were based on tenuous research findings from an evidence-based perspective. For example, the panel noted that comprehensive interdisciplinary rehabilitation treatment using individually tailored interventions provided by experienced professionals was commonly used for people with traumatic brain injury. However, they also acknowledged that this personalization of rehabilitation led to great difficulty in the scientific evaluation of its effectiveness because there was significant heterogeneity among both the people with traumatic brain injury and the comprehensive treatment programmes they received. Evidence supporting the effectiveness of comprehensive, interdisciplinary approaches was limited to one non-randomized clinical trial and uncontrolled studies. With respect to specific treatments, the levels of evidence cited to support recommendations varied markedly. The use of cognitive exercises to improve specific neuropsychological processes (attention, memory and executive skills) was supported by randomized controlled studies and case reports. Many descriptive studies and a single prospective clinical trial provided the

Table 4.2 Recommendations for rehabilitation: NIH Consensus Panel (1998)

- Rehabilitation should be matched to the needs, strengths and capacities of individuals, and modified as needs change over time

- Rehabilitation for people with moderate or severe traumatic brain injury should be interdisciplinary and comprehensive

- Rehabilitation should include cognitive and behavioural assessment and intervention

- People with traumatic brain injury and their families should have the opportunity to play an integral role in the planning and design of their rehabilitation and associated research endeavours

- People with traumatic brain injury should have access to rehabilitation through the entire course of recovery

- Substance abuse evaluation and treatment should be a component of rehabilitation

- Medications used for behavioural management can impede rehabilitation progress, and therefore should be used only in compelling circumstances

- Medications used for cognitive enhancement can be effective, but benefits should be evaluated and documented for each individual

- Community-based, non-medical services should be components of the extended care and rehabilitation available for people with traumatic brain injury

- Families and significant others should receive support

- Rehabilitation efforts should include environmental modifications to enable fuller participation

- Special programmes are needed to identify and treat people with mild traumatic brain injury

- Specialized, interdisciplinary and comprehensive programmes are necessary for young and school-age children with traumatic brain injury and for people older than age 65 with traumatic brain injury

limited support for the efficacy of behaviour modification to address the behavioural effects of traumatic brain injury. The recommendation of intervention for family members was supported solely by clinical experience as no empirical studies had evaluated the efficacy of these interventions. Neither the number nor the details of primary studies referred to as support for recommendations were provided in the report. Notwithstanding the lack of evidential detail, the review revealed that studies to support rehabilitation were relatively limited. Consequently, conclusions highlighted the following research needs:

- The completion of well-designed and controlled studies to evaluate benefits of different rehabilitation interventions.
- Replication of studies showing positive results.
- The development of innovative research methodologies.

Systematic reviews

Recently, Carney et al. (1999) and Cicerone et al. (2000) reported the results of systematic reviews undertaken to summarize the existing evidence base for cognitive rehabilitation. The cognitive rehabilitation review described by Carney et al. (1999) was a subcomponent of a larger review concerning the effectiveness of rehabilitation after traumatic brain injury. In 1999, the summary report for the entire review (Chestnut et al., 1999) was published in the *Journal of Head Trauma Rehabilitation*. Only the data specific to cognitive rehabilitation (Carney et al., 1999) are discussed here. These two reviews of cognitive rehabilitation were conducted under the direction of multidisciplinary panels and they provide essential details concerning the methodology of the reviews. Table 4.3 provides a summary of exclusionary criteria and definitions of levels of evidence applied to the primary studies that were included in both reviews. A major difference between the two reviews involved the exclusion of primary studies in which people with stroke participated. Cicerone et al. (2000) included primary studies investigating cognitive rehabilitation after stroke as well as traumatic brain injury; Carney et al. (1999) did not, thus explaining the large difference between the two reviews with respect to the number of studies included for evaluation. This difference is not inconsequential and clearly illustrates the relative strength of the research base with respect to the volume of studies that have investigated intervention effectiveness for the stroke population as compared to the traumatic brain injury population. (The findings reported by Cicerone et al. (2000) that are relevant to aphasia therapy are discussed in Chapter 3.)

Carney et al. (1999) evaluated the findings of the 32 primary studies included in their review using a framework linking cognitive rehabilitation with potential measurable benefits either directly or indirectly. Direct evidence for the effectiveness of cognitive rehabilitation came from studies that used measures of health outcomes experienced by patients in daily life, including employment. Indirect evidence came from studies using intermediate measures (for example, tests of cognitive function) as outcomes. Such studies are concerned with the question: 'Does cognitive rehabilitation improve scores on measures of cognitive function?' Indirect

Table 4.3 Exclusionary criteria and definitions of levels of evidence used by Carney et al. (1999) and Cicerone et al. (2000)

	Carney et al. (1999) Traumatic brain injury only	Cicerone et al. (2000) Traumatic brain injury and stroke
Studies identified	600	655
Exclusion criteria	Not traumatic brain injury Paediatric Pharmacological intervention Case report Instrument development Editorial or no data Alcohol/drug abuse as an outcome Review papers Stroke Acute care intervention Non-English language	Subjects other than people with TBI or stroke Paediatric Pharmacologic interventions Single-case reports without empirical data Reports not addressing intervenion Theoretical articles or descriptions of treatment approaches Review papers Intervention not adequately specified Non-peer-reviewed articles and book chapters Non-English language
Studies included	32	171
Levels of evidence	Class I: well-designed randomized controlled trials (RCTs) Class II(a): RCTs with design flaws and multicentre or population-based longitudinal (cohort) studies Class II(b): non-randomized controlled trials, case-control studies and well-designed case series Class III : case reports, uncontrolled case series and expert or consensus opinion	Class I: well-designed, prospective randomized controlled trials (RCTs) Class Ia: prospective design with a 'quasi-randomized' assignment to treatment conditions Class II: prospective, non-randomized cohort studies; retrospective, non-randomized case-control studies, or clinical series with well-designed controls that permitted between subject comparisons of treatment conditions, such as multiple baseline across subjects Class III: clinical series without concurrent controls, or studies with results from one or more single cases that used appropriate single-subject methods, such as multiple baseline across interventions with adequate quantification and analysis of results

evidence requires that the link between performance on intermediate measures and health outcomes is also evaluated. Thus, studies addressing the question: 'Do intermediate measures used to assess the effectiveness of treatment predict improvement in everyday function and employment?' also need to be evaluated.

From the perspective of direct evidence, only seven studies measuring relevant health outcomes were identified (five randomized controlled trials, one comparative study and one observational study). Three of these studies reported significant treatment effects. One small Class I study (Schmitter-Edgecombe et al., 1995) and one Class III study (Wilson et al., 1997) provided evidence of the direct effect of reminder devices on the reduction of everyday memory failures for patients with traumatic brain injury. The treatment effect evident in the study conducted by Schmitter-Edgecombe et al. (1995) was no longer evident at six-month follow-up, and follow-up results were not reported by Wilson et al. (1997). An early Class IIa study conducted by Helffenstein and Wechsler (1982) provided evidence that group treatment designed to improve interpersonal communication skills was effective. Intervention involved systematic feedback on videotaped communication interactions. The control group received the same amount (20 hours) of individual treatment with no feedback on interpersonal communication skills. Although sample size was small ($n = 16$), a significant treatment effect was found. The experimental group showed improved self-concept and interpersonal communication skills, reduced anxiety and generalization of behaviours related to effective interpersonal communication to non-therapeutic social settings. From a speech pathology perspective, the positive results evidenced by this study reinforce the clinical use of video-recording and evaluation with behavioural feedback as a strategy for the treatment of pragmatic deficits following traumatic brain injury. The remaining four studies that directly evaluated treatment using relevant health outcomes reported no significant treatment effects.

Studies providing indirect evidence included six randomized controlled trials, three comparative studies and eight observational studies. Of these, three small Class I studies (Kerner and Acker, 1985; Thomas-Stonell et al., 1994; Twum and Parente, 1994) and two Class IIb studies (Gray et al., 1992; Wood and Fussey, 1987) provided evidence that practice and computer-assisted cognitive rehabilitation improved performance on laboratory based measures of immediate recall. No studies evaluating the link between cognitive tests and health outcomes were identified. Because the eight observational studies did not meet the criteria for evidence used in this review, they did not contribute to the body of evidence about the intervention provided. Nevertheless, the results of these clinical studies were consistent with improved performance on laboratory tests following one-to-one therapeutic interaction.

Neither strong nor indeed sufficient evidence from group studies for a direct or indirect effect of cognitive intervention on health or employment was identified in the review. However, the authors stated: 'In effectively all of the studies in this review, patients improved. Although group differences were rarely observed, recovery across groups occurred' (Carney et al., 1999, p. 306). Last, based on the preliminary level of evidence in the review, two broad practice recommendations were made. The first recommended that compensatory cognitive strategies, adapted to patient groups and to individuals, be used to improve functional ability. The second recommendation acknowledged that for optimal success cognitive interventions are best delivered in the context of a broader programme that accounts for individual needs and uses various restorative and/or compensatory remediation technologies.

Cicerone et al. (2000) evaluated 171 primary studies in their systematic review of the effectiveness of cognitive rehabilitation for people with traumatic brain injury or stroke. Twenty-nine were rated as Class I studies, 35 as Class II and 107 as Class III. This relative increase in the number of studies as the strength of evidence decreases is common across most areas of practice. Thirteen studies were reviewed in the area of treatment for attention deficits, 40 in visuospatial deficits, 41 in language and communication deficits, 42 in memory deficits and 14 in executive functioning and problem-solving. Six of these studies evaluated multi-modal intervention for one or more deficits. A further 15 studies that involved a comprehensive holistic approach to cognitive rehabilitation were evaluated. Of the 29 Class I studies identified, 20 provided clear evidence to support the effectiveness of cognitive rehabilitation for people with traumatic brain injury or stroke. In most of the controlled studies that showed negative results, the intervention in question was compared with an alternative treatment, and with the exception of a single study, participants improved significantly despite evidence for a differential treatment effect being absent. Twelve of the Class I studies involving participants with traumatic brain injury evaluated the effectiveness of cognitive rehabilitation after traumatic brain injury. Overall, eight of these studies provided support for the effectiveness of cognitive remediation strategies in the treatment of attention, functional communication, memory and problem-solving after traumatic brain injury. Further, the evidence also suggested that overall improvement may be greatest when individual cognitive treatments are integrated with interpersonal therapies in comprehensive–holistic rehabilitation programmes.

As indicated earlier in this chapter, three levels of recommendations defined by the strength of associated evidence were made as a result of the review. 'Practice standards' required the strongest level of evidence and were based on at least one well-designed Class I study with an adequate sample, or overwhelming Class II evidence, that directly addressed the effectiveness of the treatment in question. 'Practice guidelines' required fair evidence to support the recommendation and were based on well-designed Class II studies with adequate samples. 'Practice options' had the lowest level of evidence and unclear clinical certainty. They were based on Class II or Class III studies and required additional grounds to support a recommendation as to whether the treatment be specifically considered. (The practice recommendations relevant to traumatic brain injury with a summary of the level of supporting evidence are presented in Table 4.4. The findings concerning language and communication deficits are discussed below.)

The committee recognized the dynamic interrelationship between linguistic and cognitive processes and reviewed treatment studies that addressed a broad scope of language-related impairments. Of the 41 studies identified to review in this area, eight were Class I studies, seven were Class II studies and 26 were Class III studies. Only 16% of these studies investigated treatment of communication disorders after traumatic brain injury; the remaining 84% of studies addressed intervention following left hemisphere stroke. Of the eight Class I studies, two involved participants with traumatic brain injury. These figures leave little doubt that the evidence base for the management of communication disorders after traumatic brain injury is substantially smaller than that available in the area of aphasia therapy.

The two Class I studies that evaluated the effectiveness of cognitive intervention for functional communication deficits after traumatic brain injury were those of Helffenstein and Wechsler (1982) and Thomas-Stonell et al. (1994). Both were also identified as providing supporting evidence in the systematic review conducted by Carney et al. (1999). In addition, Cicerone et al. (2000) identified five small Class III studies that reported benefits related to intervention for social and pragmatic communication deficits after traumatic brain injury (Gajar et al., 1984; Ehrlich and Sipes, 1985; Giles et al., 1988; Lewis et al., 1988; Milton, 1988). Although these studies all had small sample sizes, they provide support for the effectiveness of focused cognitive interventions to improve functional, interactive communication skills after traumatic brain injury. Clearly in comparison to aphasia therapy, the development and evaluation of interventions for cognitive-language disorders is in its infancy. Nevertheless, the Brain Injury-Interdisciplinary Special Interest Group of the American Congress of Rehabilitation Medicine considered that the evidence identified in their systematic review was strong enough to support the recommendation of interventions directed at improving pragmatic communication and conversational skills as a practice standard.

In summary, the four comprehensive reviews of the empirical literature on cognitive rehabilitation discussed here provide support for the

Table 4.4 Supporting evidence and practice recommendations for cognitive rehabilitation after traumatic brain injury (Cicerone et al., 2000)

Supporting evidence	Intervention
Practice standards: good evidence supports specific consideration of the following interventions for people with traumatic brain injury	
1 prospective, controlled Class I study 5 small Class III studies	Specific interventions for functional communication deficits, including pragmatic conversational skills
4 prospective, controlled Class I studies	Compensatory memory strategy training for mild memory impairments
Practice guidelines: fair evidence supports specific consideration of the following interventions for people with traumatic brain injury	
2 Class I studies 2 Class II studies	Attention training during post-acute rehabilitation. Insufficient evidence to distinguish treatment effect during acute recovery
1 prospective, controlled Class I study	Cognitive interventions for specific language impairments, such as reading comprehension and language formation
1 Class Ia study 2 Class II studies	Training in formal problem-solving strategies and their application to everyday situations and functional activities during post-acute rehabilitation
3 controlled Class II studies	Comprehensive–holistic neuropsychologic rehabilitation to reduce cognitive and functional disability
Practice options: evidence with unclear clinical certainty supports specific consideration of the following interventions for people with traumatic brain injury	
1 Class II study 8 Class III studies	Use of memory notebooks or other external aids to facilitate acquisition of specific skills and knowledge for people with moderate to severe memory impairments; should directly apply to functional activities
2 Class II studies	Verbal self-instruction, self-questioning, and self-monitoring to promote self-regulation for people with deficits in executive functioning; should incorporate detailed neuropsychologic and clinical assessment data to modify treatment on the basis of individual strengths and limitations
1 controlled Class II study	Integrated treatment, that is both individual cognitive and interpersonal therapies within the context of comprehensive–holistic neuropsychologic rehabilitation
2 Class II studies	Computer-based interventions that include active therapist involvement to foster insight into cognitive strengths and weaknesses, to develop compensatory strategies and to facilitate the transfer of skills into real life situations as part of multi-modal intervention for cognitive deficits

effectiveness of several treatments for cognitive impairments associated with traumatic brain injury. In addition, these evidence-based reviews have clearly identified gaps to be filled by future research to validate the effectiveness and utility of cognitive rehabilitation.

Conclusions: future directions

The NIH Consensus Panel drew two conclusions that were clearly supported by the state of evidence presented at the consensus conference:

- Well-designed and controlled studies are needed to evaluate benefits of different rehabilitation interventions.
- The evaluation of traumatic brain injury interventions will require innovative research methodologies (NIH, 1998, p. 28).

The conclusions themselves lead to multiple challenges for clinicians and researchers alike. Although these challenges certainly apply to the evaluation of cognitive interventions after traumatic brain injury, they are not exclusive to the area and have been identified across many of the chapters in this book. The first consideration is the questions to ask. Researchers must ask the important, not the trivial, questions and must do so with focused hypotheses. Rigorous attention must be paid to the variables under scrutiny. Research reports must include detailed operational definitions of the cognitive intervention(s) (independent variables) being evaluated. Reliable outcome measures (dependent variables) that are relevant to people with traumatic brain injury and their families, and to funding bodies need to be used and if necessary developed. Subject variables (for example, demographics, injury severity and chronicity) that underpin the hallmark heterogeneity of the traumatic brain injury population need be clearly specified and, where possible, controlled for within research designs. Further, it is important to account for the confounding variables of spontaneous recovery and a general stimulation effect versus an intervention-specific effect.

Increased research attention also needs to be paid to long-term maintenance of those gains that are achieved in rehabilitation. A recent study conducted by Sander et al. (2001) is the exception rather than the rule with respect to evaluation of maintenance in traumatic brain injury rehabilitation outcome research. The objective of this study was to determine changes in functioning from admission to discharge, and maintenance of those changes over time, for people with mild to severe traumatic brain injury involved in a comprehensive–integrated post-acute rehablitation programme ($n = 34$). The study includes a full description of the nature of the rehabilitation programme as well as reference to further sources providing additional details. Within the research design, provision was made to control statistically for time since injury. Reliable and valid outcome measures were used (Disability Rating Scale, (DRS) – Rappaport et al., 1982; Community Integration Questionnaire, (CIQ) – Willer et al., 1994) that had been developed specifically for patients with traumatic brain injury, and follow-up evaluation was carried out at two post-discharge follow-up time points. Results indicated that people who were admitted to the rehabilitation programme within eight months of injury showed substantial functional improvement (independence, social activities, productivity) from admission to discharge. Group analyses indicated that functional gains were maintained over time with no significant change being evident from discharge to either of the follow-up periods (12 months and 46 months post-discharge).

The use by Sander et al. (2001) of a multivariate repeated-measures design with the inclusion of time from injury to discharge as a covariate enabled greater confidence in attributing the improvements measured at discharge to treatment rather than simply spontaneous recovery. However, as these workers indicated, such a design does not provide evidence that maintenance of gains at follow-up was attributable only to the functional results of rehabilitation. Environmental modifications, the supporting efforts of family and friends, emotional adjustments and late neurological recovery are just some of the factors that may have contributed to follow-up results. Although the group results of this study indicated maintenance of functional gains over time, they held within them illustration of another of the dilemmas facing researchers in the field. That is, inspection of individual participants' DRS and CIQ scores at discharge and the two follow-up points indicated that many individual participants showed changes. For example, only 50% of participants obtained the same 'level of functioning' score on the DRS at discharge and the first follow-up; less than 40% obtained the same score at discharge and the second follow-up. Participants were equally likely to get better or worse at either follow-up. Such results are consistent with a conceptualization of outcome as a dynamic process characterized by positive and negative changes that reflect the impact of a multiplicity of factors. This tension between individual and group results underscores the need for efficacy research to involve research using both well-controlled single-subject experimental design and well-controlled multivariate group design. Indeed, as highlighted in all the reviews considered in this chapter, traumatic brain injury is an extremely heterogeneous disorder with regard to its neuropathology, its clinical presentation and its outcome. Consequently, group studies must face the difficult challenge of accounting for the influence of the many variables that shape an individual's response to acquired disability. Jordon (2000, p. 3123), in his editorial for the *Journal of the American Medical Association*, further emphasized this situation when he stated that 'traumatic brain injury has many unique features (i.e., cognitive and psychosocial) that are not properly addressed by data systems. Any attempt to investigate the efficacy of traumatic brain injury rehabilitation should focus on a select subset of patients with brain trauma'. Given the heterogeneity of the traumatic brain injury population and the individual nature of treatment, the use of sound single-subject research designs and controlled multiple-baseline designs across interventions and participants will significantly contribute to the evidence research base.

In conclusion, the developing evidence base for cognitive rehabilitation needs considerable growth in order for clinicians to be fully confident in their ability to provide optimal care for the many people who experience the challenge of living with the effects of traumatic brain injury. Evidence needs to be collected using a broad approach to research, including group designs, single-subject experimental designs, combined qualitative and quantitative methods and systematic replication of positive results.

References

Allen K, Linn RT, Gutierrez H, Willer BS. Family burden following traumatic brain injury. Rehabilitation Psychology 1994; 39: 29–48.

American Speech–Language–Hearing Association (ASHA). The role of speech–language pathologists in the identification, diagnosis and treatment of individuals with cognitive-communicative impairments. ASHA 1988; 30: 79.

Brooks DN. The head-injured family. Journal of Clinical and Experimental Neuropsychology 1991; 13: 155–188.

Carney N, Chestnut R, Maynard H, Mann N, Patterson P, Helfand M. Effect of cognitive rehabilitation on outcomes for persons with traumatic brain injury: a systematic review. Journal of Head Trauma Rehabilitation 1999; 14: 277–307.

Chestnut R, Carney N, Maynard H, Mann N, Patterson P, Helfand M. Summary report: evidence for the effectiveness of rehabilitation for persons with traumatic brain injury. Journal of Head Trauma Rehabilitation 1999; 14: 176–88.

Cicerone K, Dahlberg C, Kalmar K, Langenbahn D, Malec J, Bergquist T, Felicetti T, Giacino J, Harley P, Harrington D, Herzog J, Kneipp S, Laastch L, Morse P. Evidence-based cognitive rehabilitation: recommendations for clinical practice. Archives of Physical Medicine and Rehabilitation 2000; 81: 1596–1615.

Coelho C, De Ruyter F, Stein M. Treatment efficacy: cognitive-communicative disorders resulting from traumatic brain injury in adults. Journal of Speech and Hearing Research 1996; 39: 5–17.

Cooper K, Tabaddor K, Hauser A, Shulman K, Feiner C, Factor P. The epidemiology of head injury in the Bronx. Neuroepidemiology 1983; 2: 70–88.

Corrigan J, Smith-Knapp K, Granger C. Outcomes in the first 5 years after traumatic brain injury. Archives of Physical Medicine and Rehabilitation 1998; 79: 298–305.

Douglas J, Spellacy F. Indicators of long-term family functioning following severe traumatic brain injury in adults. Brain Injury 1996; 10: 819–39.

Douglas J, Spellacy F. Correlations of depression in adults with severe traumatic brain injury and their carers. Brain Injury 2000; 14: 71–88.

Ehrlich J, Sipes A. Group treatment of communication skills for head trauma patients. Cognitive Rehabilitation 1985; 3: 32–7.

Fussey K, Tyerman A. An exploration of memory retraining in rehabilitation following closed head injury. International Journal of Rehabilitation Research 1985; 8: 465-7.

Gajar A, Schloss P, Schloss C, Thompson C. Effects of feedback and self-monitoring on head trauma youths' conversational skills. Journal of Applied Behavior Analysis 1984; 17: 353-8.

Giles G, Fussey I, Burgess P. The behavioral treatment of verbal interaction skills following severe head injury: a single case study. Brain Injury 1988; 2: 75-9.

Gillis R. Traumatic Brain Injury: Rehabilitation for Speech–Language Pathologist. Boston, MA: Butterworth–Heinemann, 1996.

Gray J, Robertson I, Pentland B, Anderson S. Microcomputer-based attentional retraining after brain damage: a randomised group controlled trail. Neuropsychological Rehabilitation 1992; 2: 97-115.

Guerrero J, Thurman D, Sniezek J. Emergency department visits associated with traumatic brain injury: United States, 1995-1996. Brain Injury 2000; 14: 181-6.

Hagen C. Language disorders secondary to closed head injury: diagnosis and treatment. Topics in Language Disorders 1981; 1: 73-87.

Hagen C. Language disorders in head trauma. In: A Holland (Ed.). Language Disorders in Adults: Recent Advances. San Diego, CA: College-Hill Press, 1984.

Harrington D, Levandowski D. Efficacy of an educationally-based cognitive retraining program for the traumatically head injured as measured by LNNB pre- and post-test scores. Brain Injury 1987; 1: 65-72.

Hartley L. cognitive-communicative Abilities following Brain Injury: A Functional Approach. San Diego, CA: Singular Publishing, 1995.

Heilman K, Safran A, Geschwind N. Closed head trauma and aphasia. Journal of Neurology, Neurosurgery, and Psychiatry 1971; 34: 265-9.

Helffenstein D, Wechsler R. The use of interpersonal process recall (IPR) in the remediation of interpersonal and communication skill deficits in the newly brain injured. Clinical Neuropsychology 1982; 4: 139-43.

Hinkeldey N, Corrigan J. The structure of head-injured patients' neurobehavioural complaints: a preliminary study. Brain Injury 1990; 4: 115-34.

Hunter R. Skiing injuries. American Journal of Sports Medicine 1999; 27: 381-9.

Jordon B. Cognitive rehabilitation following traumatic brain injury. Journal of the American Medical Association 2000; 383: 3123-4.

Katz D. Neuropathology and neurobehavioural recovery from closed head injury. Journal of Head Trauma Rehabilitation 1992; 7: 1-15.

Kerner M, Acker M. Computer delivery of memory retraining with head injured patients. Cognitive Rehabilitation 1985; 3: 26-31.

Kraus J, Black M, Hessol N, Ley P, Rokaw W, Sullivan C et al. The incidence of acute brain injury and serious impairment in a defined population. American Journal of Epidemiology 1984; 119: 186-201.

Kreutzer J, Gervasio A, Camplair P. Patient correlates of caregivers' distress and family functioning after traumatic brain injury. Brain Injury 1994; 8: 211-30.

Kreutzer J, Wehman P (eds). Community Integration Following Traumatic Brain Injury. Baltimore, MD: Paul H Brookes, 1991.

Levin H, Benton A, Grossman R. Neurobehavioural Consequences of Closed Head Trauma. New York, NY: Oxford University Press, 1982.

Lewis F, Nelson J, Nelson C, Reusink P. Effects of three feedback contingencies on the socially inappropriate talk of a brain injured adult. Behaviour Therapy 1988; 19: 203-11.

Livingston M, Brooks D, Bond M. Patient outcome in the year following severe head injury and relatives, psychiatric and social functioning. Journal of Neurology, Neurosurgery and Psychiatry 1985; 48: 876-81.

Lovasik D, Kerr M, Alexander S. Traumatic brain injury research: a review of clinical studies. Critical Care Nursing Quarterly 2001; 23: 24-41.

MacDonald G. Assessing systematic reviews and clinical guidelines. In: V Moyer (Ed.). Evidence Based Paediatrics and Child Health. London: BMJ Books, 2000.

McGuffie A, Fitzpatrick M, Hall D. Golf-related head injuries in children: the little tigers. Scottish Medical Journal 1998; 43: 139-40.

Mills V, Nesbeda T, Katz D, Alexander M. Outcomes of traumatically brain injured patients following postacute rehabilitation programs. Brain Injury 1992; 6: 219-28.

Milton S. Management of subtle cognitive communication deficits. Journal of Head Trauma Rehabilitation 1988; 3: 1-12.

National Institutes of Health (NIH). Rehabilitation of Persons with Traumatic Brain Injury. NIH Consensus Statement 1998; 16: 1-41.

Pang D. Pathophysiologic correlates of neurobehavioural syndromes following closed head injury. In: M Ylvisaker (Ed.). Head Injury Rehabilitation: Children and Adolescents. Newton, MA: Butterworth-Heinemann, 1985.

Ponsford J, Sloan S, Snow P. Traumatic Brain Injury: Rehabilitation for Everyday Adaptive Living. Hove: Lawrence Erlbaum Associates, 1985.

Prigatano G. Neuropsychological Rehabilitation after Brain Injury. Baltimore, MD: Johns Hopkins University Press, 1986.

Prigatano G, Roueche J, Fordyce D. Nonaphasic language disturbances after closed head injury. Language Sciences 1985; 1: 217-29.

Rappaport M, Hall K, Hopkins K, Belleza T, Cope DN. Disability rating scale for severe head injury: coma to community. Archives of Physical Medicine and Rehabilitation 1982; 63: 118-23.

Richardson J. Clinical and Neurospychological Aspects of Closed Head Injury. Hove: Lawrence Erlbaum Associates, 1990.

Ruff R, Niemann H. Cognitive rehabilitation versus day treatment in head injured adults: is there an impact on emotional and psychosocial adjustment? Brain Injury 1990; 4: 339-47.

Ruff R, Baser C, Johnson J, Marshall L. Neuropsychological rehabilitation: an experimental study with head injured patients. Journal of Head Trauma Rehabilitation 1989; 4: 20-36.

Sander A, Roebusk T, Struchen M, Sherer M, High W. Long-term maintenance of gains obtained in postacute rehabilitation by persons with traumatic brain injury. Journal of Head Trauma Rehabilitation 2001; 16: 356-73.

Sarno M. The nature of verbal impairment after closed head injury. Journal of Nervous and Mental Disease 1980; 168: 685-92.

Schmitter-Edgecombe M, Fahy J, Whelan J, Long C. Memory remediation after severe closed head injury: notebook training versus supportive therapy. Journal of Consulting and Clinical Psychology 1995; 63: 484-9.

Snow P, Douglas J. Discourse rehabilitation following traumatic brain injury. In: S McDonald, L Togher, C Code (eds). Communication Disorders Following Traumatic Brain Injury. Hove: Psychology Press, 1999.

Snow P, Ponsford J. Assessing and managing changes in communication and interpersonal skills following TBI. In: J Ponsford, S Sloan, P Snow (eds). Traumatic Brain Injury: Rehabilitation for Everyday Adaptive Living. Hove: Lawrence Erlbaum Associates, 1995.

Sohlberg M, Mateer C. Introduction to Cognitive Rehabilitation: Theory and Practice. New York, NY: Guilford Press, 1989.

Tate R, Lulham JM, Broe GA, Strettles B, Pfaff A. Psychosocial outcome for the survivors of severe blunt head injury: the results from a consecutive series of 100 patients. Journal of Neurology, Neurosurgery and Psychiatry 1989; 52: 1128-34.

Tate R, McDonald S, Lulham J. Incidence of hospital-treated traumatic brain injury in an Australian community. Australian and New Zealand Journal of Public Health 1998; 22: 419-23.

Thomas-Stonell N, Johnson P, Schuller R, Jutai J. Evaluation of a computer based program for cognitive-communication skills. Journal of Head Trauma Rehabilitation 1994; 9: 25-37.

Twum M, Parente R. Role of imagery and verbal labeling in the performance of paired associates tasks by persons with closed head injury. Journal of Clinical and Experimental Neuropsychology 1994; 16: 630-9.

Wang C, Schoenberg B, Li S, Yang Y, Cheng X, Bolis L. Brain injury due to head trauma. Epidemiology in urban areas of the People's Republic of China. Archives of Neurology 1986; 43: 570-572.

Willer B, Ottenbacher K, Coad M. The Community Integration Questionnaire. American Journal of Physical and Medical Rehabilitation 1994; 73: 103-7.

Wilson B, Evans J, Emslie H, Malinek V. Evaluation of Neuropage: a new memory aid. Journal of Neurology, Neurosurgery and Psychiatry 1997; 63: 113-5.

Wood R. Brain Injury Rehabilitation: A Neurobehavioural Approach. London: Croom-Helm, 1987.

Wood R, Fussey I. Computer based cognitive retraining: a controlled study. International Disability Studies 1987; 9: 149-53.

Ylvisker M, Feeney T. Collaborative Brain Injury Intervention: Positive Everyday Routines. San Diego, CA: Singular Publishing, 1998.

Ylvisaker M, Szekeres S, Feeney T. Communication disorders associated with traumatic brain injury. In: R Chapey (Ed.). Language Intervention Strategies in Aphasia and Related Neurogenic Communication Disorders. New York, NY: Lippincott Williams & Wilkins, 2001.

Ylvisaker M, Hanks R, Johnson-Greene D. Perspectives on rehabilitation of individuals with cognitive impairment after brain injury: rationale for reconsideration of theoretical paradigms. Journal of Head Trauma Rehabilitation 2002; 17: 191-209.

CHAPTER 5

The evidence base for the treatment of stuttering

SUSAN BLOCK

Introduction: stuttering in context

This chapter reviews the nature of stuttering, its aetiology and the evidence underpinning the diagnosis and treatment of stuttering in children and adults. Although it is beyond the scope of this chapter to discuss all aspects of stuttering comprehensively, it alerts clinicians to the presence and quality of the available evidence, and provides practical ways of applying evidence to clinical practice and decision-making.

Sackett and Haynes (1995) outlined the essential steps in the emerging science of evidence-based medicine (these are discussed in detail in Chapter 1):

- Formulating the problem into answerable questions.
- Finding the best evidence with which to answer these questions.
- Critically appraising the evidence to assess its validity and usefulness.
- Implementing the results of this appraisal in clinical practice.
- Evaluating performance.

These steps are as relevant in the area of stuttering as they are in any area of medicine and health care, and should become automatic procedures for clinicians working in the area of stuttering.

Clinicians need to focus on evidence to ensure a close and responsible relationship between research and clinical practice. The potentially devastating problem of stuttering demands state-of-the-art (or science) evidence-based treatment if the most serious implications of the disorder are to be prevented.

The nature of stuttering

Stuttering is generally agreed upon as disorder of rhythm (Wingate, 1964) and it is a disorder often described as 'multi-faceted'. Although the most commonly described aspect is that of the speech characteristics (repetition, blocking), other aspects range from overt secondary symptoms (excessive eye blinking, facial grimacing) to feelings of embarrassment or moments of extreme anxiety. Van Riper (1982, p. 15) proposed what he considered to be a comprehensive or more valid definition of stuttering as what 'occurs when the forward flow of speech is interrupted by a motorically disrupted sound, syllable, or word or by the speaker's reaction thereto'.

Stuttering is prevalent in approximately 1% of the population (Bloodstein, 1987). It occurs more frequently in young children than in adults, and Bloodstein concluded from a literature review that there is an incidence of 4-5%. The condition occurs in far greater numbers in males than in females (3-4:1). Stuttering can have a sudden or gradual onset. It can occur with no significantly-related events and it can also remit spontaneously. Most stuttering begins in early childhood – often in the second or third year of life (Yairi and Ambrose, 1992; Onslow et al., 1993) – and can have devastating effects on individuals and their families. Such effects may range from limiting the length of sentences used or avoiding words or situations, to school refusal and severe anxiety or depression. In adulthood, stuttering can present as a chronic (or ongoing) condition. Although treatment for children who stutter is generally shorter and often less complex (that is, not directly changing the manner in which speech is produced), for adults it may be more complex and take significantly longer. Because of the length of time the adult has had the problem, there may be also resultant effects on self-esteem, levels of anxiety and general well-being that complicate management.

The complex implications and effects of stuttering often lead individuals and their families to seek their own information about stuttering and its treatment; rapid changes in technology have allowed increased and faster access to this information. Some clients (or their families) may have more up-to-date information about aspects of stuttering or its treatment, or may have read more widely than some of our colleagues, for whom stuttering may form only a small component of the caseload. If clinicians are to inform themselves more responsibly and then inform their clients about evidence and best practice, they must be aware of the issues involved.

Aetiology of stuttering

Stuttering has been investigated from a variety of perspectives, and as a result, people who stutter have been exposed to a wide variety of treatments, often with little theoretical basis or empirical support. It has been contended that stuttering is caused by parents' misdiagnoses (Johnson, 1961), was the result of cerebral imbalance (Travis, 1931), learnt behaviour (Shames, 1975), a role conflict (Sheehan, 1970), a neurological inco-ordination/reflex (Schwartz, 1976), an unconscious conflict/ego dysfunction (Glauber, 1982) or a physical abnormality for which many devices have been designed (Katz, 1977). Most theories of the aetiology of stuttering fall into the basic categories of physiological or psychological models. Manning (1996, pp. 31–2) contends, 'one thing remains clear. In nearly all cases, stuttering is a multidimensional problem' with 'some measure of support as well as conflicting evidence for nearly all theories of stuttering onset'. Recent literature presents changing views on aetiology (Curlee and Siegal, 1997; Bernstein Ratner and Healey, 1999). Neurological and biological aspects of causation are being investigated and advances in neural imaging (for example, positron emission tomography – PET), cerebral blood flow technologies and magnetic resonance imaging (MRI) are providing opportunities for investigation not previously available (Ingham, 1998).

Similarly, advances in genetic analysis and investigation are providing opportunities that may lead to different directions for stuttering management. The implications of findings relating to the specifics of genetic transmission, risk factors and potential for recovery from stuttering have been discussed by Cox et al. (1984), Yairi et al. (1996) and Smith and Kelly (1997). Felsenfeld (1998, p. 52) further explains that if a genetic link can be identified, there will be implications in terms of 'responsiveness to therapeutic management, probability of spontaneous recovery, and long-term outcome'.

Speech motor control is another area that has received increased attention in recent times. Ingham (1998) provides not only an historical overview of the area, but a well-reasoned discussion of the implications of the research in the area. The research is founded in the premise that stuttering is a neurophysiological disorder affecting the speech motor system. Voice initiation timing (Adams and Hayden, 1976), hemispheric processing (Moore and Haynes, 1980), voicing differences (Janssen and Wieneke, 1987), and respiratory changes (Johnston et al., 1993) are some of the aspects that have been considered. Variability in linguistic stress has also been proposed (Packman and Lincoln, 1996) and is one of the most recent attempts to discuss causation. Changes in fluency resulting from changes in speech motor production (for example, following auditory feedback masking) have also been considered (Martin et al., 1985; Block et al., 1996) as have changes resulting from altering feedback frequency (Kalinowski et al., 1993; Ingham et al., 1997).

One of the most perplexing questions raised by this general area of research is whether the speech motor control differences discerned in many of the studies are fundamental differences between individuals who stutter and fluent speakers, or whether they are differences that result either from treatments or from individuals' self-imposed attempts to achieve fluency. Ingham (1998) alludes to three potentially profitable clinical areas of speech motor control research that may have been underestimated:

- An understanding of the motor variables that may be responsible for the prolonged speech effect.
- The role of respiration.
- The relationship of auditory factors in treatment.

Further investigation of these areas has the potential to increase our understanding of both stuttering and aspects of treatment. However, further evidence is required before we can confidently confirm the true basis of the relationship of this area to stuttering aetiology.

Despite these advances, there is not yet one theory of stuttering that could be said to meet all the criteria for acceptable evidence-based support. This is despite the fact that the disorder has been traced back to the time of Moses (Van Riper, 1971, p. 201) and it has been studied from an enormous range of perspectives (Curlee and Perkins, 1984; Curlee and Siegel, 1997). There is some consistency in the view that stuttering is a multidimensional disorder. Van Riper (1982) delineated four 'tracks' of stuttering development. Wall and Myers (1984) differentiated psycholinguistic, psychosocial and physiological factors. Adams (1990) and Starkweather et al. (1990) proposed a 'demands and capacities' model of stuttering. Perkins (1996) evaluated the theories of stuttering and contended that many of the theories lack a scientific base. He outlined six criteria for evaluating the theories. To date no one theory fulfils each of Perkins' (1996) criteria. Thus, if the basic theories of stuttering lack a clear and credible scientific evidence base, the evidence base for the diagnostic methods and treatment approaches might also be deficient.

Diagnosis of stuttering

The diagnosis of stuttering in adults and older children is less problematic than in the pre-school age group. The former groups usually present with descriptions of what they do when they stutter and usually consider themselves to be stuttering. In other words, they bring the diagnosis with them. Pre-school children, however, are usually brought for a consultation by their parents with the query about whether they are indeed stuttering. Although this may be a straightforward process in most cases, there is discussion about the evidence that suggests that confirmation of moments of stuttering, especially in young children, may be subject to disagreement, thus confusing the issue of differential diagnosis (Perkins, 1990). Perkins (1990, p. 370) describes a diagnostic method of validating authentic stuttering. He contends that the 'most definitive evidence about any aspect of stuttering is that listeners are unable to judge unit-by-unit occurrences of it acceptably'. Perkins (1990, p. 374) considers that literature reviews 'provide consistent evidence that listeners apparently do not have enough information about the essence of stuttering to make accurate judgements of whether or not what they hear as stuttering is authentic'.

Perkins (1990, p. 376) defined stuttering as 'the involuntary disruption of a continuing attempt to produce a spoken utterance' supporting the earlier evidence of Kelly and Conture (1988) that stuttering is involuntary. Moore and Perkins (1990) produced evidence (albeit from one subject) that stuttering was involuntary. This questions clinical reliance on perceptual impressions of what is thought to be stuttering and confirms the fact that the most valid evidence of whether or not stuttering has occurred rests with the individual who is stuttering. Perkins (1990) considers that this is the reason that studies looking for listener agreement of stuttering fail – as they are not reflecting what he feels is the evidence of the true nature of stuttering. If, as Perkins (1990) contends, the difference between stuttered and non-stuttered speech is involuntary or voluntary disruption, the task at hand is to devise a clinically useful tool to recognize or measure the disruption and the nature of the disruption itself.

Lewis (1994) reported on a survey of articles over a five-year period on reports of observer agreement of stuttering. Fifty-five studies were identified, and Lewis (1994) concludes that the evidence is varied and confounded by variations in procedural and reporting variations. Similar sentiment to that of Perkins (1990) is reflected in the conclusion that:

> When used as indices of observer agreement, the five procedures repeatedly relied upon in the current stuttering literature, (i.e., Sander's Agreement Index [Sander, 1961], Pearson product–moment correlation coefficient, Mean difference scores, tests of deviation from known distributions, and Point-by-point percentage agreement) have serious shortcomings. (Lewis, 1994, p. 273)

Thus, not only is there concern about convincing evidence supporting individual theories of stuttering, but concern exists regarding the accurate recognition of stuttering itself. Such concern has led to the recommendation that, rather than rely solely on questionable means of differentially diagnosing stuttering in young children, intervention should be considered when children are reacting negatively to their stuttering, when parents want their child treated, and if the child is more than five years old (Curlee and Yairi, 1997). Similarly, Packman and Onslow (1998) state that in the absence of clear guidelines for instigating treatment, intervention should begin immediately where the child and/or parent indicates distress. Hence, the decision to commence treatment is based on factors other than, or in addition to, speech characteristics.

The various disfluency taxonomies such as those of Gregory and Hill (1980), Yairi and Lewis (1984), Conture (1997) and Yairi (1997) make the description and measurement of stuttering, in particular in children, a confusing process. Such descriptions and measurements range from descriptions of disfluencies (Gregory and Hill, 1984; Packman and Onslow, 1998) to percentages of syllables stuttered (Ingham and Andrews, 1973) and ratings of reactions or levels of anxiety (Andrews and Cutler, 1974).

Packman and Onslow (1998) devised 'the behavioural data language of stuttering' in an attempt to provide clinicians and researchers with a valid and reliable data language of stuttering and to increase agreement about moments of stuttering. These authors described 29 types of stuttering behaviours (Packman and Onslow, 1998, p. 40). These were refined to three main categories: repeated movements, fixed postures and superfluous behaviours. Although this is certainly a step towards clinical utility and possibly a more reliable measure, it would not satisfy all of Perkins' (1990) concerns. The contribution of Packman and Onslow (1998) is to provide a descriptive language of the visible and perceivable signs of stuttering but there is no inclusion of acoustic, auditory or self-report/rating measures.

The study by Yairi and Lewis (1984), differentiating stuttering children from non-stuttering children, concluded that stuttering children had more part-word repetitions and more repetitive units than the non-stuttering children. Following this, Hubbard and Yairi (1998) found that stuttering children showed evidence of more clusters of disfluencies. Although both these studies used control subjects, the small subject numbers (10 and 15 subjects, respectively) make generalizations difficult. In addition, a factor compounding clinical decision-making was that these authors (Hubbard and Yairi, 1998) found that non-stuttering children exhibited all the disfluency types that stuttering children exhibited. In attempting to clarify the differentiation between stuttered and non-stuttered speech in young children, Onslow (1996) presents a summary of the results of previous studies, most of which would be classified as cohort studies of the speech of stuttering and non-stuttering pre-school children. Onslow (1996) indicates that these studies provide some evidence for differentiation that may be useful for clinicians.

Onslow's (1996, p. 28) summary includes the following results:

- Stuttering pre-school children generally have more disfluencies than their non-stuttering counterparts.
- Part-word repetitions of sounds and syllables and sound prolongations are

common in stuttering pre-school children. Part-word repetitions are probably the most distinctive feature of early stuttering.

- Part-word repetitions and prolongations may occur in the speech of non-stuttering children, but it is not clear to what extent these resemble the part-word repetitions and prolongations of stuttering pre-school children.
- Stuttering pre-school children may show more 'clusters' of disfluencies when compared to non-stuttering children.
- Stuttering children may have more repetition units in disfluencies than non-stuttering children, and they may have a greater range of repetition units per disfluency. However, at present the matter is open to question because there has been one report which found no differences.
- Stuttering and non-stuttering pre-school children may not be distinguishable by the durations of their disfluencies. However, this finding has yet to be replicated.
- Early stuttering may involve head, face or body movements.

Although the points outlined above are taken from a variety of research findings, Onslow (1996) states that there are flaws limiting the confidence with which all of the findings can be viewed. These flaws include lack of replication, small subject numbers, few long-term evaluations and poorly defined descriptions of stuttering. This leads to concern about the accuracy of judgements of the stutters themselves – an issue discussed previously in this section. Reports by Cordes and Ingham (1996) and Yairi (1996) also reflect the concern that this debate has raised. Thus, the area of the accurate description of stuttering (and therefore its diagnosis) falls short of acceptable levels of evidence (Briggs, 2001).

The extreme variability and inconsistency of stuttering is confounding for clinicians. People may stutter to a greater or lesser degree at different times, or in different situations. This makes reliable diagnosis, accurate speech descriptions and impressions of the degree of impact of the disorder problematic, as speech samples may not always be representative of the person's usual speech. Ingham (1984) addressed this issue of representative measurement comprehensively.

Because of the variability of stuttering, in particular with regard to young children, diagnosis may be a difficult and precarious process. Much of the literature is characterized by suggestions or recommendations for managing this process rather than providing a strong evidence-base for the diagnosis itself. Authors such as Yaruss et al. (1998) describe useful findings to guide clinicians in the evaluation process. However, at present most clinicians will continue to rely on the summary above provided by Onslow (1996) as it is clinically relevant, easy to apply and has consensus from other authorities.

Treatment of stuttering

One of the most frustrating factors in clinical practice with people who stutter is the fact that there are many treatments available, and the majority are recommended with little or no supporting evidence (Cordes and Ingham, 1998). Even where there are data, there is no consensus about what should be the approach taken or what should be the focus of treatment (for example, stutter-more-fluently, speak-more-fluently, attitude change; Gregory, 1979). Similarly, there is a lack of consensus on what outcomes should be evaluated in stuttering treatment (that is, speech measures such as speech rate and percentage of syllables stuttered, speech naturalness and self-reports and/or communicative effectiveness). It is evident that there is no agreement on how stuttering behaviour should be measured and similarly, there is no agreement on what should be measured to confirm the success of treatment.

In 1995, the Special Interest Division of the American Speech–Language–Hearing Association (ASHA) on fluency and fluency disorders contended 'the field lacked standards for the treatment of stuttering' (ASHA, 1995, p. 26). 'Preferred practice patterns' had been developed for the assessment of stuttering, but the area of treatment had been neglected. Some general guidelines for treatment were provided but some of the more specific treatment strategies recommended lack well-substantiated evidence for their effectiveness.

An enormous variety of treatments have been used to manage stuttering (Van Riper, 1973; Dalton, 1983; Ingham, 1984; Ham, 1986, 1990; Peters and Guitar, 1991; Onslow, 1996; Rustin et al., 1996; Shapiro, 1999). The earliest forms of stuttering treatment often involved suggestion or persuasion, relaxation or changes in speech rate and rhythm (Van Riper, 1973). Symptom reduction followed, and in the 1960s, behaviour therapies emerged (Van Riper, 1973; Ham, 1986). More recent trends have been to integrate different approaches (Bloodstein, 1995; Menzies et al., 1999). The recent growth of the self-help movement has also added another dimension to treatment for stuttering – particularly in terms of support, well-being and fluency maintenance.

The fundamental approaches to treatment have been classified as either speak-more-fluently approaches or stutter-more-fluently approaches (Gregory, 1979). The focus in the former is to retrain speech motor co-ordination to prevent the stuttering from occurring. An example of this is prolonged speech (Ingham, 1984). In the latter approach, the focus is to change the stuttering as soon as the individual becomes aware of a stutter. Hence, ideally, only the stuttered component of the speech is changed. Techniques such as 'pull outs' or 'cancellation' (Van Riper, 1973) exemplify this approach. When selecting treatments, clinicians should consider which of these two philosophical approaches they will follow, as the implications of each for the person who stutters are very different.

Irrespective of the approach taken, treatments have varied for children and adults and range from very indirect treatment (for example, *'I remember very clearly my mother driving me every Friday afternoon to see a speech therapist who lived in the city. I would spend an hour playing with toys while the therapist "talked" to my mother. I do not think this helped my mother much and it was certainly little help to me'* [Tunbridge, 1994, p. 3]); to more speech-focused direct treatment (that is, 'Good treatment means first learning a skill...The exact technique that you learn varies with the treatment program that you enter, but skill in dealing with your inefficient speech control system is the important first step,' [Neilson in Tunbridge, 1994, p. x]).

Direct speech-focused treatments

Direct speech-focused treatments have been described by Culatta and Goldberg (1995) as having any or all of the following seven elements.

- Reduced utterance length at beginning of treatment.
- Reduced speech rate at beginning of treatment.
- Controlled breathing patterns.
- Easy onsets to sounds, words or phrases.
- Altered vocalization.
- Gentle or modified articulatory gestures.
- Any verbal or other consequence that immediately follows a stutter.

Attanasio (1999) contends that it is important to consider the goals of the person who stutters, as well as their daily communicative needs. The issue of treatment goals is important clinically, as there may be times during the treatment process when the clinician and the client do not have the same goals for treatment or when the goals change. This is exemplified, particularly for an adult, who may be satisfied with an increase in fluency, and at other times may desire help, for example, decreasing anxiety about speaking rather than having a focus on the fluency itself. This is often observed or reported when people who stutter must give a formal presentation to a large audience. They may be so overwhelmed by the prospect that unless they have some strategies to manage or reduce their anxiety it is almost futile to attempt to gain some focus on fluent speech production.

This leads to the question of how and when goals are established. Stuttering can become a chronic condition in adults; something for which they may require ongoing treatment at various stages of their adult life, so it is probable that treatment goals may change from time to time. This may depend on the effectiveness of the treatment strategies, the priorities of individuals at the time and their physical or psychological state. Attanasio (1999) recommends consideration of the daily communication needs of the person who stutters, confirming the need for a very individual focus in treatment. There is enormous variation in the type as well as the amount of speaking people do each day.

Stages of treatment

The treatment process may be described as having three stages: 'instatement', 'transfer' and 'maintenance'. To ensure a positive treatment outcome in terms of long-term maintenance of fluency gains, it is recommended that the latter two stages be incorporated into the first (instatement). It should be acknowledged here that this is not such a significant issue in the pre-school stuttering population. Onslow (1996, p. 78) reports 'generalization of stutter-free speech in preschool children is not thought to be the problem that it is for adults'. Indeed, Onslow's preferred treatment option for young children, the Lidcombe Program, (Lincoln and Harrison, 1999) has an essential component which requires parents to administer the treatment in the home environment. Thus, this incorporates aspects of generalization into the early stages of the fluency instatement very directly.

If clinicians consider these stages in the treatment process for adults who stutter, it may well be the case that optimal treatment outcome could be compromised because of the balance given to each stage. For example, it is frequently the case that clinicians spend the bulk of their time teaching specific fluency strategies to adults who stutter and then spend very little time working with them directly on facilitating the transfer and maintenance of fluency. If the stages were viewed as a triangle, the bulk of the effort would be at the top and little formal treatment would be at the base. It may be preferable, in terms of ensuring better treatment outcome, to reverse the triangle and put the bulk of treatment effort into the final two stages. Certainly, the issue of relapse has been identified as one of the significant problems with many treatments.

This may well be a reason for the increase in interest in the self-help movement that will be discussed later in this chapter. Bloodstein (1995, p. 445) states, 'of all the problems that limit the effectiveness of therapy, the one that has made the greatest claim on the attention of clinical researchers is relapse'. For this reason, maintenance procedures are now routinely being incorporated into treatment programmes and will continue to be refined in an attempt to address individual differences in responses to treatment and to enhance the likelihood of long-term maintenance.

Treatment of children

The literature reveals that the treatment of stuttering in childhood and adolescence lacks specific research and attention. Several landmark studies reported promising results with small numbers of children under experimental conditions (Martin et al., 1972; Peters, 1977; Reed and Godden, 1977; Costello, 1995). These results were obtained using operant conditioning (that is, positive reinforcement, punishment and time-out). Despite the positive indications, further substantial evidence (such as increased subject numbers, replication) was not forthcoming. Costello Ingham and Riley (1998) contend that there is a 'pressing need to document treatment efficacy for young children who stutter'. In recent studies which have incorporated aspects of the earlier operant investigations (Onslow et al., 1990a; Onslow et al., 1990b; Lincoln and Onslow, 1997), the results of the Lidcombe Program, a parent-administered, operant, non-programmed stuttering treatment for pre-school children (Lincoln and Harrison, 1999), indicate promising results. Long-term results indicate near-zero levels of stuttering maintained from two to seven years after treatment. Again, although the evidence is not from randomized controlled studies, it is from well-designed, cohort, long-term investigations with several types of objective measures (Briggs' (2001) level of evidence III.1). Jones et al. (2001) make reference to a randomized controlled trial that is currently underway to provide further evidence for the Lidcombe Program and the results are eagerly awaited.

A clinical, multi-site controlled trial was reported by Craig et al. (1996) who compared intensive smooth speech (a derivative of prolonged speech), intensive EMG (electromyographic) feedback and home-based smooth speech in a group design experimental model. The findings were that home-based smooth speech and EMG feedback were superior to the intensive smooth speech. Although different treatment centres administered different treatments, a shortcoming of the design of the study, other aspects of the design render the results worthy of further attention. The level of evidence provided by this study would be classified as III.1 and III.2 (Briggs, 2001).

Treatment of adults

In 1980, Andrews and colleagues undertook a meta-analysis of the effects of stuttering treatment. Their literature search of 100 publications in four journals found poor consensus of long-term treatment effectiveness and poor consensus of which treatments were most effective. It would seem somewhat contradictory, therefore, that Andrews et al. (1980) concluded that prolonged speech, gentle onsets, attitude therapy and airflow techniques were the superior treatments with prolonged speech and gentle onsets demonstrating better gains in both the short and long term.

Andrews et al. (1980) found that adults typically received 80 hours of treatment. Although these authors searched recent books, periodicals, conference proceedings and dissertations, they could calculate effect sizes in only 29 of 100 publications. They did, however, conclude that, overall, a 'large proportion of the studies were therefore well designed, used reliable and appropriate measures, employed an adequate follow-up interval, and had a low rate of client loss' (Andrews et al., 1980, p. 294). The 'large proportion' lacks definition and despite the confidence in the design of the studies, most of them at best would be allocated to the Briggs (2001) levels III.2 and III.3. The conclusion was that:

> Data suggest that substantial improvement needs at least 100 hours of treatment in which a variant of the prolonged speech technique is used at a slow rate to establish control over stuttering, with the resulting fluent speech shaped to normal speech by a defined schedule. (Andrews et al., 1980, p. 304)

Andrews et al. (1980) also concluded that systematic transfer of the new speech into the real world appears beneficial, and some clients may need counselling to improve their attitude. Some may benefit if their family and friends offer support as they seek to generalize their fluent speech. Lastly, the clinic 'may need to offer a planned maintenance program to consolidate all these activities' (Andrews et al., 1980, p. 304). These conclusions were based on replicated findings, not necessarily on well-controlled or well-designed studies.

The analysis of Andrews et al. (1980) also revealed two areas that lacked research data. These were: the treatment of younger children (where there were no appropriately documented results of treatment), previously discussed; and the paucity of information relating to the components of the treatments – thus facilitating our understanding of why individual treatments actually work.

Continued acknowledgement of the importance of evidence in the field of stuttering is apparent through the publication of articles such as the review of research findings by Andrews et al. (1983). Following the earlier meta-analysis (Andrews et al., 1980), Andrews and colleagues (1983) went on to scan the literature for treatment strategies that were supported by robust findings, which had been replicated. Findings supported by two or more research studies were replicated in two or more research centres, and with no negative reports, were designated as 'Class A' facts. These would correspond with a Briggs (2001) level of evidence of III.1 or III.2. Andrews and colleagues also reported classes B, C and D facts, which revealed conflicting reports, replication within the same centre, or a combination of both these features. The aim in the review 'was to provide a guide to the literature for both students and researchers' (Andrews et al., 1983, p. 226). These authors not only provided a guide to the literature itself but also provided a way of drawing conclusions about the published data and of evaluating the evidence. However, none of the studies reported demonstrated unequivocal evidence at sufficiently high levels, that is, they were not randomized controlled trials (Briggs level of evidence I or II). Rather, they were usually cohort or case-control studies, or more non-scientific case reports.

Andrews et al. (1983) reported a number of conditions that either eliminated or reduced stuttering, based on the criteria outlined above. (These are described in Box 5.1.)

Box 5.1

Conditions reported to eliminate or reduce stuttering (Andrews et. al., 1983)

- Conditions that *immediately eliminate* stuttering (frequency of stuttering is reduced by 90–100%):

    - Chorus reading
    - Prolonged speech and delayed auditory feedback (DAF)
    - Shadowing
    - Slowed speech
    - Lipped speech
    - Rhythmic speech
    - Singing

- Conditions that *gradually eliminate* stuttering (stuttering is progressively reduced and can reach zero):

    - Response-contingent stimulation of stuttering

- Conditions that *immediately reduce* stuttering (frequency of stuttering is reduced by 50–80%):

    - Speaking alone
    - DAF (50–150 ms)
    - Change in pitch
    - Speaking in time to rhythmic movement
    - Masking
    - Whispering

- Conditions that *gradually reduce* the stuttering (frequency of stuttering is decreased progressively but is not eliminated):

    - Haloperidol
    - EMG (Electromyographic) feedback from speech muscles

Andrews et al. (1983) commented that a problem with the earlier meta-analysis (Andrews et al., 1980) was that only studies that reported outcome data in terms of means and standard deviations could be assessed. Thus, for the wider review they included Bloodstein's (1981) criteria. Incorporating these criteria, Andrews et al. (1983, p. 234) concluded, 'only the prolonged speech and precision shaping strategies have reported sufficient data to meet the majority of these requirements'. This confirmed the earlier finding of Andrews et al. (1980). The later landmark study by Boberg and Kully (1994) continued to provide evidence supporting prolonged speech for the treatment of adults and adolescents. This study was noteworthy as it was one of the first to provide repeated measures over a long time period (12–24 months), thus fulfilling the Briggs levels of evidence at III.1.

Andrews et al. (1980) referred to the fact that in addition to treatment for children, another area requiring more investigation was that of the components of treatments. When investigating the components of prolonged speech, Harrison et al. (1998) report some interesting preliminary data from a one-day programme. In their search for best practice, these authors state that the results indicate that there may be aspects of the original prolonged speech programmes that do not contribute to the resulting fluency. Further developments of this research may indicate changes in service delivery that will have substantial benefits for both clinicians and clients. In a later study by O'Brien et al. (2001), the authors extended the search for simplifying prolonged speech instruction and presented the results of a trial with three subjects, challenging many of the assumptions upon which many prolonged speech programmes are based. This has particular relevance for intensive programming, such as that described by Boberg and Kully (1994) and Craig et al. (1996). Although the results presented by O'Brien et al. (2001) are experimental (that is, laboratory rather than clinical) and preliminary, evidence from their continued development may provide interesting evidence for changes in clinical practice.

In her review of the stuttering treatment literature, Cordes (1998, p. 118) reports that, 'the methodological problems are actually so pervasive in the stuttering treatment literature that it was, to a great extent, not possible to complete a straightforward summary of reported treatment outcomes'. (For this reason, an extensive description of all the treatment literature will not be provided here. However, a range of treatments investigated [Cordes, 1998] are outlined.) Cordes (1998) selected peer-reviewed articles from several sources and included studies that were published between 1965 and 1996, and where they 'clearly represented an assessment of a stuttering treatment technique with the implicit or explicit goal of change beyond experimental conditions' (Cordes, 1998, p. 119). The following treatments were included:

- Play therapy.
- Acupuncture.
- Reinforce therapy.
- Self-recording.
- Precision fluency shaping.
- Parent-administrative operant.
- Other packages.
- Punishment.
- Rhythmic speech.
- Desensitization/cognitive.
- Response-contingent time-out.
- Recorded self-models.
- Delayed auditory feedback.
- Electromyographic feedback.
- 'Programmed traditional'.
- Prolonged speech plus cognitive.
- Parental change.
- Masking.
- Graduated length and complexity of utterance (GILCU)/extended length of utterance (ELU).
- Airflow and regulated breathing.
- Prolonged/smooth speech.

Cordes (1998) expressed concern that the treatments that were most often recommended in the treatment studies reviewed (64 papers looking at 81 different treatments) were not the treatments that had been researched most comprehensively. Nor were they the treatments that were currently in widespread use, indicating a gap between research and clinical application. Consequently, Cordes (1998) extended the literature search, with the result that a further 24 references recommended 27 treatments for stuttering. Table 5.1 lists the recommended treatments that maintain stuttering below 1% and are supported by research. Such treatments warrant ongoing consideration (from Cordes, 1998, p. 136), as they are the few that satisfy most of the methodological and measurement criteria already discussed. Only prolonged speech reaches the criteria for best practice described earlier. However, further substantiation of the evidence base is required as results from randomized controlled trials are still lacking (Briggs (2001) levels of evidence I or II).

The recent meta-analysis of Thomas and Howell (2001) met some harsh criticism. These workers evaluated studies published since 1993 in an attempt 'to provide an impartial look at studies of efficacy across treatments of stuttering' (Thomas and Howell, 2001, p. 313). They aimed to critically

Table 5.1 Numbers (per cent) of research articles that met three measurement and design criteria (from Cordes, 1998, p. 136)

Measurement and design criteria	Research articles reporting maintained stuttering <1%	Prolonged speech*	Cognitive/ emotional*	Combined*
Data on stuttering frequency and speech rate reported	6/8 (75)	7/14 (50)	0/6 (0)	0/3 (0)
Repeated measurements taken on at least two occasions before and after treatment	8/8 (100)	9/14 (64.3)	1/6 (16.7)	2/3 (66.7)
Stuttering measurements outside clinic environment	7/8 (87.5)	6/14 (42.9)	0/6 (0)	0/3 (0)

*Articles related to the most frequently recommended treatments – papers reporting any data on stuttering frequency and speech rate.

address measurement issues, treatment integrity, design issues, specification of treatment and tests of treatment outcome. When applying their criteria Thomas and Howell (2001) conclude that only eight studies fulfilled their requirements: Craig and Kearns, 1995; Ryan and Van Kirk Ryan, 1995; Stager et al., 1995; Onslow et al., 1996; Druce et al., 1997; Ingham et al., 1997; Eichstadt et al., 1998; Hancock et al., 1998). Storch (2002) rebuke the authors for their selection of these studies, indicating that they have omitted several significant contributions to the field, most notably Boberg and Kully, (1994) and all the studies relating to the Lidcombe Program (Onslow et al., 1994). Additionally, Thomas and Howell (2001) classified experimental trials as treatment studies and as a consequence of these factors (and other shortcomings), Storch (2002) believes that they have not conducted a meta-analysis and 'any conclusions reached from a review of these eight papers is severely compromised by what appears to have been an all but arbitrary method of selecting papers.'

However, there is an interesting issue raised by both Ingham and Bothe (2002) and Thomas and Howell (2001): the importance of considering the evidence from treatment failures. This may reveal important information for researchers and clinicians and is worthy of attention in considering all aspects of the evidence base. Indeed, an area of interest and promise was that of the role of pharmacology in stuttering. Discussion of lack of success of drug trials, in particular in the long-term (Stager et al., 1995) reveals valuable information (for example, about compliance) and exemplifies the reason for Bloodstein's (1995) Criteria 10: the importance of not ignoring dropouts.

In the appendix to his book, Bloodstein (1995) summarized the results of treatments reported in 164 studies using his criteria (Bloodstein, 1981, 1995). Although Bloodstein remarks that the results must be viewed with caution, he considers that:

> it is evident we are able to offer many stutterers a considerable amount of help...
> It is unmistakable that a great variety of methods are capable of bringing about what a clinician may regard in good faith as a successful outcome of therapy in a large proportion of cases. (Bloodstein, 1995, p. 438)

This is somewhat at odds with Cordes' (1998) contention, although she is referring to specific scientific research design issues and Bloodstein (1995) is referring to his more clinically based criteria for use by clinicians as well as researchers.

Conclusions: future directions

It is important to ensure that the speech pathology profession is encouraged to make use of the information clinicians have – to inform them of appropriate, substantiated evidence of effective clinical practice. It is also important that relevant clinical evidence is not discarded solely because it does not fulfil the highest standards of evidence-based practice described in the first two chapters of this book. Rather, clinical evidence should be further developed and properly researched to ensure it fulfils all the necessary criteria to inform responsible clinical practice.

When discussing the relationship between research and clinical practice Perkins (1996) outlined six criteria for the evaluation of theories of stuttering. Perkins (1996) contends that many of the theories lack a scientific base for the following six reasons.

1 They do not explain cause and effect.
2 They do not involve theory construction and empirical testing.
3 They do not account for all defining characteristics.
4 They do not permit contradictory predictions.
5 They must be subject to empirical disproof.
6 They are not valid until their predictions have been verified experimentally.

Not only has the evidence base for the theories of stuttering been questioned, but the evidence base for treatments has been similarly discussed. As early as 1981, Bloodstein developed criteria or 'tests' by which stuttering treatments should be evaluated before they could be considered successful. Bloodstein expanded the number of his criteria to 12 in 1995; these have become benchmarks for researchers and form fundamental principles for students and clinicians when making treatment choices and decisions.

Bloodstein's criteria are as follows:

1 The method must be shown to be effective with an ample and representative group of stutterers.
2 Results must be demonstrated by objective measures of speech behaviour such as frequency of stuttering or rate of speech and by judges' ratings of severity.
3 Reports of therapeutic success must be based on repeated evaluations and adequate samples of speech.
4 Improvement must be shown to carry over to speaking situations outside the clinical setting.
5 The stability of results must be demonstrated by long-term follow-up investigations.
6 Suitable control groups or control conditions must be used to show that reductions in stuttering are the result of treatment.

7 Subjects' speech must sound natural and spontaneous to listeners.
8 Subjects must be free from the necessity to monitor their speech.
9 Treatment must remove not only stuttering, but also the fears, the anticipations, and the person's self-concept as a stutterer.
10 The success of a program should not be inflated by ignoring dropouts.
11 The method must be shown to be effective in the hands of essentially any qualified clinician, including those without unusual status, prestige, or force of personality.
12 The method must continue to be successful when it is no longer new and the initial wave of enthusiasm over it has died away. (Bloodstein, 1995, p. 439)

Onslow (2001) discussed treatment outcomes in an evidence-based framework and suggested that the scientific evidence for stuttering treatments should meet the following criteria.

1 At least 10 published cases in the peer-reviewed scientific literature.
2 Incorporate a pre-treatment assessment and
3 Several post-treatment assessments.
4 Those assessments should occur over a clinically meaningful post-treatment period and
5 Should incorporate objective speech data from
6 Everyday speaking situations that
7 Show reductions in stuttering severity of greater than 70%. (Onslow, 2001, p. 2)

The recommendations made by Bloodstein (1995) and Onslow (2001) have many things in common: representative measures, repeated measures and consideration of factors other than fluency. Indeed, many other authors have proposed similar criteria for the evaluation of treatment efficacy in stuttering (Ingham, 1984; Watson, 1994; Yaruss, 1998; Attanasio, 1999; Ingham and Cordes, in press). Despite this, Onslow (2001) contended that the evidence base in stuttering treatment is still quite modest and Briggs (2001) confirmed 'we still await the publication of a truly randomized controlled trial'. Acknowledgement of the gold standard for evidence has been the motivation for providing information to educate clinicians in evaluating research and indeed in designing research. The contributions of Ingham (1993), Moscicki (1993) and Jones et al. (2001, 2002) are attempts to discuss and clarify the processes involved in the research paradigms rather than solely investigate outcomes themselves.

Perhaps a more fundamental issue related to evidence and best practice is defining exactly what constitutes treatment itself. Bernstein Ratner (1997) summarizes the issues, including what constitutes treatment, how success is defined, when treatment is warranted (in particular, in young children) as well as the use of data to improve decision-making. Bernstein Ratner's (1997) concluding comments reflect Bloodstein's (1995) opinions. She comments that counting stuttering alone is not a sufficient indicator of either the severity of the problem or of therapeutic success. A scientific balance is required by making well-informed judgements and implementing effective therapeutic approaches when they appear warranted.

It is also important that the evidence is considered from the point of view of the person who stutters. People who stutter may have very different opinions about what constitutes 'successful' treatment and to what types of treatment they are prepared to subject themselves, that is, speak-more-fluently versus stutter-more-fluently approaches. They also know their speech intimately and know what is their primary focus of concern at any time. Clinicians are well cautioned to listen to consumers. Bloodstein (1995, p. 449) notes, 'the growth of the stutterers' self-help movement in recent years has added a new dimension to the outlook for the betterment of stutterers' lives'. If members of the speech pathology profession are grappling with the issues of evidence, how much more likely is it that members of these groups may also be uninformed about best practice and thus may be giving advice that may be inappropriate or at worst, harmful? Therefore, it is important that we address the many aspects of evidence and promote the evidence to all the stakeholders, in particular to our clients, or potential clients. Clinicians need to be mindful of the opinions of their clients. If they do not like the treatments clinicians offer, it is irrelevant what the supporting evidence is; people will not choose to use them. Clinicians must always keep their focus on the person with the problem, not on the problem alone.

Curlee and Yairi (1998, p. 20) discuss the fact that, 'dialogues arising from the questions, concerns, and disagreements of respected colleagues are critical to the integrity of scientific disciplines and the health professions whose clinical practice rests on the knowledge base of those disciplines'. It needs to be acknowledged, however, that much of the dialogue and disagreement of researchers or specialists in any field may diminish the confidence of non-specialists who do much of the treatment, in this case, of stuttering. Cordes and Ingham (1998) highlighted this in the preface to their book:

> Many of the gaps in our discipline (i.e., stuttering) are not between researchers and clinicians at all, but are instead among those who would prefer to approach stuttering from a certain point of view, whether for research or for treatment; thus, we have divisions among those who approach stuttering scientifically, personally, emotionally, socially, behaviorally, cognitively, physiologically, acoustically, or through some combination of these. (Cordes and Ingham, 1998, p. viii)

It is imperative that student clinicians are trained to evaluate evidence from a wide variety of sources, such as research studies, reviews, assessments and outcome evaluations, and are then actively encouraged to put that evidence into practice. They must be able to form their own opinions if the researchers and so-called specialists are not demonstrating best practice or are not confirming evidence (especially if established by competing researchers). However, student clinicians must also be aware that not only do they need to be cognisant of the evidence for treatment selection, they must also think carefully about how they implement the treatment. They need to be aware of the many aspects of stuttering and an individual's reaction to them.

It is apparent that treatments have evolved which address the problem of stuttering in a variety of ways. Some treatments address single aspects of the disorder (such as speech production or anxiety) and others attempt to address the needs of the individual more comprehensively (such as cognitive behavioural therapy combined with smooth/prolonged speech).

In consideration of the above, Onslow (2001) concluded that the evidence for best practice in the treatment of stuttering in pre-school children supports the Lidcombe Program. For school-age children the evidence supports the use of smooth speech and computerized EMG biofeedback. There is a paucity of evidence for the adolescent population; however, there is some support for intensive smooth speech programmes. In adults, smooth speech, a derivative of prolonged speech (Ingham, 1984), offers evidence of controlling stuttered speech. Although none of these are supported by Briggs' (2001) highest level of evidence, all are supported by well-controlled studies with demonstrably robust clinical findings and thus, should be front-line treatments of choice.

Cordes (1998) states, that if clinicians disregard evidence, self-help groups are indeed justified in professing a 'help-yourself' philosophy rather than supporting and promoting treatments that have a poor outcome either in terms of speech fluency, anxiety management or whatever else the individuals presenting for help may wish to change. Clinicians need to consider carefully the philosophical approaches they take in treatment and consider stuttering intervention to be a collaborative journey (Shapiro, 1999). The challenge for the speech pathology profession is to recognize that people who stutter may often have sought much information about their disorder before presenting for an assessment or treatment. If their questions are not answered accurately and thoroughly, they will have little confidence in speech pathology. Evidence-based best practice necessitates ongoing learning, problem solving and scrutiny of the scientific body of literature related to all aspects of stuttering. It necessitates flexible service delivery, a variety of treatment options and open discussion with the stakeholders in the treatment process. Evidence-based clinical practice will enable these factors to occur as well as ensuring the maximum community respect for the speech pathology profession and the best possible outcome for people encumbered by what is at times, the truly wretched disorder of stuttering.

References

Adams M. The demands and capacities model: 1. Theoretical elaborations. Journal of Fluency Disorders 1990; 15: 135-41.

Adams M, Hayden P. The ability of stutterers and nonstutterers to initiate and terminate phonation during production of an isolated vowel. Journal of Speech and Hearing Research 1976; 19: 290-6.

American Speech-Language-Hearing Association (ASHA). Guidelines for practice in stuttering treatment. ASHA 1995; 37 (Suppl. 14): 26-35.

Andrews G, Cutler J. Stuttering therapy: the relation between changes in symptom level and attitudes. Journal of Speech and Hearing Disorders 1974; 39: 312-19.

Andrews G, Guitar B, Howie M. Meta-analysis of the effects of stuttering treatment. Journal of Speech and Hearing Disorders 1980; 44: 287-307.

Andrews G, Craig A, Feyer A, Hoddinott S, Howie P, Neilson M. Stuttering: a review of research findings and theories circa 1982. Journal of Speech and Hearing Disorders 1983; 48: 226-246.

Attanasio J. Treatment of early stuttering: some reflections. In: Onslow M, Packman A. The Handbook of Early Stuttering Intervention. San Diego, CA: Singular Publishing Group, 1999; Chapter 10.

Bernstein Ratner N. Leaving Las Vegas: clinical odds and individual outcomes. American Journal of Speech–Language Pathology 1997; 6: 29-33.

Bernstein Ratner N, Healey EC (Eds) Stuttering Research and Practice: Bridging the gap. Mahwah, NJ: Lawrence Erlbaum Assoc,1999.

Block S, Ingham R, Bench R. The effects of the Edinburgh Masker on stuttering. Australian Journal of Human Communication Disorders 1996; 24: 11-19.

Bloodstein O. A Handbook on Stuttering. Chicago, IL: National Easter Seal Society, 1981.

Bloodstein O. A Handbook on Stuttering (fourth edition). Chicago, IL: National Easter Seal Society, 1987.

Bloodstein O. A Handbook on Stuttering (fifth edition). Chicago, IL: National Easter Seal Society, 1995.

Boberg E, Kully D. Long-term results of an intensive treatment program for adults and adolescents who stutter. Journal of Speech and Hearing Research 1994; 37: 1050-1059.

Briggs J. Levels of Evidence. The Joanna Briggs Institute for Evidence Based Nursing and Midwifery, 2001.

Conture E. Evaluating childhood stuttering. In: Curlee RF, Siegel GM (eds). Nature and Treatment of Stuttering: New Directions (second edition). Needham Heights, MA: Allyn & Bacon, 1997; 239-256.

Cordes A. Current status of the stuttering treatment literature. In: Cordes A, Ingham RJ (eds). Treatment Efficacy for Stuttering. A Search for Empirical Bases. San Diego, CA: Singular Publishing, 1998; Chapter 10.

Cordes A, Ingham RJ. Time-interval measurement of stuttering: establishing and modifying judgment accuracy. Journal of Speech and Hearing Research 1996; 39: 298-310.

Cordes A, Ingham RJ (eds). Treatment Efficacy for Stuttering. A Search for Empirical Bases. San Diego, CA: Singular Publishing, 1998.

Costello J. The establishment of fluency with time-out procedures: three case studies. Journal of Speech and Hearing Disorders 1995; 40: 216-31.

Costello Ingham J, Riley G. Guidelines for documentation of treatment efficacy for young children who stutter. Journal of Speech, Language and Hearing Research 1998; 41: 753-70.

Cox N, Kramer P, Kidd K. Segregation analyses of stuttering. Genetic Epidemiology 1984; 1: 245-253.

Craig A, Kearns M. Results of a traditional acupuncture intervention for stuttering. Journal of Speech and Hearing Research 1995; 38: 572-578.

Craig A, Hancock K, Chang E, McCready C, Shepley A, McCaul A et al. A controlled clinical trial for stuttering in persons aged 9 to 14 years. Journal of Speech and Hearing Research 1996; 39: 808-826.

Culatta R, Goldberg SA. Stuttering Therapy: An Integrated Approach to Theory and Practice. Boston, MA: Allyn & Bacon, 1995.

Curlee R, Perkins W (eds). Nature and Treatment of Stuttering. New Directions. San Diego, CA: College-Hill Press, 1984.

Curlee R, Siegel G (eds). Nature and Treatment of Stuttering. New Directions (second edition). Needham Heights, MA: Allyn & Bacon, 1997.

Curlee R, Yairi E. Treatment of early childhood stuttering: advances and research needs. American Journal of Speech–Language Pathology 1998; 7: 20-2.

Dalton P (ed.) Approaches to the Treatment of Stuttering. London: Croom Helm, 1993.

Druce T, Debney S, Byrt T. Evaluation of an intensive treatment program for stuttering in young children. Journal of Fluency Disorders 1997; 22: 169-86.

Eichstadt A, Watt N, Gibson J. Evaluation of the efficacy of a stutter modification program with particular reference to two new measures of secondary behaviours and control of stuttering. Journal of Fluency Disorders 1998; 23: 231-46.

Felsenfeld S. What can genetics research tell us about stuttering treatment issues? In: Cordes A, Ingham R (eds). Treatment Efficacy for Stuttering. A Search for Empirical Bases. San Diego, CA: Singular Publishing Group, 1998; Chapter 3.

Glauber P (edited by Glauber H). Stuttering – A Psychoanalytic Understanding. New York, NY: Human Sciences Press Inc., 1982.

Gregory H. Controversies about Stuttering Therapy. Baltimore, MD: University Park Press, 1979.

Gregory H, Hill D. Stuttering therapy for children. Seminars in Speech, Language and Hearing 1980; 1: 351-63.

Ham R. Techniques of Stuttering Therapy. Englewood Cliffs, NJ: Prentice-Hall, 1986.

Ham R. Therapy of Stuttering. Preschool through Adolescence. Englewood Cliffs, NJ: Prentice-Hall, 1990.

Hancock K, Craig A, McCready C, McCaul A, Costello D, Campbell K et al. Two-to-six-year controlled-trial stuttering outcomes for children and adolescents. Journal of Speech, Language and Hearing Research 1998; 41: 1242-52.

Harrison E, Onslow M, Andrews C, Packman A, Webber M. Control of stuttering with prolonged speech: preliminary outcome of a one-day instatement program. In: Cordes A,

Ingham RJ (eds). Treatment Efficacy for Stuttering: A Search for Empirical Bases. San Diego, CA: Singular Publishing Group, 1998; Chapter 9.

Hubbard C, Yairi E. Clustering of disfluencies in the speech of stuttering and nonstuttering preschool children. Journal of Speech and Hearing Research 1998; 31: 228-33.

Ingham RJ. Stuttering and Behavior Therapy. Current Status and Experimental Foundations. San Diego, CA: College-Hill, 1984; Chapter 10.

Ingham RJ. Stuttering treatment efficacy: paradigm dependent or independent? Journal of Fluency Disorders 1993; 18: 133-49.

Ingham RJ. Learning from speech-motor control research. In: Cordes A, Ingham RJ (eds). Treatment Efficacy for Stuttering: A Search for Empirical Bases. San Diego, CA: Singular Publishing, 1998; Chapter 4.

Ingham R, Andrews G. Details of a token economy stuttering therapy program for adults. Australian Journal of Human Communication Disorders 1973; 1: 13-20.

Ingham RJ, Cordes AK. On watching a discipline shoot itself in the foot: some observations on current trends in stuttering treatment research. In: Healey C, Ratner N (eds). Stuttering Treatment Efficacy. New York, NY: Lawrence Erlbaum, in press.

Ingham R, Moglia R, Frank P, Ingham J, Cordes A. Experimental investigations of the effects of frequency-altered auditory feedback on the speech of adults who stutter. Journal of Speech, Language, and Hearing Research 1997; 40: 349-60.

Janssen P, Wieneke P. The effects of fluency-inducing conditions on the variability in the duration of laryngeal movements during stutterers' fluent speech. In: Peters H, Hulstijn W (eds). Speech Motor Dynamics in Stuttering. New York, NY: Springer-Verlag, 1987; 337-44.

Johnson W. Stuttering and What You Can Do About It. Minneapolis, MN: The University of Minnesota 1961.

Johnston S, Watkin K, Macklem P. Lung volume changes during relatively fluent speech in stutterers. Journal of Applied Physiology 1993; 75: 696-703.

Jones M, Gebski V, Onslow M, Packman A. Design of randomised controlled trials. Principles and methods applied to a treatment for early stuttering. Journal of Fluency Disorders 2001; 26: 247-267.

Jones M, Gebski V, Onslow M, Packman A. Statistical power in stuttering research: a tutorial. Journal of Speech, Language, and Hearing Research 2002; 45: 243-55.

Kalinowski J, Armson J, Roland-Mieszkowski M, Stuart A, Gracco V. Effects of alterations in auditory feedback and speech rate on stuttering frequency. Language and Speech 1993; 36: 1-16.

Katz M. Survey of patented anti-stuttering devices. In: Rieber R. The Problem of Stuttering: Theory and Therapy. New York, NY: Elsevier, 1977.

Kelly E, Conture E. Acoustic and perceptual correlates of adult stutterers' typical and imitated stutterings. Journal of Fluency Disorders 1988; 13: 233-52.

Lewis K. Reporting observer agreement on stuttering event judgements: a survey and evaluation of current practice. Journal of Fluency Disorders 1994; 19: 269-84.

Lincoln M, Harrison E. The Lidcombe Program. In: Onslow M, Packman A (eds). The Handbook of Early Stuttering Intervention. San Diego, CA: Singular Publishing, 1999; Chapter 5.

Lincoln M, Onslow M. Long-term outcome of early intervention for stuttering. American Journal of Speech-Language Pathology 1997; 6: 51-8.

Manning W. Clinical Decision Making in the Diagnosis and Treatment of Fluency Disorders. Albany, NY: Delmar Publishers, 1996.

Martin R, Kuhl P, Haroldson S. An experimental treatment with two preschool stuttering children. Journal of Speech and Hearing Research 1972; 15: 743–52.

Martin R, Johnson L, Siegel G, Haroldson S. Auditory stimulation, rhythm and stuttering. Journal of Speech and Hearing Research 1985; 28: 487–95.

Menzies R, Onslow M, Packman A. Anxiety and stuttering: exploring a complex relationship. American Journal of Speech-Language Pathology 1999; 8: 3–10.

Moore W, Haynes W. Alpha hemispheric asymmetry and stuttering: some support for segmentation dysfunction hypothesis. Journal of Speech and Hearing Research 1980; 23: 229–247.

Moore S, Perkins W. Validity and reliability of judgements of authentic and simulated stuttering. Journal of Speech and Hearing Disorders 1990; 55: 383–391.

Moscicki EK. Fundamental methodological considerations in controlled clinical trials. Journal of Fluency Disorders 1993; 18: 183–196.

O'Brien S, Cream A, Onslow M, Packman A. Reliable, non-programmed, instrument-free method for the control of stuttering with prolonged speech. Asia Pacific Journal of Speech, Language and Hearing 2001; 6: 9–96.

Onslow M. Behavioral Management of Stuttering. San Diego, CA: Singular Publishing, 1996.

Onslow M. Stuttering Treatment in 2001: Evidence, Innovation and Controversies. Invited presentation at the annual conference of the Speech Pathology Association of Australia, Melbourne, 2001.

Onslow M, Andrews C, Costa L. Parental severity scaling of early stuttered speech: four case studies. Australian Journal of Human Communication Disorders 1990a; 18: 47–61.

Onslow M, Costa L, Rue S. Direct early intervention with stuttering: some preliminary data. Journal of Speech and Hearing Disorders 1990b; 55: 406–16.

Onslow M, Harrison E, Jones A. Early Stuttering: Onset, Treatment and Recovery. Paper presented at the annual conference of the Australian Association of Speech and Hearing, Darwin, 1993.

Onslow M, Andrews C, Lincoln M. A control/experimental trial of an operant treatment for early stuttering. Journal of Speech and Hearing Research 1994; 37: 1244–59.

Onslow M, Costa L, Andrews C, Harrison E, Packman A. Speech outcomes of a prolonged-speech treatment for stuttering. Journal of Speech and Hearing Research 1996; 39: 734–49.

Packman A, Lincoln M. Early stuttering and the V model. Australian Journal of Human Communication Disorders 1996; 24: 45–55.

Packman A, Onslow M. The behavioral data language of stuttering. In: Cordes A, Ingham RJ (eds). Treatment Efficacy for Stuttering. A Search for Empirical Bases. San Diego, CA: Singular Publishing Group, 1998; Chapter 2.

Perkins W. What is stuttering? Journal of Speech and Hearing Disorders 1990; 55: 370–382.

Perkins W. Stuttering and Science. San Diego, CA: Singular Publishing Group, 1996.

Peters A. The effect of positive reinforcement on fluency: two case studies. Language, Speech and Hearing Services in Schools 1977; 8: 15–22.

Peters T, Guitar B. Stuttering: An Integrated Approach to its Nature and Treatment. Baltimore, MD: Williams & Wilkins, 1991.

Reed C, Godden A. An experimental treatment using verbal punishment with two preschool stutterers. Journal of Fluency Disorders 1977; 2: 225-33.

Rustin L, Botterill W, Kelman E. Assessment and Therapy for Young Dysfluent Children: Family Interaction. London: Whurr Publishers, 1996.

Ryan B, Van Kirk Ryan B. Programmed stuttering treatment for children: comparison of two establishment programs through transfer, maintenance, and follow-up. Journal of Speech and Hearing Research 1995; 38: 61-75.

Sackett DL, Haynes B. On the need for evidence-based medicine. Evidence-Based Medicine 1995; 1: 4-5.

Sander EK. Reliability of the Iowa speech disfluency test. Journal of Speech and Hearing Disorders 1961; (Monograph Suppl. 7): 21-30.

Schwartz M. Stuttering Solved. London: Heinemann, 1976.

Shames G. Operant conditioning and stuttering. In: Eisenson J. Stuttering. A Second Symposium. New York, NY: Harper & Row, 1975; Chapter 4.

Shapiro D. Stuttering Intervention: A Collaborative Journey to Fluency Freedom. Austin, TX: Pro-Ed, 1999.

Sheehan J. Stuttering: Research and Therapy. New York, NY: Harper & Row, 1970.

Smith A, Kelly E. Stuttering: a dynamic multifactorial model. In: Curlee R, Siegel G (eds). Nature and Treatment of Stuttering: New Directions (second edition). Needham Heights, MA: Allyn & Bacon, 1997; 204-217.

Stager S, Ludlow C, Gordon C, Cotelingam M, Rappaport J. Fluency changes in persons who stutter following a double blind trial of clomipramine and desipramine. Journal of Speech and Hearing Research 1995; 38: 516-525.

Starkweather W, Gottwald S, Halfond M. Stuttering Prevention: A Clinical Method. Englewood Cliffs, NJ: Prentice-Hall, 1990.

Storch EA. Incorporating effectiveness research in assessing the validity of stuttering treatments. (Letter to the Editor.) Journal of Fluency Disorders 2002; 27: 175-6.

Thomas C, Howell P. Assessing efficacy of stuttering treatments. Journal of Fluency Disorders 2001; 26: 311-333.

Travis L. Speech Pathology. New York, NY: Appleton–Century, 1931.

Tunbridge N. The Stutterer's Survival Guide. Sydney: Addison–Wesley, 1994.

Van Riper C. The Nature of Stuttering. Englewood Cliffs, NJ: Prentice-Hall, 1971.

Van Riper C. The Treatment of Stuttering. Englewood Cliffs, NJ: Prentice-Hall, 1973.

Van Riper C. The Nature of Stuttering (second edition). Englewood Cliffs, NJ: Prentice-Hall, 1982.

Wall M, Myers F. Clinical Management of Childhood Stuttering. Austin, TX: Pro-Ed Inc., 1984.

Watson J. Improving the effectiveness of stuttering intervention: the journey continues. Folia Phoniatrica Logopaedia 1994; 46: 214-22.

Wingate M. A standard definition of stuttering. Journal of Speech and Hearing Disorders 1964; 29: 484-9.

Yairi E. Applications of disfluencies in measurements of stuttering. (Letter to the Editor.) Journal of Speech and Hearing Research 1996; 39: 402.

Yairi E. Disfluency characteristics of childhood stuttering. In: Curlee RF, Siegel GM (eds). Nature and Treatment of Stuttering: New Directions (second edition). Needham Heights, MA: Allyn & Bacon, 1997; 49-78.

Yairi E, Ambrose N. Onset of stuttering in preschool children. Selected factors. Journal of Speech and Hearing Research 1992; 35: 782-8.

Yairi E, Lewis B. Disfluencies at the onset of stuttering. Journal of Speech and Hearing Research 1984; 27: 145-54.

Yairi E, Ambrose N, Cox N. Genetics of stuttering: a critical review. Journal of Speech and Hearing Research 1996; 39: 771-84.

Yaruss S. Treatment outcomes in stuttering: finding value in clinical data. In: Cordes A, Ingham RJ (eds). Treatment Efficacy for Stuttering. A Search for Empirical Bases. San Diego, CA: Singular Publishing, 1998; Chapter 10.

CHAPTER 6

The evidence base for the management of individuals with voice disorders

JENNI OATES

Introduction: voice disorders in context

The aim of this chapter is to place the literature on the evaluation and treatment of vocal disorders in the context of evidence-based practice. This introductory section provides an overview of the nature and prevalence of voice disorders, the significance of voice disorders for individuals and society, and the historical development of the management of voice disorders. The second section of the chapter outlines and evaluates the available evidence for speech pathologists' management of clients with voice disorders. Throughout this chapter the focus is on disorders of phonation (that is, disorders of resonance are not considered).

The nature and prevalence of voice disorders

Human speech is achieved through a synergy of respiration, phonation, resonance and articulation. Voice encompasses phonation and resonance powered by respiration and forms an integral component of speech and human communication. The perceptual parameters of voice (pitch, loudness, quality and resonance) vary to enhance the linguistic content of thoughts and ideas and the expression of feelings and emotions (Titze, 1994; Russell, 1999).

Traditionally, voice has been considered disordered when the production of one or more of its perceptual parameters are notably dissimilar to those of people of the same age, sex and culture (Boone and McFarlane, 1988; Aronson, 1990). Stemple et al. (1995) introduced the perspective of the individual speaker and stated that voice is disordered when it no longer meets the voicing requirements previously available to the speaker. Similarly, Aronson (1990) and Sataloff and Abaza (2000) state that a definition of a disordered voice must encompass the ability of the voice to fulfil the speaker's social and occupational requirements.

A variety of reported and observable symptoms accompany voice disorders. Clients may report symptoms relating to physical sensations and/or perceptual aspects of the voice. These include: feelings of a lump in the throat; a frequent need to clear the throat; sensations of discomfort associated with phonation (pain or soreness, vocal fatigue); and reports of a voice characterized by atypical pitch or loudness, hoarseness or weakness (Colton and Casper 1996; Harris, 1998). Harris (1998) classifies symptoms into three categories: voice quality (for example, hoarse); comfort (degree of discomfort or pain when speaking); and stamina (length of speaking time prior to onset of negative voice change).

Similarly, signs or characteristics that may be observed or tested in clients with voice disorders (Colton and Casper, 1996; Oates and Russell, 1998) include impairment in pitch, loudness and quality, and their acoustic correlates. Changes in respiration, such as audible inspiration and inadequate breath support resulting in reduced phrase length, may also be a sign of voice disorder.

Observable changes to the larynx associated with voice disorders include mucosal changes, such as the presence of nodules, polyps, contact ulcers, mucous retention and epidermoid cysts, oedema, erythema, haemorrhage and vocal fold scar. Physiological impairment of the larynx may include hyperadduction of the vocal folds, ventricular fold compression, anterior-posterior compression, impairments in amplitude, phase and regularity of vocal fold vibration, and reduction in vocal fold mobility, mucosal wave and glottal closure.

There is no universally accepted classification system for voice problems. However, the traditional approach has been broadly based on a functional versus organic dichotomy (Fawcus, 2000a). Most systems remain aetiologically based (for example, Aronson, 1990) adhering to the premise that such a system facilitates a better understanding of voice disorders. Titze (1994) contributes to the determination of a classification system by proposing three major divisions:

- Congenital (structural) voice disorders.
- Disorders related to tissue change.
- Disorders related to neurological or muscular change.

A fourth division, vocal fatigue, is more speculative. Verdolini (1994) proposes a classification system that combines symptomatology and aetiology. Verdolini's (1994) system includes four categories: discrete mass lesions; distributed tissue changes; organic movement disorders; and non-organic disorders. Although recent contributions to the establishment of a classification system overcome in part the difficulties of earlier dichotomous systems, confusion remains. Inconsistent terminology and the illusive nature of some voice disorders where the cause, the presenting symptoms and maintenance factors overlap, continue to thwart attempts to establish a universally accepted classification system (Fawcus, 2000a).

Until recently, data on the prevalence of voice disorders have been scarce. The fact that voice disorders do not, as a rule, constitute a threat to life and do not often lead to severe reductions in speech intelligibility may account in part for the paucity of prevalence data. In addition, the multiple methods available for identifying voice disorders (for example, self-report, perceptual, acoustic and physiological measurement and laryngeal examination) and the aetiological and diagnostic confusions that abound make the design of prevalence studies difficult. There are no current data available on voice disorders in children, although earlier reports estimate conservatively that 6% of children have voice disorders at any given moment (Aronson, 1990). Verdolini and Ramig (2001) suggest that the prevalence of voice disorders in the general adult population of the USA lies between 3% and 9%. A recent prevalence study on a large sample of adults from the general population in Australia provides a prevalence rate of 4% (Russell, 1999).

Prevalence data for certain sub-groups of people whose voices are 'at risk' by virtue of an occupational reliance on voice, for example, school teachers and singers, are more readily available. Again, the way in which voice disorders are measured in these prevalence studies (for example, self-report survey versus direct examination of the larynx) appears to influence prevalence figures. In general, however, recent research has demonstrated consistently that teachers, singers and other professional voice users are at significantly higher risk of voice disorder than are members of the general population (see, for example, Smith et al., 1997; Russell et al., 1998; Smith et al., 1998).

The significance of voice disorders for individuals and society

'Voice problems are common and they matter' (Verdolini and Ramig, 2001, p. 37), particularly in contemporary Western societies where a large proportion of people rely on their voice as a critical requirement of their occupation. The impact of a voice disorder on an individual will vary according to the severity of the problem and the reliance of the individual on voice as a communication tool within the home, social, educational and working environment. However, a voice disorder is highly likely to result in significant restrictions in social and occupational activity and participation as well as compromised emotional well-being (Sataloff and Abaza, 2000; Verdolini and Ramig, 2001). Individuals with voice problems may experience frustration, anxiety, depression, social isolation, reduced speech intelligibility, quality of life, occupational productivity, economic and social status, loss of self-esteem and general personality changes (Smith et al., 1996; Rosen and Sataloff, 1997; Roy and Bless, 2000).

At a societal level, the cost of voice disorders can also be high. Although there are no reported studies providing data on the societal impact of vocal problems, Verdolini and Ramig (2001, p. 43) estimate that if we consider only time away from work and health care costs, 'voice disorders may result in societal losses in the billions of dollars in the US alone'.

The historical development of the management of individuals with voice disorders

In the nineteenth century, management of those with voice disorders was the domain of general medical practitioners and laryngologists. Medico-surgical approaches were therefore the primary focus of diagnosis and treatment. Psychiatrists also played a part in managing people with voice problems at that time, although mainly for problems considered to be other than medical conditions (that is, those voice problems labelled as 'psychoneuroses'). Early in the twentieth century, these professionals were joined by singing teachers and speech correctionists who based their management on traditional breathing and singing techniques aimed at enhancing the normal voice. The medico-surgical and psychological approaches were thus extended to include a more symptomatic approach to evaluation and intervention. In the middle of the twentieth century, the profession of speech pathology developed. Speech pathologists became key professionals involved in the management of people with voice problems and their work resulted in a more holistic approach with greater integration of medical, psychological and symptomatic methods. More recently, speech pathologists have also promoted a direct physiological approach to voice therapy (Stemple et al., 1995; Casper and Murry, 2000). Today, the work of speech pathologists remains central to the management of clients with voice disorders, although it is increasingly recognized that effective evaluation and treatment requires a team approach involving a range of professionals, including otolaryngologists and other medical specialists, singing and voice teachers, psychologists and psychiatrists. The recognition of the importance of a team approach to voice disorders has lead to the recent evolution of specialist multidisciplinary voice clinics throughout the world.

Since the 1970s the evaluation and treatment of voice disorders by speech pathologists has made a quantum leap from an art to a science. Clinicians no longer rely only on perceptual analysis of the voice and static views of the vocal folds for voice evaluation and treatments based on intuition and singing teaching methods. These methods have been augmented by technology which permits instrumental measurement of the dynamic voicing process, greater understanding of normal and impaired voice production, increased knowledge of the causes and contributing factors of voice disorders, and a clearer rationale for therapeutic interventions and prevention techniques (Baken, 1998). Indeed, there is now growing debate as to whether clinical specialization in voice is required to enable speech pathologists to keep abreast of scientific advances and to facilitate the efficient management of voice-disordered clients.

The evidence base for speech pathologists' management of clients with voice disorders

The following section considers three key questions that must be answered in our quest to apply the principles of evidence-based practice in voice management.

1 What domains of voice do we need evidence about?
2 How useful is the available evidence?
3 What future developments could improve the evidence base underlying the management of our clients with voice disorders?

What domains of voice do we need evidence about?

Before speech pathologists attempt to apply the principles of evidence-based practice to the management of clients with voice disorders, it is important to establish a framework that can underpin best practice in the voice field. A framework can guide the search for evidence so that clinicians do not become lost in the exponentially increasing volume of literature and opinion concerned with vocal dysfunction and its management. So, what domains of voice require scrutiny in order for speech pathologists to make informed decisions about the care of individual clients with voice disorders? The following framework of five domains has been adopted throughout this chapter. Speech pathologists aiming to provide the best possible care for their clients with voice disorders would be wise to search for the best available evidence in each of the five domains listed here.

- The basic science of normal voice:
    - vocal tract anatomy and histology
    - physiological mechanisms and biomechanics of voice production
    - neurological substrates of voice production
    - genetic influences on the vocal mechanism.

- Mechanisms of causation for different voice disorders:
    - vocal technique and voice use patterns
    - disease processes and general health factors
    - psychological processes
    - environmental contributors.

- Voice evaluation methods:
    - physiologic
    - acoustic
    - aerodynamic
    - perceptual.

- Intervention methods:
    - direct voice therapy
    - indirect voice therapy and education
    - medico-surgical treatments
    - psychological interventions
    - alternative therapies.

- Prevention of voice disorders.

The search for this evidence can be a daunting task, but most of the valuable literature will be located through the medical and paramedical electronic data bases MEDLINE and CINHAL, as well as through Psyclit. Searching for literature through these electronic databases can be supplemented by hand searching through the respected journals in the voice field (for example, *American Journal of Speech Language Pathology*; *Annals of Otology, Rhinology and Laryngology*; *Archives of Otolaryngology*; *International Journal of Language and Communication Disorders*; *Folia Phoniatrica*; *Journal of Laryngology and Otology*; *Journal of Medical Speech–Language Pathology*; *Journal of Speech, Language, and Hearing Research*; *Journal of Voice*; *Laryngoscope*; *Logopedics Phoniatrics Vocology*).

How useful is the available evidence in the domains of basic voice science, causal mechanisms, evaluation, intervention and prevention of voice disorders?

Basic science of normal voice

The last two decades have seen enormous advances in our understanding of the anatomy, physiology, neurology and genetics of normal voice (Larson, 1992; Titze, 1994; Sataloff, 1995; Fawcus, 2000a; Hammarberg, 2000). This increased understanding has come through multidisciplinary cooperation among voice scientists with backgrounds in anatomy, histology, neurosciences, genetics, physics, speech science, computer engineering, medicine and speech pathology. Basic biological research using human and animal tissue and computer modelling has yielded a great deal of descriptive data on the structure and functioning of the vocal folds as well as respiratory, neurological and genetic mechanisms underlying voice production (for example, Hirano and Kurita, 1986; Gray et al., 1993; Titze et al., 1993; Davis et al., 1996; Iwarrson et al., 1998; Gray, 2000; Jiang et al., 2000). This new knowledge has, in turn, provided practising clinicians with improved rationales for the development and selection of voice evaluation tools as well as intervention and prevention methods for clients with vocal dysfunction. No longer do clinicians need to depend solely on incomplete models of voice production in the design of their management programmes; instead it is now possible for clinicians to adopt a more rational basis for their evaluation and intervention (Stemple, 1993; Sataloff, 1995; Colton and Casper, 1996).

Although information derived from basic science research can provide some of the evidence to underpin best clinical practice (Sackett et al., 1998), this is far from a sufficient basis for evidence-based practice in the voice field. Clinicians will also need to evaluate the applicability of such information to particular patients and voice disorders and to evaluate the available evidence concerned with the causes of voice disorders, diagnostic methods, intervention techniques and prevention approaches.

Mechanisms of causation for different voice disorders

A large number of textbooks and journal papers concerned with the management of clients with voice problems contain discussions of the supposed causes of the myriad of known voice disorders. Clinicians are alerted to the possibility that their clients' vocal problems may arise from aetiologies, such as ineffective vocal technique and voice use patterns, disease processes and general health factors, genetic influences, psychological processes and personality factors, and environmental contributors, such as noise levels and air quality. Much of this literature presents causal information as if it was supported by high levels of evidence, yet closer examination reveals that a good deal of the evidence is anecdotal or derived from case reports and incompletely tested theoretical propositions (see for example, Boone and McFarlane, 1988; Hillman et al., 1989; Aronson, 1990; Weiner et al., 1995; Morrison et al., 1999). Fortunately, there has been an increase in the number of well-designed case-control and causal modelling studies reported in the last decade, so that clinicians now have access to some research findings at moderate levels of evidence in this important area (see, for example, Green, 1989; Russell, 1999; Roy and Bless, 2000; Roy et al.,

2000). Although randomized controlled trials and cohort studies would provide the strongest evidence for causal mechanisms in voice disorders (Sackett et al., 1998; Greenhalgh, 2001), there are no examples of such studies in the voice literature. Accordingly, systematic reviews of randomized controlled trials and cohort studies are non-existent.

Let us explore some of the evidence concerned with the aetiologies of the most common voice disorders encountered by speech pathologists: the so-called 'functional' disorders. At the anecdotal and expert opinion level, a great deal has been written about the importance of both vocal hyperfunction and psychological factors, such as personality and anxiety, as causal agents for voice disorders, including vocal fold oedema, vocal nodules and functional dysphonia (see, for example, Aronson, 1990, Morrison and Rammage, 1994; Stemple et al., 1995; Colton and Casper, 1996). The underlying proposition for the role of vocal hyperfunction is that use of excess laryngeal and respiratory muscle tension, force and constriction will lead to biomechanical changes, such as vocal ligament strain, increased vocal fold tissue viscosity, structural damage to the cover of the vocal folds, and respiratory muscle fatigue (Titze, 1994; Oates, 2000). Similarly, emotional factors are said to lead to functional voice disorders by increasing affected individuals' tendency to use hyperfunctional voicing patterns, such as hyperadduction of the vocal folds and/or ventricular folds (Oates, 2000). Some efforts have been made to formulate propositions such as theoretical models of functional voice disorders. Hillman et al. (1989), for example, postulated that the type of vocal hyperfunction that leads to vocal fatigue and subsequently to mucosal changes, such as vocal nodules, is of the 'adducted' type where increased muscle tension and collision forces along with tightly adducted vocal folds cause injury to the vocal fold cover. In contrast, the 'non-adducted' type of vocal hyperfunction characterized by increased laryngeal muscle tension but incomplete closure of the vocal folds results in functional dysphonia without mucosal change. Turning to psychological mechanisms underlying functional voice disorders, Butcher (1995) proposed, for example, that intrapsychic conflict and/or life stresses and interpersonal problems in people who are predisposed to difficulties expressing their emotions would lead to excessive musculo-skeletal tension associated with voice production.

These expert opinions and theoretical models are certainly of value to speech pathologists searching for causal mechanisms in functional voice disorders, but the search for evidence must extend at least to case-control studies (Sackett et al., 1998; Greenhalgh, 2001). Earlier case-control studies concerned with the aetiologies of functional voice disorders were limited by inadequate definition of patients and control or comparison groups; failure to ensure that comparison groups were similar to patient groups on all key factors apart from the proposed causal agents; and failure to adequately describe the nature, severity and duration of the voice disorder in the patient groups (Oates, 2000; Roy and Bless, 2000). These design limitations meant that there was no clear evidence of a direct link between vocal hyperfunction, psychological processes and functional voice disorders. The advent of better designed case-control studies in recent years has, however, provided stronger evidence that vocal hyperfunction and emotional factors are likely to lead to functional voice disorders (see, for example, Green, 1989; Masuda et al., 1993; Smith et al., 1998; Roy et al., 2000). One of the best examples of such research is the landmark study reported by Roy et al. (2000). These investigators compared four groups of patients with voice disorders (37 participants with vocal nodules, 45 with functional dysphonia, 35 with spasmodic dysphonia and 23 with unilateral vocal fold palsy) and a group of vocally normal participants (37 participants) on multiple measures of personality, anxiety, depression and self-reported vocal disorder. Stepwise logistic discriminant analyses demonstrated that the functional dysphonia and vocal nodule groups differed from one another, from the other disorder groups, and from the vocally normal control subjects. The functional dysphonia group was characterized by high levels of neuroticism, anxiety and introversion, whereas the vocal nodule group was characterized by high levels of disinhibition and extraversion. The findings generally supported the theoretical model of Roy and Bless (2000) of a dispositional basis for functional dysphonia and vocal nodules. It must be noted, however, that not all individual patients conformed to the overall group findings and that the study used only self-report measures of psychological factors and vocal disorder. Further, it should be remembered that case-control studies of this type cannot provide direct evidence of causal mechanisms. At best, such research demonstrates associations between hypothesised aetiological factors and voice disorders (Greenhalgh, 2001). Cohort studies and randomized controlled trials will be required before causal factors can be identified with confidence (Sackett et al., 1998; Greenhalgh, 2001).

Voice evaluation methods

For more than a century after Garcia devised the method of indirect laryngoscopy in 1854 (Von Leden, 1982), clinical evaluation of voice involved little more than perceptual assessment of clients' voice characteristics, simple measurement of phonatory parameters such as maximum phonation time and the relatively crude technique of mirror examination of the larynx (Stemple, 1993; Sataloff, 1995). A variety of perceptual rating protocols were used, most of which were supported by very low levels of evidence because evaluations of their validity and reliability had not been conducted. Since the late 1970s, however, there has been a virtual explosion of voice evaluation methods and diagnostic instruments. This growth in evaluation techniques shows no sign of slowing as technological advances continue into the twenty-first century. Speech pathologists, phoniatricians and laryngologists are now faced with an enormous array of techniques and instruments for the measurement of perceptual, phonatory, vibratory, aerodynamic, acoustic and electro-myographic aspects of vocal function. No longer is instrumental measurement of voice the exclusive domain of the research scientist; clinicians now have far easier access to 'relatively inexpensive, increasingly precise and ever-more-user-friendly' evaluation methods and instruments (Baken and Orlikoff, 1997, p. 147).

Despite the enormous advances in diagnostic methods in the voice field over the past 30 years, clinicians are left with the task of deciding which of the vast array of measures and instruments provide the most useful indications of vocal functioning. In order to make these decisions and to select the evaluation tools to be used in clinical practice, clinicians need to be clear on the purposes of voice evaluation and then to examine the available evidence about the utility, validity and reliability of each voice measurement technique. First, let us consider the rationale for voice evaluation. The critical purposes of voice evaluation are to establish the causal and contributing factors for the vocal disorder and to characterize the underlying physiological impairment in vocal tract functioning (Baken and Orlikoff, 1997). This information provides the key to successful management of the vocal disorder; intervention must be designed to eliminate or reduce the impact of aetiological factors and to alter the physiological mechanism of voice production (Stemple, 1993; Colton and Casper, 1996; Baken and Orlikoff, 1997). It follows that clinicians should select voice evaluation methods and measures that conform to this rationale. Voice measurements for which little or no relationship to underlying vocal tract functioning has been established, then, will have a limited role in the evaluation process. If a voice measure has no impact on treatment decisions, its value must be seriously questioned.

The second consideration in selecting evaluation methods is the need for compelling evidence that measures of vocal functioning have satisfactory utility and are valid and reliable. Such evidence is best provided through cross-sectional studies which apply the evaluation methods in question to a broad spectrum of people with a range of voice disorders and with no vocal dysfunction (Sackett et al., 1998; Greenhalgh, 2001). The long-established tenets of test and measurement theory as well as currently espoused evidence-based practice principles for evaluating diagnostic tests provide clinicians with considerable guidance here (see, for example, Sackett et al., 1998; Polgar and Thomas, 2000; Greenhalgh, 2001).

Clinicians need to examine the available evidence to determine whether specific tests of vocal functioning conform to the following specifications.

- The measure should have a known or at least highly likely relationship with vocal tract physiology.
- The measure should be reproducible over time and across and within observers.
- The relationship between expectation bias of the observer and the measure should have been established.
- Normative data for the measure across a broad spectrum of people without voice disorders should have been determined.
- The measure should have been applied to a wide range of people with different voice disorders and different degrees of severity of disorder.
- The measure should be associated with acceptable specificity, sensitivity and accuracy.

Proponents of evidence-based practice in health care would add to these specifications that new diagnostic tests should have been compared with a gold standard measure (Sackett et al., 1998; Greenhalgh, 2001). This principle is not easy to apply in the field of voice where gold standard measures are in short supply and where the purpose of voice evaluation is more concerned with establishing underlying vocal tract physiology than diagnosing medical conditions. In this situation where there is no absolute gold standard, voice clinicians need to assess new tests against a combination of existing voice measures that have well established utility, reliability and validity (Greenhalgh, 2001). Many scientists, clinicians and people with voice disorders consider that the perceptual features of voice constitute a gold standard and that instrumental measures of vocal functioning should therefore show a clear relationship with voice features that are obvious to the ear (Sataloff, 1995). Because the perceptual features of a voice disorder do have psychological reality for both clinician and client, this is a reasonable expectation (Gerratt et al., 1993; Kreiman et al., 1993) – that is, as long as those auditory perceptual measures can be shown to be valid and reliable.

Auditory perceptual evaluation of voice

Debate has raged for the past three decades concerning the value of perceptual measures of voice (see for example, Kreiman et al., 1993; Carding, 2000; Kreiman and Gerratt, 2000). Auditory perceptual methods have been criticized because of inadequate reliability between and within judges, because the relationships between perceptual measures and acoustic and physiological measures have not been clearly established, because of sensitivity and specificity limitations, and because there is no universally accepted perceptual analysis system (Ludlow, 1981; Fex, 1992; de Krom,

1995; Kreiman and Gerratt, 2000). Despite such criticism and the exponentially increasing array of alternative instrumental measures of voice, auditory perceptual measurement remains the most often used voice evaluation method in the clinic (Hammarberg, 2000). Perceptual measures are also used frequently as the standard against which instrumental measures are compared (Gerratt et al., 1993). Popular perceptual systems include the GRBAS scale (Hirano, 1981), Laver's Vocal Profile Analysis (Wirz and Mackenzie Beck, 1995), Hammarberg's Stockholm Voice Evaluation Approach (Hammarberg and Gauffin, 1995) and the Oates and Russell Perceptual Voice Profile (Oates and Russell, 1998).

The jury is still out on the utility, validity and reliability of these and other perceptual systems, partly because well-designed validation and reliability studies have been scarce (Kreiman et al., 1993; Baken and Orlikoff, 1997; Wuyts et al., 1999). The small number of studies reported have typically applied perceptual measurement to small numbers of subjects with a narrow range of voice disorders and a limited range of severity of disorder. It has also been common for subjects with normal voices to be omitted from such research and for inappropriate statistical analyses to be used. Further, the measures of vocal functioning selected for comparison with perceptual evaluations have most often been restricted to acoustic measures so that the relationship between perceptual measures and underlying vocal physiology is insufficiently specified. Fortunately, there has been a recent resurgence of interest in developing and validating better approaches to auditory perceptual evaluation. Several researchers have reported cross-sectional research that provides good evidence concerning the reliability of different types of scales for perceptual ratings (for example, Wuyts et al., 1999; Hammarberg, 2000; Zraick and Liss, 2000) and the influences of factors such as listener experience, type of speech sample and degree of severity and complexity of vocal impairment on perceptual judgements (for example, Revis et al., 1999; Kreiman and Gerratt, 2000; Wolfe et al., 2000). It is now clearer that terminology in common usage for describing voice quality features is associated with reasonable validity in terms of its relationship with underlying vocal tract physiology and acoustic features (Hammarberg, 2000; Kreiman and Gerratt, 2000). Similarly, it has been demonstrated that reliability can be enhanced through various strategies such as providing anchored voice stimuli and using computer-based rating systems that allow judges to continually compare and adjust their ratings (for example, Granqvist, 1996; Zraick and Liss, 2000).

Instrumental measures of voice

Just as there is debate about the diagnostic value of auditory perceptual ratings of voice, so there is considerable controversy surrounding the utility, validity and reliability of virtually all instrumental measures of vocal functioning (for recent reviews, see Hammarberg, 2000; Carding, 2000). As concluded recently by Wuyts et al. (2000, p. 797), 'Voice research so far has not led to the construction or a consensus about a sensitive measure that unambiguously quantifies voice quality'. Let us take the example of acoustic analysis, another common evaluation approach used in voice clinics. The easy availability of low-cost user-friendly acoustic analysis software and hardware along with the recognition that acoustic analysis is quick and non-invasive has meant that this seemingly objective method of voice evaluation has become increasingly popular. Acoustic analysis systems provide automatic extraction of a large number of vocal parameters, such as fundamental frequency, intensity, dynamic range and frequency range, jitter, shimmer and harmonic-to-noise ratio. These systems also allow the clinician to extract, although not automatically, other acoustic features of the power spectrum, such as level of the first formant relative to the level of the fundamental.

Unfortunately, the ease of obtaining acoustic indices is not matched by clear evidence of the value of many of these parameters. The quality of research investigating the validity and reliability of acoustic measurement has been limited by failure to examine sufficient numbers of subjects with a wide range of disorder types, voice quality characteristics and dysphonia severities (Carding, 2000). Further, there is considerable evidence demonstrating that clinicians should be cautious in their application of acoustic analysis. Measures such as 'jitter' and 'shimmer', for example, suffer from many shortcomings, including inadequate correspondence with perceptual ratings and physiological measures, large inter-subject variability, inability to differentiate normal from impaired voice quality, lack of normative data and wide variations across different analysis systems (Baken and Orlikoff, 1997; Wuyts et al., 2000). In addition, many acoustic analysis instruments are associated with unacceptable measurement error in the case of moderate to severe pathological voice quality, and most systems cannot yet reliably analyse voice quality parameters in connected speech (Baken and Orlikoff, 1999).

The outlook for acoustic analysis is not as bleak as it may first appear, however. Clinicians now have access to clinical standards and guidelines for acoustic analysis, guidelines that are underpinned by at least moderately strong evidence. Titze (1995), for example, has published a summary statement arising from an international workshop sponsored by the National Center for Voice and Speech in Colorado in 1994. This workshop was conducted with leading scientists in the field to reach consensus on the purpose and methods of acoustic voice analysis. Similarly, for the first time, several recent texts devoted to measurement of voice and speech provide well-researched guidelines and summaries of relevant research (for example, Baken and Orlikoff, 1999; Kent and Ball, 1999). Further, new approaches to describe the acoustic features of voice have begun to appear in the journals over the past year. These innovative approaches take a multi-dimensional view of vocal acoustics and have abandoned the earlier dependence on isolated acoustic measures (for example, Fröhlich et al., 2000; Wuyts et al., 2000). The result has been the development of promising measures with considerably improved utility, reliability and validity.

Examination of the evidence base for other instrumental approaches to voice analysis (for example, videostroboscopy, high speed imaging, flow glottography, phonetography, electromyography, electroglottography, and aerodynamic measurement) is beyond the scope of this chapter. However, just as is the case for perceptual and acoustic measurement, there is a growing trend towards evidence based research in all of these evaluation methods.

Intervention methods

There is no shortage of descriptions in the literature of voice therapy techniques for clients with a wide range of hyperfunctional, psychogenic and organic voice disorders. Specific voice therapy techniques are outlined in many of the well-known textbooks published over the last 20 years (for example, Wilson, 1987; Boone and McFarlane, 1988; Greene and Mathieson, 1989; Aronson, 1990; Morrison and Rammage, 1994; Andrews, 1995; Stemple et al., 1995; Colton and Casper, 1996; Harris et al., 1998; Fawcus, 2000b). Many journal papers that provide general descriptions of therapy methods have also been published in that time (see Pannbacker, 1998; Ramig and Verdolini, 1998). The volume of information on voice therapy available to the clinician is certainly impressive. A critical question remains to be answered, however. To what extent can clinicians confidently select those intervention methods that are most likely to result in improved vocal functioning for clients with particular voice disorders?

In 1993 Joseph Stemple reviewed the previous 25 years of literature on voice therapy and concluded that, 'the more things change, the more they appear to stay the same' (Stemple, 1993, p. 293). Stemple acknowledged that there had been enormous advances in our understanding of the basic science of voice production, aetiologies of voice disorders and voice evaluation techniques, but he decided that the same intervention techniques had been used by speech pathologists for decades with little attempt to scientifically evaluate their efficacy and effectiveness. This same view of the status of voice therapy has been espoused by many prominent scientists and clinicians (for example, Moore, 1977; Reed, 1980; Perkins, 1985; Hillman et al., 1990; Enderby and Emerson, 1995), with the most recent reviews repeating essentially the same message (for example, Pannbacker, 1998; Ramig and Verdolini, 1998; Carding, 2000).

Between them, the most recent overviews, published by Pannbacker (1998, 1999), Ramig and Verdolini (1998) and Carding (2000), unearthed 80 data-based articles that have evaluated the effectiveness of voice therapy. These 80 papers were published between 1960 and 1999, and most focused on adults with hyperfunctional voice disorders. Pannbacker (1998, 1999) and Ramig and Verdolini (1998) did not specify the sources of the literature they reviewed, whereas Carding (2000) stated that he gathered the literature from the reference lists of earlier review papers (for example, Ramig and Verdolini, 1998), cross-referencing from the original articles, and database searches by use of MEDLINE and Psyclit. Because these three recent reviews have not cited the same papers, clinicians will need to consult each review to be confident that they have accessed all of the available research papers for that period. The author's own database and hand searching strategy for the same time period yielded only two studies that were not cited in these three reviews (see Benninger and Jacobson, 1995; Kelchner et al., 1999). For the period following 1999, no overviews are provided the literature. The author has uncovered five further research papers published between 1999 and 2001 (see Rosen et al., 2000; Roy et al., 2000; Ylitalo and Hammarberg, 2000; MacKenzie et al., 2001; Roy et al., 2001), giving a grand total of 87 articles on evaluation of voice therapy published since 1960.

Because Pannbacker (1998, 1999), Ramig and Verdolini (1998) and Carding (2000) have already provided comprehensive reviews of virtually all of the treatment evaluation studies in the voice field, the focus of the remainder of this chapter is to place the literature on the efficacy and effectiveness of voice therapy in the context of evidence-based practice. (Detailed reviews of the findings of the various studies are not given here.)

The traditional hierarchy of evidence puts systematic reviews and meta-analyses at the pinnacle of the hierarchy (Guyatt et al., 1995; Greenhalgh, 2001). Alas, there are no reports of this type in the literature concerned with voice therapy. There are certainly literature reviews as outlined earlier, but these fall far short of being either reviews conducted according to rigorous, predetermined criteria (systematic review) or an integration of numerical or qualitative data from more than one study (meta-analysis).

So to the next level down the hierarchy, the randomized controlled trial (Guyatt et al., 1995; Greenhalgh, 2001). Overall, voice therapy evaluations do not fare well at this level either, although the small number of randomized controlled trials that have been reported do provide some valid evidence for the effectiveness of therapy. Only 12 of the 87 published studies can be categorized as randomized controlled trials. Over half of these randomized controlled trials have investigated treatment methods (mainly Lee Silverman

Voice Therapy [LSVT]) for patients with Parkinson's disease (for example, Johnson and Pring, 1990; Ramig et al., 1995; Ramig and Dromey, 1996; Ramig et al., 1996). The remainder have evaluated the accent method in patients with various aetiologies (Basiouny, 1998), vocal function exercises in subjects with normal voices and teachers (Stemple et al., 1994; Roy et al., 2001), and direct and indirect therapy for patients with a variety of non-organic dysphonias (Carding et al., 1999; MacKenzie et al., 2001). Randomized controlled trials in voice therapy have either compared two treatment methods (for example, Ramig et al., 1996; Basiouny, 1998), a treatment approach with no treatment or a placebo (for example, MacKenzie et al., 2001) or two treatment methods with no treatment within the same study (for example, Carding et al., 1999; Roy et al., 2001). It is important to remember here that comparisons between two treatments only tell us whether or not one technique is superior to the other; this type of study does not inform us whether a particular therapy is more effective than no therapy. Only one of the studies has used double-blinding (Stemple et al., 1994), although this would not have been feasible in most investigations of patients with dysphonia. Subject numbers have been reasonably large in the majority of the randomized controlled trials (26–204 participants). Only two studies have investigated smaller numbers of subjects (12–18 participants) where questions could be raised concerning the power of the statistical analyses. Patient inclusion and exclusion criteria have generally been clearly specified, systematic biases with the possible exception of performance bias and subject attrition have been avoided, and treatment outcomes have mostly been measured multi-dimensionally by use of reliable methods. Only one of these studies (see MacKenzie et al., 2001) reported confidence intervals for the results and none reported the clinical significance of the findings, thus reducing the strength of the evidence they provide. In general, however, the randomized controlled trials used strong designs and provided good evidence for the effectiveness of the voice therapy approaches under examination. Table 6.1 provides a summary of the available evidence derived from the randomized controlled trials. This table displays information on the participants and vocal disorders examined, the study design, voice measures, main findings and level of evidence (as used by the Joanna Briggs Institute for Evidence Based Nursing and Midwifery).

Although the evidence provided by prospective controlled trials without randomization, and by empirical single-case designs, is considered lower on the evidence hierarchy than randomized controlled trials (Howard, 1986; Guyatt et al., 1995; Greenhalgh, 2001), such studies can make an important contribution (Greenhalgh, 2001). Surprisingly, only a small number of studies evaluating voice therapy have taken either of these moderately strong approaches to research design. Andrews et al. (1986), Murry and Woodson

Table 6.1 Evidence for the efficacy or effectiveness of voice therapy as derived from randomized controlled trials

Voice disorder	Source	Design	Participants	Measures	Results	Evidence level
Non-organic dysphonias	MacKenzie et al. (2001)	RCT	204 adults with hoarseness, two groups: 1 Symptomatic voice therapy with indirect therapy 2 No treatment	1 Perceptual ratings and self-report 2 Amplitude and frequency perturbation 3 SF-36 4 Anxiety, depression and quality of life	Voice therapy associated with significant improvements on perceptual measures, amplitude perturbation, but no significant effect on psychological factors or quality of life.	II
Non-organic dysphonias	Carding et al. (1999)	RCT	45 dysphonic adults, three groups: 1 Symptomatic and indirect voice therapy 2 Indirect voice therapy 3 No treatment	1 Perceptual ratings and self-report 2 Laryngoscopy findings 3 Lx wave 4 Acoustic measures of fundamental frequency jitter and shimmer, s/n ratio	Patients who had symptomatic voice therapy showed greatest gains with significant change on most measures. 93% of this group showed significant improvement. Indirect therapy less effective, but 46% improved.	II
Teachers with variety of dysphonias	Roy et al. (2001)	RCT	58 dysphonic teachers, three groups: 1 Vocal function exercises 2 Vocal hygiene 3 No treatment	1 Vocal handicap index 2 Self-report of perceived benefit	The vocal function exercise (VFE) group was the only group that showed a significant reduction in vocal handicap. The VFE group also reported more overall improvement and greater ease and clarity of voice after treatment than the vocal hygiene group.	II

			groups:			
varying functional and organic aetiologies	(1998)		1 Accent method and vocal hygiene 2 Vocal hygiene	2 Laryngoscopy findings 3 Acoustic measures 4 Aero-dynamics 5 Flow glottogram	made significantly greater improvements on majority of measures than did the group receiving only vocal hygiene advice.	
Parkinson's disease	Johnson and Pring (1990)	RCT	12 adults in two groups: 1 'Traditional' speech therapy 2 No treatment	1 Frenchay dysarthria assessment 2 Acoustic measures of fundamental frequency and intensity	Treatment group showed significant improvement on all measures. Control group showed either no change or deterioration.	II
Parkinson's disease	Ramig and Dromey (1996)	RCT	17 adults in two groups: 1 LSVT 2 Respiration therapy	1 SPL on vowels, syllables, reading and monologue 2 Ps 3 Maximum flow declination rate 4 Relative vocal fold adduction	LSVT group achieved significant improvements on all measures. The respiration therapy group did not improve on any measure apart from SPL in monologue.	II
Parkinson's disease	Ramig et al. (1996)	RCT (within stratified groups)	35 adults in two groups: 1 LSVT 2 Respiration therapy	1 SPL 2 Average fundamental frequency 3 Fundamental frequency variability 4 Forced vital capacity (FVC)	LSVT group showed significant improvement in SPL and fundamental frequency variability, whereas respiration therapy group showed no improvement.	II
Parkinson's disease	Ramig et al. (1995)	RCT (within stratified groups)	45 adults in two groups: 1 LSVT 2 Respiration therapy	1 Perceptual ratings and self-report 2 Acoustic measures (average fundamental frequency, fundamental frequency variability, SPL) 3 Maximum phonation time and FVC 4 Depression and sickness impact profile	LSVT group showed significant improvement on more voice measures than the respiration therapy group. LSVT group also showed greater and more consistent voice gains than the respiration group. LSVT group improved on sickness impact whereas the respiration therapy group did not.	II

(1995), Verdolini-Marston et al. (1994) and Verdolini-Marston et al. (1995) are the only groups of investigators to have undertaken prospective comparisons of alternative treatment methods. Andrews et al. (1986) compared laryngeal EMG biofeedback and progressive relaxation training using five matched pairs of patients with hyperfunctional dysphonia. Murry and Woodson (1995) compared botulinum toxin (Botox) injections alone with Botox in combination with behavioural voice therapy in 27 patients with adductor spasmodic dysphonia. Verdolini-Marston et al. (1995) compared the effectiveness of 'confidential voice therapy' and 'resonant voice therapy' against a no-treatment control for 13 women with vocal nodules, whereas Verdolini-Marston et al. (1994) evaluated hydration treatment against a placebo for six women with vocal nodules. Although the study by Andrews et al. (1986) was well controlled, with clear patient inclusion and exclusion criteria, and multi-dimensional measurement of voice outcomes, systematic selection bias could not be prevented, the number of participants was very small and the study could not determine whether EMG biofeedback and/or relaxation therapy were any better than no treatment. The study reported by Verdolini-Marston et al. (1995) was also reasonably well controlled despite the lack of random assignment, but participant numbers were very small and the groups were not equivalent in terms of severity of vocal dysfunction. The study by Murry and Woodson (1995) had similar strengths and weaknesses, but was even more vulnerable to selection bias because patient preference was used in assigning patients to the two groups. A particular strength of the evaluation of hydration treatment for vocal nodules conducted by Verdolini-Marston et al. (1994) was the use of double blinding, although, again, the sample size was very small.

Turning to empirical case designs, again these are rare in the voice therapy literature. Blood (1994) reports the only study of this type. Blood (1994) evaluated a treatment protocol using a computer-assisted biofeedback device with two adults with vocal nodules. The patients underwent a programme comprised of multiple baseline measures, an alternating treatment design incorporating traditional therapy for hyperfunction, computer-assisted respiratory training and relaxation therapy (12 sessions in total), and follow-up assessments over three months after termination of treatment. This study was well designed and documented and has provided preliminary evidence of treatment effectiveness (Carding, 2000). Table 6.2 provides a summary of the available evidence derived from this empirical single-case design and from the prospective controlled trials without randomization.

We are now down to the lowest levels of the evidence hierarchy, but are left with 70 of the total of 87 studies unaccounted for. This means that the majority of published evaluations of voice therapy have used research designs that can provide only the weakest levels of evidence for treatment

Table 6.2 Evidence for the efficacy or effectiveness of voice therapy as derived from prospective controlled studies without randomization and empirical single-case designs

Voice disorder	Source	Design	Participants	Measures	Results	Evidence level
Hyperfunctional dysphonias	Andrews et al. (1986)	PCT	10 adults, two matched groups: 1 EMG bio-feedback 2 Progressive relaxation	1 Surface laryngeal tension (EMG) 2 Fundamental frequency contour 3 Perceptual ratings and self-report	Both EMG biofeedback and relaxation were associated with reduced laryngeal tension, improved fundamental frequency control, improved voice quality (self-report and perceptual ratings).	III.1
Adductor spasmodic dysphonia	Murry and Woodson (1995)	PCT (but based on patient choice)	27 adults, two groups: 1 Botox 2 Botox and voice therapy	1 Mean airflow rate 2 Acoustic measures of jitter, shimmer, signal to noise ratio 3 Time between injections	Botox and voice therapy group showed significantly higher airflow rates, better acoustic outcomes, and greater duration between injections than Botox only group.	III.1
Vocal nodules	Verdolini-Marston et al. (1994)	PCT (within-subject design)	Six adult women each received hydration and placebo in counter-balanced order	1 Phonation threshold pressure 2 Acoustic measures of jitter, shimmer, signal to noise ratio 3 Laryngoscopy findings 4 Perceptual ratings of voice quality 5 Self-rated vocal effort	Significantly greater benefits of hydration treatment than placebo for all measures except signal to noise ratio. However, some benefits were also seen for the placebo condition.	III.1

(contd)

Table 6.2 (contd)

Voice disorder	Source	Design	Participants	Measures	Results	Evidence level
Vocal nodules	Verdolini-Marston et al. (1995)	PCT	13 adult women matched alternating assignment to three groups: 1 Resonant voice therapy 2 Confidential voice therapy 3 Vocal hygiene only	1 Self-rated vocal effort 2 Perceptual ratings of voice quality 3 Laryngoscopy findings	Both therapy groups improved, but there was no significant difference in outcomes between the two types of therapy. The vocal hygiene group showed no significant improvement.	III.1
Vocal nodules	Blood (1994)	ESCD (multiple baseline, alternative treatment design)	2 adult women alternating between voice therapy and voice therapy plus relaxation	1 Self-ratings 2 Perceptual ratings of voice quality 3 Laryngoscopy findings 4 Acoustic measures and maximum phonation time	All measures improved in both women and nodules were eliminated. Relaxation did not enhance treatment effects.	III.3

efficacy and effectiveness (that is, levels III.2, III.3 and IV according to the Joanna Briggs Institute framework). These studies are of four main types:

- Prospective studies of a single group of patients before and after treatment (for example, Kotby et al., 1991; Roy and Leeper, 1993).
- Prospective reviews of treatment programmes (for example, Andersson and Schalén, 1998).
- Retrospective reviews of therapy methods or intervention programmes (for example, Ylitalo and Hammarberg, 2000).
- Case reports (for example, Glaze, 1996).

Case reports yielding the weakest evidence of all made up the largest proportion of this research in the 1960s and 1970s, but have been far less common over the last 20 years. Prospective programme reviews have been very rare. Single-group studies and retrospective reviews, however, remain common in the current literature. None of these 70 studies used randomization or blinding of investigators or subjects; none used any experimental control of factors that may influence voice outcomes; none compared treatment results against no-treatment or placebo conditions, and none reported on the clinical significance of their findings. Despite these serious limitations, several design strengths are evident in some of the more recent prospective single-group studies and programme reviews. Adequate subject numbers, clear descriptions of patient characteristics and intervention procedures, consistent application of treatment procedures and outcome measures, multi-dimensional and reliable outcome measurement, reasonable follow-up times, little or no loss of subjects, and appropriate statistical analysis have been the positive features of several studies (for example, Roy et al., 1997; Andersson and Schalén, 1998). Such studies provide evidence of positive treatment effects and, in the absence of a large body of research using controlled trials or empirical case designs, clinicians can derive reasonable guidance for the design of voice therapy programmes from this research.

Prevention of voice disorders

Although there has been a prodigious amount of work published on the effectiveness of voice therapy, the same cannot be said about programmes designed to prevent voice problems. The research and clinical literature contains few references to primary prevention (Marge, 1991). Apart from cursory comments about prevention in the major texts on voice disorders (for example, Morrison and Rammage, 1994; Colton and Casper, 1996), only four discussion papers and five research reports on primary prevention of vocal dysfunction could be tracked down in the journals. This lack of attention to prevention issues is surprising when we know that large numbers of voice disorders and their underlying causes ought to be preventable (Marge, 1991). Flynn (1983), Kahane and Mayo (1989), Johnson (1991) and Marge (1991) have all written about the rationale and objectives of prevention programmes, principles of primary prevention, prevention strategies, and implementation and evaluation of prevention programmes. There are, however, no examples of systematic reviews or randomized controlled trials of prevention programmes in the voice literature and there is only one report of a study that has made some attempt to introduce an element of control into the research (see Chan, 1994). Chan (1994) implemented a vocal hygiene programme with 12 kindergarten teachers over a two-month period and compared acoustic and electroglottographic measures of voice before and after testing with the same features in 13 teachers who did not undergo the vocal hygiene education. Although Chan (1994) demonstrated that the experimental group improved their vocal characteristics while there was no change in the voices of the control group, there was little attempt to control other factors that could have influenced outcomes. The remaining four evaluation studies also targeted vocal hygiene knowledge and voice care behaviours in groups such as school children, teachers and cheerleaders, but none of these studies made comparisons with control groups (see Cook et al., 1979; Nilson and Schneiderman, 1983; Aaron and Madison, 1991; Nickel et al., 1992). Further, these studies all provide very low levels of evidence for the effectiveness of the prevention strategies because of their narrow focus on vocal hygiene, because the outcomes measured were limited to participants' knowledge of vocal hygiene and because follow-up measurement was rarely conducted.

Although the preceding discussion has shown that the overall quality of evidence relevant to clinical practice in voice has improved considerably in the past five years, much of the evidence is at a level lower on the evidence hierarchy than is ideal. We therefore turn to the last of our three questions.

What future developments could improve the evidence base underlying the management of our clients with voice disorders?

Over the past decade the evidence base available for clinicians managing clients with voice disorders has improved considerably in level, quality and statistical precision. We now have access to several well-designed case-control studies of relevance to causal mechanisms in voice disorders (for example, Roy et al., 2000), cross-sectional studies that support particular perceptual and instrumental voice evaluation methods (for example, Kreiman and Gerratt, 2000; Wuyts et al., 2000) and randomized controlled trials and prospective comparisons that support a number of intervention approaches (for example, Ramig et al., 1996; Carding et al., 1999; MacKenzie et al., 2001; Roy et al., 2001). However, the number of relevant published studies remains very small, the range of voice disorders and patients investigated is limited, confidence intervals and clinical significance of research findings for nearly all published studies are not specified, and evidence at the highest levels, systematic reviews and meta-analyses, is non-existent in the voice field. In relation to studies of treatment efficacy in particular, it is also clear that the important comparisons of treatment methods with no treatment conditions have rarely been conducted. That systematic reviews and meta-analyses have not been reported is not surprising. Until the number of studies of at least moderate levels of evidence increases, until a wider range of disorders and patients are studied, until non-treatment comparisons are incorporated into effectiveness research, and until researchers routinely report on confidence intervals and effect sizes, there will continue to be an inadequate database on which to conduct such high-level work.

The application of evidence-based health care principles to clinical practice in voice disorders is certainly beginning to affect the care of patients with voice problems. Evidence-based practice formulations assist clinicians to develop relevant, searchable questions, to search the literature effectively and efficiently, and to appraise the evidence critically. It is, however, at the stage of implementation of the results of such appraisal that clinicians may reach an impasse. The research evidence is not yet of sufficient quantity or at a sufficiently high level to allow direct application to clinical practice across a wide range of disorders and patients.

Carding (2000) proposes a way forward to increase the amount and quality of treatment effectiveness research that may redress some of the limitations of the available evidence for treatment efficacy and effectiveness in voice disorders. He outlines an approach to research design that essentially follows the randomized controlled trial model. Whether this approach to efficacy research in the voice field will be shown to be useful and feasible is a moot point. Other chapters in this text take up this issue in more detail, but voice researchers will need to consider carefully the ethical problems in setting up no treatment conditions, the difficulties in designing intervention methods that are not confounded by variability in patient- and clinician-specific factors, and the difficulty of designing ecologically valid effectiveness studies when it is known that the most prevalent voice disorders are associated with multi-factorial causal and contributing factors.

Acknowledgement

To my academic colleague at La Trobe University, Georgia Dacakis, for her invaluable suggestions and support in the preparation of this chapter.

References

Aaron VL, Madison CL. A vocal hygiene program for high-school cheerleaders. Language, Speech, and Hearing Services in Schools 1991; 22: 287-90.

Andersson K, Schalén L. Etiology and treatment of psychogenic voice disorder: results of a follow-up study of thirty patients. Journal of Voice 1998; 12: 96-106.

Andrews ML. Manual of Voice Treatment. Pediatrics through Geriatrics. San Diego, CA: Singular Publishing Group, 1995.

Andrews S, Warner J, Stewart R. EMG biofeedback and relaxation in the treatment of hyperfunctional dysphonia. British Journal of Disorders of Communication 1986; 21: 353-69.

Aronson AE. Clinical Voice Disorders (third edition). New York, NY: Thième, 1990.

Baken RJ. Foreword. In: Harris T, Harris S, Rubin JS, Howard DM (eds). The Voice Clinic Handbook. London: Whurr Publishers, 1998.

Baken RJ, Orlikoff RF. Voice measurement: is more better? Logopedics Phoniatrics Vocology 1997; 22: 147-51.

Baken RJ, Orlikoff RF. Clinical Measurement of Speech and Voice. San Diego, CA: Singular Publishing Group, 1999.

Basiouny S. Efficacy of the accent method of voice therapy. Folia Phoniatrica et Logopaedica 1998; 50: 146-64.

Benninger MS, Jacobson B. Vocal nodules, microwebs, and surgery. Journal of Voice 1995; 9: 326-31.

Blood GW. Efficacy of a computer-assisted voice treatment protocol. American Journal of Speech-Language-Pathology 1994; 3: 57-66.

Boone DR, McFarlane SC. The Voice and Voice Therapy (fourth edition). Englewood Cliffs, NJ: Prentice-Hall, 1988.

Butcher P. Psychological processes in psychogenic voice disorder. European Journal of Disorders of Communication 1995; 30: 467-74.

Carding P. Evaluating Voice Therapy. Measuring the Effectiveness of Treatment. London: Whurr Publishers, 2000.

Carding P, Horsley IA, Docherty GJ. A study of the effectiveness of voice therapy in the treatment of 45 patients with nonorganic dysphonia. Journal of Voice 1999; 13: 72-104.

Casper JK, Murry T. Voice therapy methods in dysphonia. Otolaryngologic Clinics of North America: Voice Disorders and Phonosurgery II 2000; 33: 983-1002.

Chan RWK. Does the voice improve with vocal hygiene education? A study of some instrumental voice measures in a group of kindergarten teachers. Journal of Voice 1994; 8: 279-91.

Colton R, Casper JK. Understanding Voice Problems. A Physiological Perspective for Diagnosis and Treatment (second edition). Baltimore, MD: Williams & Wilkins, 1996.

Cook JV, Palaski DJ, Hanson WR. A vocal hygiene program for school-age children. Language, Speech, and Hearing Services in Schools 1979; 10: 21-6.

Davis P, Zhang SP, Bandler R. Midbrain and medullary control of respiration and vocalisation. Progress in Brain Research 1996; 107: 315-25.

Enderby P, Emmerson R. Does Speech and Language Therapy Work? A Review of the Literature. London: Whurr Publishers, 1995.

Fawcus M. The causes and classification of voice disorders. In: Freeman M, Fawcus M (eds). Voice Disorders and their Management (third edition). London: Whurr Publishers, 2000a.

Fawcus R. The physiology of phonation. In: Freeman M, Fawcus M (eds). Voice Disorders and their Management (third edition). London: Whurr Publishers, 2000b.

Fex S. Perceptual evaluation. Journal of Voice 1992; 6: 155-8.

Flynn PT. Speech-language pathologists and primary prevention: from ideas to action. Language, Speech and Hearing Services in Schools 1983; 14: 99-104.

Fröhlich M, Michaelis D, Werner Strube H, Kruse E. Acoustic voice analysis by means of the hoarseness diagram. Journal of Speech, Language and Hearing Research 2000; 43: 706-20.

Gerratt BR, Kreiman J, Antonanzas-Barroso N, Berke GS. Comparing internal and external standards in voice quality judgements. Journal of Speech and Hearing Research 1993; 36: 14-20.

Glaze LE. Treatment of voice hyperfunction in the pre-adolescent. Language Speech and Hearing Services in Schools 1996; 27: 244-56.

Granqvist S. Enhancements to the visual analogue scale, VAS, for listening tests. TMH -Quarterly Progress and Status Reports 1996; 4: 61-5.

Gray SD. Cellular physiology of the vocal folds. Otolaryngologic Clinics of North America: Voice Disorders and Phonosurgery 2000; 33: 679-97.

Gray SD, Hirano M, Sato K. Molecular and cellular structure of vocal fold tissue. In: Titze IR (Ed.). Vocal Fold Physiology: Frontiers in Basic Science. San Diego, CA: Singular Publishing Group, 1993.

Green G. Psycho-behavioral characteristics of children with vocal nodules: WPBIC ratings. Journal of Speech and Hearing Disorders 1989; 54: 306-12.

Greene M, Mathieson L. The Voice and its Disorders (fifth edition). London: Whurr Publishers, 1989.

Greenhalgh T. How to Read a Paper. The Basics of Evidence Based Medicine. London: BMJ Books, 2001.

Guyatt GH, Sackett DL, Sinclair JC, Hayward R, Cook DJ, Cook RJ. Users' guides to the medical literature. IX. A method for grading health care recommendations. Journal of the American Medical Association 1995; 274: 1800-4.

Hammarberg B. Voice research and clinical needs. Folia Phoniatrica et Logopaedica 2000; 52: 93-102.

Hammarberg B, Gauffin J. Perceptual and acoustic characteristics of voice quality differences in pathological voices as related to physiological aspects. In: Fujimura O, Hirano M (eds). Vocal Fold Physiology: Voice Quality Control. San Diego, CA: Singular Publishing Group, 1995.

Harris S. Speech therapy for dysphonia. In: Harris T, Harris S, Rubin JS, Howard DM (eds). The Voice Clinic Handbook. London: Whurr Publishers, 1998.

Harris T, Harris S, Rubin JS, Howard DM (eds). The Voice Clinic Handbook. London: Whurr Publishers, 1998.

Hillman RE, De Lassus C, Hargrave J, Walsh M, Bunting MS. The efficacy of speech-language pathology intervention: voice disorders. Seminars in Speech and Language 1990; 11: 297-309.

Hillman RE, Holmberg EB, Perkell JS, Walsh M, Vaughan C. Objective assessment of vocal hyperfunction: an experimental framework and initial results. Journal of Speech and Hearing Research 1989; 32: 373-92.

Hirano M. Clinical Examination of Voice. New York, NY: Springer, 1981.

Hirano M, Kurita S. Histological structure of the vocal fold and its normal and pathological variations. In: Kirchner JA (Ed.). Vocal Fold Histopathology: A Symposium. San Diego, CA: College-Hill Press, 1986.

Howard D. Beyond randomised controlled trials; the case for effective case studies of the effects of treatment in aphasia. British Journal of Disorders of Communication 1986; 21: 89-103.

Iwarrson J, Thomasson M, Sundberg J. Effects of lung volume on the glottal voice source. Journal of Voice 1998; 12: 424-33.

Jiang J, Lin E, Hanson DG. Vocal fold physiology. Otolaryngologic Clinics of North America: Voice Disorders and Phonosurgery 2000; 1: 699-718.

Johnson TS. Principles and practices of prevention as applied to voice disorders. Seminars in Speech and Language 1991; 12: 14-22.

Johnson JA, Pring TR. Speech therapy in Parkinson disease: a review and further data. British Journal of Disorders of Communication 1990; 25: 183-94.

Kahane JC, Mayo R. The need for aggressive pursuit of healthy childhood voices. Language, Speech, and Hearing Services in Schools 1989; 20: 102-7.

Kelchner LN, Stemple JC, Gerdeman B, Le Borgne W, Adam S. Etiology, pathophysiology, treatment choices, and voice results for unilateral adductor vocal fold paralysis: a 3-year retrospective. Journal of Voice 1999; 13: 592-601.

Kent RD, Ball MJ. The Handbook of Voice Quality Measurement. San Diego, CA: Singular Publishing Group, 1999.

Kotby MN, El-Sady SR, Basiouny SE, Abou-Rass YA, Hegazi MA. Efficacy of the accent method of voice therapy. Journal of Voice 1991; 5: 316-20.

Kreiman J, Gerratt BR. Sources of listener disagreement in voice quality assessment. Journal of the Acoustical Society of America 2000; 108: 1867-76.

Kreiman J, Gerratt BR, Kempster GB, Erman A, Berke G. Perceptual evaluation of voice quality: review, tutorial, and a framework for future research. Journal of Speech and Hearing Research 1993; 36: 21-40.

de Krom G. Some spectral correlates of pathological breathy and rough voice quality for different types of vowel segments. Journal of Speech and Hearing Research 1995; 38: 794-811.

Larson CR. Brain mechanisms involved in the control of vocalisation. Journal of Voice 1992; 2: 301-11.

Ludlow C. Research needs for the assessment of phonatory function. ASHA Reports 1981; 11: 3-8.

MacKenzie K, Millar A, Wilson JA, Sellars C, Dreary IJ. Is voice therapy an effective treatment for dysphonia? A randomised controlled trial. British Medical Journal 2001; 323: 658-61.

Marge M. Introduction to the prevention and epidemiology of voice disorders. Seminars in Speech and Language 1991; 12: 48-73.

Masuda T, Ikeda Y, Manako H, Komiyama S. Analysis of vocal abuse: fluctuations in phonation time and intensity in four groups of speakers. Acta Otolaryngologica 1993; 113: 547-52.

Moore GP. Have the major issues in voice disorders been answered by research in speech science? A 50 year retrospective. Journal of Speech and Hearing Disorders 1977; 42: 152-60.

Morrison M, Rammage L. The Management of Voice Disorders. San Diego, CA: Singular Publishing Group, 1994.

Morrison M, Rammage L, Emami AJ. The irritable larynx syndrome. Journal of Voice 1999; 13: 447-55.

Murry T, Woodson G. Combined modality treatment of adductor spasmodic dysphonia with botulinum toxin and voice therapy. Journal of Voice 1995; 9: 460-5.

Nickel DG, Middleton GF, Brand MN. The effectiveness of a vocal health program for the elementary classroom. Rocky Mountain Journal of Communication Disorders 1992; Fall: 21-6.

Nilson H, Schneiderman CR. Classroom program for the prevention of vocal abuse and hoarseness in elementary school children. Language, Speech, and Hearing Services in Schools 1983; 14: 121-7.

Oates J. Voice disorders associated with hyperfunction. In: Freeman M, Fawcus M (eds). Voice Disorders and their Management (second edition). London: Whurr Publishers, 2000.

Oates JM, Russell A. Learning voice analysis using an interactive multi-media package: development and preliminary evaluation. Journal of Voice 1998; 12: 500-12.

Pannbacker M. Voice treatment techniques: a review and recommendations for outcome studies. American Journal of Speech-Language Pathology 1998; 7: 49-64.

Pannbacker M. Treatment of vocal nodules: options and outcomes. American Journal of Speech-Language Pathology 1999; 8: 209-17.

Perkins W. Assessment and treatment of voice disorders: state of the art. In: Costello J (Ed.). Speech Disorders in Adults. San Diego, CA: College Hill, 1985.

Polgar S, Thomas SA. Introduction to Research in the Health Sciences. Edinburgh: Churchill Livingstone, 2000.

Ramig L, Dromey C. Aerodynamic mechanisms underlying treatment-related changes in SPL in patients with Parkinson disease. Journal of Speech and Hearing Research 1996; 39: 798-807.

Ramig LO, Verdolini K. Treatment efficacy: voice disorders. Journal of Speech, Language, and Hearing Research 1998; 41: S101-S116.

Ramig L, Countryman S, Thompson L, Horii Y. A comparison of two forms of intensive speech treatment for Parkinson disease. Journal of Speech and Hearing Research 1995; 38: 1232-51.

Ramig L, Countryman S, O'Brien C, Hoehn M, Thompson L. Intensive speech treatment for Parkinson disease: short- and long-term comparison of two techniques. Neurology 1996; 47: 1496-1504.

Reed CG. Voice therapy: a need for research. Journal of Speech and Hearing Disorders 1980; 45: 157-69.

Revis J, Giovanni A, Wuyts F, Triglia J. Comparison of different voice samples for perceptual analysis. Folia Phoniatrica et Logopaedica 1999; 51: 108-16.

Rosen DC, Sataloff RT. Psychology of Voice Disorders. San Diego, CA: Singular Publishing Group, 1997.

Rosen CA, Murry T, Zinn A, Zullo T, Sonbolian M. Voice handicap index change following treatment of voice disorders. Journal of Voice 2000; 14: 619-23.

Roy N, Bless DM. Personality traits and psychological factors in voice pathology: a foundation for future research. Journal of Speech, Language and Hearing Research 2000; 43: 737-48.

Roy N, Leeper HA. Effects of the manual laryngeal musculoskeletal tension reduction technique as a treatment for functional voice disorders: perceptual and acoustic measures. Journal of Voice 1993; 7: 242-9.

Roy N, Bless DM, Heisey D, Ford CN. Manual circumlaryngeal therapy for functional dysphonia: an evaluation of short- and long-term treatment outcomes. Journal of Voice 1997; 11: 321-31.

Roy N, Bless DM, Heisey D. Personality and voice disorders: A superfactor trait analysis. Journal of Speech, Language and Hearing Research 2000; 43: 749-68.

Roy N, Ryker KS, Bless DM. Vocal violence in actors: an investigation into its acoustic consequences and the effects of hygienic laryngeal release training. Journal of Voice 2000; 14: 215-30.

Roy N, Gray SD, Simon M, Dove H, Corbin-Lewis K, Stemple JC. An evaluation of the effects of two treatment approaches for teachers with voice disorders: a prospective randomized clinical trial. Journal of Speech, Language, and Hearing Research 2001; 44: 286-96.

Russell A. Voice problems in teachers: prevalence and prediction. Unpublished doctoral dissertation, La Trobe University, Victoria, Australia, 1999.

Russell A, Oates J, Greenwood KM. Prevalence of voice problems in teachers. Journal of Voice 1998; 12: 467-79.

Sackett DL, Richardson WS, Rosenberg W, Haynes RB. Evidence-based Medicine. How to Practice and Teach EBM. Edinburgh: Churchill Livingstone, 1998.

Sataloff RT. Rational thought: the impact of voice science upon voice care. Journal of Voice 1995; 9: 215-34.

Sataloff RT, Abaza MM. Impairment, disability, and other medical-legal aspects of dysphonia. Otolaryngologic Clinics of North America: Voice Disorders and Phonosurgery II 2002; 33: 1143-53.

Smith E, Verdolini K, Gray S, Nichols S, Lemke J, Barkmeier J et al. Effect of voice disorders on quality of life. Journal of Medical Speech-Language Pathology 1996; 4: 223-44.

Smith E, Gray S, Dove H, Kirchner HL, Heras H. Frequency and effects of teachers' voice problems. Journal of Voice 1997; 11: 81-7.

Smith E, Lemke J, Taylor M, Kirchner HL, Hoffman H. Frequency of voice problems among teachers and other occupations. Journal of Voice 1998; 12: 480-8.

Stemple JC. Voice research: so what? A clearer view of voice production, 25 years of progress; the speaking voice. Journal of Voice 1993; 7: 293-300.

Stemple JC, Glaze LE, Gerdeman BK. Clinical Voice Pathology: Theory and Management (second edition). San Diego, CA: Singular Publishing Group, 1995.

Stemple JC, Lee L, D'Amico B, Pickup B. Efficacy of vocal function exercises as a method of improving voice function. Journal of Voice 1994; 8: 271-8.

Titze IR. Principles of Voice Production. Englewood Cliffs, NJ: Prentice-Hall, 1994.

Titze IR. Workshop on Acoustic Voice Analysis. Summary Statement. Iowa City, IO: National Center for Voice and Speech, 1995.

Titze IR, Baken RJ, Herzel H. Evidence of chaos in vocal fold vibration. In: Titze IR (Ed.). Vocal Fold Physiology: Frontiers in Basic Science. San Diego, CA: Singular Publishing Group, 1993.

Verdolini K. Voice disorders. In: Tomblin JB, Morris HL, Spriestersbach DC (eds). Diagnosis in Speech-language Pathology. San Diego, CA Singular Press, 1994.

Verdolini K, Ramig LO. Review: occupational risks for voice problems. Logopedics Phoniatrics Vocology 2001; 26: 37-46.

Verdolini-Marston K, Burke MK, Lessac A, Glaze L, Caldwell E. Preliminary study of two methods of treatment for laryngeal nodules. Journal of Voice 1995; 9: 74-85.

Verdolini-Marston K, Sandage M, Titze IR. Effect of hydration treatments on laryngeal nodules and polyps and related voice measures. Journal of Voice 1994; 8: 30-47.

Von Leden H. The cultural history of the human voice. In: Lawrence VL (Ed.). Transcripts of the Eleventh Symposium: Care of the Professional Voice. Part II. New York, NY: The Voice Foundation, 1982.

Weiner GM, Batch AJG, Radford K. Dysphonia as an atypical presentation of gastro-esophageal reflux. Journal of Laryngology and Otology 1995; 109: 1195-6.

Wilson DK. Voice Problems of Children (third edition). Baltimore, MD: Williams & Wilkins, 1987.

Wirz SL, Mackenzie Beck J. Assessment of voice quality: the vocal profile analysis scheme. In: Wirz S (Ed.) Perceptual Approaches to Communication Disorders. London: Whurr Publishers, 1995.

Wolfe VI, Martin DP, Palmer CI. Perception of dysphonic voice quality by naïve listeners. Journal of Speech, Language, and Hearing Research 2000; 43: 697-705.

Wuyts FL, De Bodt MS, Van de Heyning PH. Is the reliability of a visual analog scale higher than an ordinal scale? An experiment with the GRBAS scale for perceptual evaluation of dysphonia. Journal of Voice 1999; 13: 508-17.

Wuyts FL, De Bodt MS, Molenberghs G, Remacle M, Heylen L, Millet B, Van Lierde K, Raes J, Van de Heyning PH. The dysphonia severity index: an objective measure of vocal quality based on a multiparameter approach. Journal of Speech, Language, and Hearing Research 2000; 43: 796-809.

Ylitalo R, Hammarberg B. Voice characteristics, effects of voice therapy, and long-term follow-up of contact granuloma patients. Journal of Voice 2000; 14: 557-66.

Zraick RI, Liss JM. A comparison of equal-appearing interval scaling and direct magnitude estimation of nasal voice quality. Journal of Speech, Language, and Hearing Research 2000; 43: 979-88.

CHAPTER 7

The evidence base for the management of dysphagia

SHEENA REILLY

Introduction: dysphagia in context

The purpose of this chapter is to summarize and guide readers to the best available evidence for the assessment and management of dysphagia. This introduction will address a number of issues fundamental to the evolution of dysphagia management. In the remainder of the chapter the evidence for 'best practice' in dysphagia will be presented and evaluated.

Defining dysphagia

Dysphagia, derived from the Greek words *dys* ('with difficulty') and *phagia* ('to eat'), is the term used to describe difficulty in eating and swallowing. Dysphagia is prevalent and is a debilitating and costly disorder in terms of social distress to patients and families, and admissions or re-admissions to hospital (Martin-Harris, 1999). A surprisingly large population of children and adults (up to 10 million people in the USA) are said to be affected by dysphagia (NIH Publication No. 97-3217). In Table 7.1 the literature from a variety of sources has been critically appraised, collated and the data summarized to illustrate current dysphagia prevalence estimates in a variety of clinical populations. The population with dysphagia includes individuals of all ages, from birth to senescence. Dysphagia may occur as a congenital or acquired condition. The resulting problems may be structural, neuromuscular or functional, or a combination of all three. Dysphagia is commonly associated with stroke, brainstem or cortical tumours, cerebral palsy, cranio-facial anomalies, traumatic brain injury, neuro-degenerative disease or cancers of the head and neck and their treatment. Children and adults share some of the same underlying aetiologies associated with dysphagia.

Table 7.1 Prevalence of dysphagia, source and population examined

Population	Source*	Dysphagia prevalence range %
Hospital patients (adult)	Groher and Bukatman (1986)	12.5
Nursing home residents	Siebens et al. (1986)	26-30
Elderly - community	Baum and Bodner (1983)	13-15**
Diagnostic groups		
Stroke ***	Nilsson et al. (1998) Daniels et al. (1997, 1998)	19-90
Neuromuscular disorders (e.g., spinal muscular atrophy, myotonic dystrophy, myasthenia gravis)	Willig et al. (1994)	34.9
Parkinson's disease	Coates and Bakheit (1997) Hartelius and Svensson (1994)	23-81
Poliomyelitis	Coelho and Ferranti (1991) Cosgrove et al. (1987)	20-27
Progressive supranuclear palsy	Litvan et al. (1997)	55.6
Multiple sclerosis	Hartelius and Svensson (1994) Mayberry and Atkinson (1986)	13-73
Motor neuron disease (BP, PMA, ALS)	Leighton et al. (1994)	29-71
Alzheimer's disease	Volicer et al. (1989)	32-84
Huntington's disease	Kagel and Leopold (1992)	100
Head-injured children	Morgan et al. (2003)	5.3
Head-injured adults	Cherney and Halper (1996)	42
Cerebral palsy	Reilly et al. (1996)	91
	Sullivan et al. (2000)	89
	Dahl et al. (1996)	60
	Thomessan et al. (1991)	50
Head and neck cancer	List et al. (1999)	33
Down syndrome	Frazier and Friedman (1996) Spender et al. (1996)	84
Rett syndrome	Morton et al. (1997) Reilly and Cass (2001)	100
Cleft lip and palate	Trenouth and Campbell (1996) Jones (1988)	25-50

* Source provided for lowest and highest prevalence rate given.
** Gender variation reported.
*** Diagnostic methods highly variable.

Development of the field from an historical perspective

Recent surveys show that 47% of speech pathologists work with clients with dysphagia (ASHA, 2001a). In hospital and residential healthcare settings this proportion rises to 92% and 100%, respectively (ASHA, 2001a). Not surprisingly against this background, the assessment and management of dysphagia has been the focus for research and clinical expenditure. An appraisal of the literature revealed a lack of substantial information on many aspects of what constitutes normal swallowing, including the development of oral and pharyngeal function from birth to maturity. In paediatrics for example, clinicians and researchers are usually surprised to find that one of the most frequently quoted studies on normal development of oral function is based on the longitudinal observations of just three infants (Evans-Morris and Dunn Klein, 1987).

In the drive to meet an increasing 'clinical need', there has been little time devoted to the description and measurement of normal swallowing. Instead, energies have been directed at attempts to measure abnormalities in swallowing.

In 1989 Martin Bax (Editor of *Developmental Medicine and Child Neurology*) examined the bibliography of the journal for publications on infant feeding. In the previous 10 years there had been few publications: one paper in 1986; none in 1987 and two in 1988. As a result, Bax (1989, p. 285) issued a challenge to all health professionals involved in paediatrics to 'pay increased attention to infant feeding'. In the last 12 years the situation has changed: numerous specialist textbooks devoted to the management of dysphagia (both adults and children) have emerged, as has the publication of a specialist journal devoted to dysphagia and a plethora of refereed journal articles. In 2001, Reilly and Perry reported a dramatic increase in the number of dysphagia-related publications, which these authors demonstrated by a simple search of just two databases (MEDLINE and CINAHL) by use of the keyword *dysphagia*. The search results for a 20-year period (1980–2000) revealed a more than five-fold increase.

Prevalence/incidence

Collation of prevalence data raised a number of interesting issues. First, the prevalence of dysphagia in some syndromes or disorders is unknown. Second, the accuracy of the available data was beset by poor methodology. Few studies observed basic epidemiological principles for determining prevalence (see Bower, 2000, pp 17–23 for further details). For example, samples were not representative and did not include the full spectrum of the disease or disorder. In addition, sample size tended to be small and the sample drawn from clinical or referred series of cases. Third, the definition of dysphagia used in the majority of studies varied and the methods by which the diagnoses of dysphagia were confirmed were not consistent. (The figures presented in Tables 7.1 and 7.2 are prevalence ranges rather than single figures because of the wide variability in the reported prevalence rates.)

Of note was the finding that a range of diagnostic methods were used to confirm the presence of dysphagia, including:

- self-report
- clinical observation
- clinical examination
- specific diagnostic investigations (for example, videofluroscopic swallowing study, VFSS).

Closer examination of two clinical populations (stroke and Parkinson's disease) revealed that reported prevalence rates varied depending on the

Table 7.2 Variable prevalence rates quoted for dysphagia in stroke (19%–74%) and Parkinson's disease (18-81%) according to the diagnostic method employed

Source	Diagnostic method	Prevalence (%)*
Stroke		
Nilsson et al. (1998)	Self-report	19
Smithard et al. (1996)	Survey	50
Gottlieb et al. (1996)	Clinical examination and water test	28
Barer (1989)	Clinical examination	29
Axelsson et al. (1989)	Observation	30
Kidd et al. (1993)	VFSS and water test	42
Gordon et al. (1987)	Water swallow test	45
DePippo et al. (1994a)	Clinical examination	59
Daniels et al. (1997, 1998)	Clinical examination and VFSS	65–80
Parkinson's disease		
Hartelius and Svensson (1994)	Self-report	18–21
Singer et al. (1992)	Questionnaire	23
Bushman et al. (1989)	Questionnaire, VFSS	35–75
Fuh et al. (1997)	VFSS	63
Wintzen et al. (1994)	Questionnaire, VFSS	72–81
Edwards et al. (1994)	Gastrointestinal exam, video-oesophagram	77
Coates and Bakheit (1997)	Clinical examination	81

* Prevalence rates have been rounded to nearest whole figure.

** Rates vary as to when prevalence measured after stroke (for example, 67%, Hinds and Wiles, 1998), within seven days (for example, 43% Wade and Hewer 1997) or six months' post-stroke (for example, 50%, Mann et al., 2000).

diagnostic method that was used in the study. For example, in stroke, Nilsson et al. (1998), using self-report as the diagnostic method, reported a prevalence rate of 19%, whereas Daniels et al. (1997, 1998), using a combination of VFSS and clinical examination, reported a prevalence rate of 90%. However, even when two studies used the same diagnostic method (for example, clinical examination) prevalence rates varied from 29% (Barer, 1989) to 59% (DePippo et al., 1994a). (Later in this chapter some possible explanations for these variations in reported prevalence rates will be explored further.)

In responding to rapidly developing clinical needs, dysphagia has become a specialism that is not necessarily underpinned by basic science. Management programmes for individuals with dysphagia have been developed in the absence of adequate knowledge about normal function. The available prevalence data in dysphagia are weakened by study designs that are not grounded in the principles of epidemiology, by unclear and inappropriate use of definitions and by inconsistency in measurement. Why should this be so problematic? First, because without such data it is impossible to ensure that the appropriate and necessary clinical resources are allocated and available for identifying and managing individuals with dysphagia. Second, data are important for the development of research – without internationally agreed standards and definitions it is impossible to make comparisons and draw conclusions from studies. How can speech pathologists know what the extent of the problem is if they cannot agree on how to measure the problem? This has broader implications in that the design of intervention studies, and the comparison of results from such studies, will be impossible if we are unable to measure accurately the characteristics of dysphagia and the main outcomes of interest.

Establishing best practice

When establishing what is best practice in the evaluation and management of individuals with dysphagia, three questions were posed:

- What is current best practice in the evaluation of dysphagia?
- Is there any evidence that screening for dysphagia is effective?
- What is current best practice in the treatment of dysphagia?

Each of these will be addressed in turn in the remainder of this chapter.

What is current best practice in the evaluation of dysphagia?

Typically, there are two parts to evaluating swallowing function: the non-instrumental (reviewing the history, undertaking a clinical assessment and a mealtime observation); and the instrumental examination (for example, endoscopy, videofluroscopy). Although great variety exists in the structure and content of these examinations, the non-instrumental examination usually involves four components: case history; medical note review; patient observation; and clinical examination (sometimes by use of standardized protocols; for example, the 5 ml 'water test' (Di-Pippo et al., 1994b) and the *Schedule of Oral Motor Assessment* (Reilly, Skuse and Wolke, 2000a)).

Non-instrumental evaluation

Case history or medical note review

The case history or medical note review is an information-gathering process. There are several published versions of the case history examination for dysphagia and these vary according to the dysphagia population being examined (for example, Groher, 1987; Logemann, 1998; Reilly, Skuse and Wolke, 2000b). Many of the items clinicians routinely include in the case history, and believe to be significant, have not undergone rigorous scrutiny to discover whether such signs, symptoms or behaviours are indeed predictive of, or associated with, dysphagia. Furthermore, the generalizability of these items to different populations is also unknown (for example, paediatrics versus adults, neurological versus structural abnormalities).

A recent systematic review by the Joanna Briggs Institute for Evidence Based Nursing and Midwifery (www.joannabriggs.edu.au) highlighted the inconsistent use of terminology. The reviewers (Ramritu et al., 2000) appraised the signs and symptoms associated with dysphagia in people with neurological impairment (many of these included items obtained during a case history) and assigned levels of evidence to each. The evidence underpinning each sign or symptom was generally low (Level III.3 case studies) with a few examples of stronger evidence from well designed cohort or case-control studies (Level III.2 and Level III.3). Most noticeable was the fact that the majority of the available evidence (in particular in children) did not originate from scientific studies, but rather, came from the opinions of respected authorities, based on clinical experience and the reports of expert committees (Level IV).

The review highlighted that there was marked inconsistency in the use of terminology and definitions in the papers appraised. Numerous systems were used and these included the following descriptions.

- Individual oral and pharyngeal behaviours (for example, decreased mouth and tongue movements).
- The consequences of dysphagia (for example, drooling, coughing, choking).

- The morbidity associated with dysphagia (for example, respiratory problems such as pneumonia) or diet restriction.

These descriptors refer to very different aspects of dysphagia, including *impairment* (for example, restricted tongue movement), *disability* (for example, inability to chew), *handicap* (for example, restricted diet) and the effect on individuals' quality of life (for example, cannot eat in public). Furthermore, there was another group of behaviours that represented health outcomes (for example, weight loss, dehydration, aspiration pneumonia). These findings highlight the fact that there was little consensus about the use of terminology across populations and wide variation in the definitions used by clinicians and researchers. Consequently, it is difficult to make valid comparisons between studies and to benchmark across studies and clinical services. Although it could be argued that the inconsistency described above demonstrates the multi-dimensional nature of dysphagia, it is also possible that this jumble of definitions reflects a lack of precision in exactly what is being measured, and furthermore, exactly how to measure. It is not surprising, perhaps, that the field lacks valid and reliable measurement tools.

Patient observation or clinical evaluation

Observation and clinical evaluation is the main method used to evaluate dysphagia. Typically, clinical evaluation includes some specific assessment protocols, such as an oral peripheral or structural assessment, as well as observation of individuals' eating and drinking skills (ASHA, 2001b). Clinicians combine this information with the case history data to:

- make inferences about the function of the oral and pharyngeal stages of swallowing
- make judgements regarding the adequacy of airway protection
- make judgements about the coordination of respiration and swallowing
- postulate whether the patient can swallow safely.

Because there is no universally agreed or standardized format for clinical evaluation, there are almost as many versions as there are adults and children with dysphagia. Those that do exist were developed to observe and rate abnormality, and often little attention has been paid to what is normal. Logemann (1983) demonstrated that clinicians could not reliably predict from the results of clinical evaluation which patients would aspirate on VFSS. They were only correct about 40% of the time. Thus, the accuracy of the inferences made from clinical evaluation, to identify individuals who can swallow safely or those with an oral stage and/or pharyngeal stage disorder, remains an inexact science. Furthermore, the significance or contribution of the different components that make up clinical evaluation is unknown. McCullough et al. (1999) recently demonstrated that fewer than 50% of the measures clinicians typically employ during the clinical examination are rated with sufficient inter- and intra-judge reliability.

Summary: non-instrumental evaluation

To summarize, the combination of the case history, review of medical notes, clinical examination and observation serve as 'stage one' of the diagnostic process for individuals with dysphagia who present to speech pathologists. In the first instance the results are used to determine if further investigation is required (providing these facilities are available). Those not requiring further investigation enter a treatment or a non-treatment group. The dilemma for the dysphagia clinician is knowing how accurate and reliable their inferences are and whether their decision to investigate (based on clinical information and observation) affects patient outcomes. Despite the fact that many versions of the non-instrumental examination exist, few have undergone adequate statistical validation, nor have they been shown to be reliable when replicated with other dysphagia populations and across clinicians. Williams and Mellis (2000, p. 100), discussing general paediatric practice, state that, 'we should try to develop and understand the evidence base for issues that have previously been defined as "art", such as communication with families, history taking and examination, and teaching'. Powerful evidence of the need to do so, comes from a survey sent to 300 speech pathologists in the USA practising in dysphagia (McCullough et al., 1999). The aim of the survey was to determine examination and measures used by clinicians to assess swallowing; measures were divided into four sections (history, oral motor, voice and trial swallows). The majority of respondents worked with dysphagic adults who had neurogenic disorders.

Despite a poor return rate of 20%, the survey results were interesting, indicating that clinicians varied in their clinical bedside methods and measures used to assess swallowing. Individual beliefs and preferences played a large part in practice – even when there was no research to support the use of a particular measure. McCullough et al. (1999) compared clinicians' preferences and practices with research support (that is, there was some demonstrated utility for detecting dysphagia) for each measure. All the history measures ($n = 10$) were preferred and practised by the clinicians; eight history measures were supported by research. Interestingly, the two most preferred and practised were the two measures not supported by research. Ten of 15 oral motor measures were preferred and practised, yet just three had research support. Clinicians said they preferred and practised six of the seven voice measures; four of the voice measures had research support. Lastly, of the trial swallow measures, 15 of 21 received preference and practice ratings from the clinicians surveyed. Just eight of the 15 measures had research support.

McCullough et al. (1999) concluded that clinicians prefer and practise a number of clinical bedside measures that have no research support, indicating that they rely heavily on their experience, what they have been taught through in-service courses and workshops even though the utility of some of these may not have been demonstrated. The challenge in dysphagia is to move the non-instrumental evaluation of dysphagia beyond 'art' towards science.

Instrumental evaluation

The use of instrumentation to evaluate dysphagia has developed historically from diagnostic tools or tests used for other purposes in medicine, which allow direct visualization of oral, pharyngeal and oesophageal cavities (for example, endoscopy has developed into fibro-optic endoscopic evaluation of swallowing (FEES); the barium swallow was modified to become videofluroscopic swallowing study (VFSS)). It is possible that this historical use has ensured their ready acceptance into clinical practice without prior evaluation.

Selecting instrumental evaluations

Selection of the appropriate investigation is dependent on the clinical question being posed, the availability of the procedure and, in some populations, the invasive nature – and therefore tolerance – of the procedure (this can be an important consideration with children). Each diagnostic investigation differs in the information it provides for clinicians. For example, both VFSS and a salivagram will determine if aspiration has occurred, however, a salivagram will not provide information about the type of aspiration (food or liquid versus regurgitated stomach contents) nor inform clinicians as to when the aspiration occurred in the swallowing cycle (before, during or after the swallow was triggered).

Is there any evidence that the results of instrumental examinations such as VFSS enhance the diagnostic process? Logemann (1983) provided the first strong evidence to support the view that investigation, via VFSS, was an important component of the assessment process. The results of this landmark study demonstrated that clinicians were poor at predicting the outcome of dysphagia investigations (namely aspiration) from clinical bedside evaluation. The results from a study by Arvedson et al. (1994) support these findings in children, where 26% of children with neurological disorders who underwent VFSS were found to aspirate (mainly liquids) and that the aspiration was silent in 94%. In another study, Logemann et al. (1992) demonstrated that swallow rehabilitation outcomes were affected by the type of evaluation procedure adopted. These workers compared results from patients undergoing a bedside examination to those receiving VFSS. The sample of 103 patients with partial laryngectomy, was unevenly distributed to the bedside arm of the study ($n = 21$) and the VFSS arm of the study ($n = 82$). Data were collected weekly and all subjects received VFSS follow-up at three months. Although a non-randomized study, significantly better results were found in the patients who underwent VFSS. Mean time to achieve oral food intake was slower in the bedside examination group and overall swallow measures (transit times and swallow efficiencies) were much improved in the VFSS group. Similar results supporting the role of instrumental investigation have been obtained in studies on children (Tanaguchi and Moyer, 1994). In a more recent study, Martin-Harris et al. (2000) examined the clinical utility of VFSS. Specifically, these workers set out to evaluate the clinically relevant information obtained from the examination and to determine if this had an effect on patient management. Approximately 608 VFSS examinations were reviewed and only 1.4% were classified as normal; aspiration occurred in just over a third. Individuals with swallowing abnormalities did not always aspirate (no aspiration was recorded in just over half the studies). The authors studied five outcome variables of interest, including referrals made to other specialties, the effectiveness of compensatory strategies, treatment recommendations and if the mode of intake and diet grade changed. They found that there was a high percentage of change in all variables of interest which they claimed indicated the high clinical utility of VFSS and demonstrated that VFSS was more than a tool for identifying aspiration. It should be noted that the available evidence comes primarily from studies that have used VFSS rather than other instrumental examinations.

This fact raises a further important question. Of the investigative procedures available and in use, is there any evidence that one technique yields better results than another? Furthermore, what are the benefits in terms of improved patient outcomes, cost and ease of usage? These very questions were posed as part of the evidence report/technology assessment, *Diagnosis and Treatment of Swallowing Disorders (Dysphagia) in Acute Care Stroke Patients* (ACHPR, 1999). The report describes each instrumental procedure in full, reports the advantages and disadvantages of each procedure, and compares the sensitivity and specificity of each. The report concluded that, 'neither videofluoroscopy nor fiberoptic endoscopy' are 'perfect gold standards for the detection of aspiration, because each yields false-negative and false-positive results' (ACHPR, 1999, p. 9). Furthermore, the report went on to say that a further reason why there were no conclusive data was because of the small sample sizes of the studies reviewed with limited statistical power to detect effects of interest. Readers are directed to this excellent review for further discussion (www.ahcpr.gov).

Just one paediatric study that compared the results from VFSS to FEES was located. Leder and Karas (2000) set out to investigate the diagnostic usefulness of FEES in children. These authors studied 30 subjects, described as children ranging in age from 11 days to 20 years (mean age 10 years 4 months). As described, seven subjects were randomly assessed by use of both FEES and VFSS, and 23 subjects received FEES only. Blinded ratings were made from the investigations. At the same time the authors also investigated if the procedure (VFSS or FEES) affected the rehabilitative strategy recommended. The authors reported 100% agreement between the blinded diagnostic results and the rehabilitative strategies recommended after FEES and VFSS. They concluded that FEES may be used to routinely diagnose and treat paediatric patients with dysphagia. It is worth noting that the sample in this study was very small and it is not clear if there was true randomization (Level III.2).

VFSS

VFSS is the investigation most commonly used in clinical practice and therefore it will be discussed in further detail. For a detailed description of the VFSS procedure, readers are directed to Logemann (1983). The results from VFSS are used as a basis for management and prognosis for recovery of dysphagia; it is crucial, therefore, that the claims made about its diagnostic usefulness are critically appraised. As discussed earlier, Logemann (1983) found that the use of VFSS 'added value' to the assessment process by demonstrating that aspiration could not be detected reliably solely from clinical evaluation. Schmidt et al. (1994) studied the risk of developing pneumonia, dehydration and death in stroke patients. The case records of 26 patients undergoing VFSS were examined and compared to 33 randomly selected case-matched dysphagic control subjects who did not undergo VFSS. The results, summarized below in Box 7.1, demonstrated that the information obtained from VFSS regarding the material aspirated (this information could not be reliably obtained from clinical evaluation alone) did have a direct effect on the development of pneumonia and on mortality (two of the primary outcomes of interest) but not hydration. In Box 7.1 the odds ratios for developing pneumonia, death and dehydration are illustrated according to the aspiration observed. Dehydration was unrelated to aspiration. Patients who aspirated (any texture) ran a 7.6 times greater chance of developing pneumonia than those who did not aspirate. Patients who aspirated thickened consistencies ran a 5.6 times greater risk of developing pneumonia than those who did not aspirate or those who aspirated thin liquids only.

Box 7.1

VFSS (odds ratio) – obtained for aspirators as compared to non-aspirators and/or aspirators of thin liquids only

- Development of pneumonia:
    - aspiration – any consistency   7.6
    - aspiration – thickened liquids/solids   5.6
- Death:
    - aspiration – thickened liquids/solids   9.2

These results, with the results from studies such as those conducted by Logemann et al. (1994), Schmidt et al. (1994), Tanaguchi and Moyer (1994) and Schwartz et al. (2001), provide moderate to strong evidence (Level III.1 and level II) to support the view that the use of diagnostic techniques (such as VFSS) contribute essential diagnostic information and result in improved patient outcomes (for example, reducing the risk of developing pneumonia).

This is essential evidence, because life-changing decisions, such as the need to eliminate 'non-safe' consistencies from a diet and the need for alternative (non-oral, tube) feeding, are made based on these results (Reilly and Perry, 2001). However, further work on the predictive validity and reliability of instrumental measures is required. Some recent studies have attempted to address the reliability of interpretations of VFSS (Scott et al., 1998; McCullough et al., 2001). However, although the procedure itself may be standardized the interpretation of the study in most clinical situations remains largely an unvalidated procedure.

Although VFSS has been referred to by clinicians and researchers as the 'gold standard' for assessing swallowing, however, this proposition reveals a limited understanding of the statistical requirements of a gold standard. The gold standard is a diagnosis obtained from an acknowledged standard, such as an investigative test (biopsy), or from long-term follow-up. Any newly developed test or diagnostic procedure would be compared and judged against the gold standard. Does the information obtained from VFSS provide a definitive diagnosis and has it been judged against other standards? The evidence report/technology assessment, *Diagnosis and Treatment of Swallowing Disorders (Dysphagia) in Acute Care Stroke Patients* (AHCPR, 1999, p. 110) concluded that 'measuring the performance of diagnostic tests for dysphagia is difficult because of the lack of a gold standard'. Following a critical appraisal of the literature, this publication reported that no test was 100% accurate, that is, with perfect sensitivity and specificity, and it was not possible to 'demonstrate any significant advantage of one test over another' (AHCPR, 1999, p. 110). These findings were later supported in a randomized prospective study by Aviv (2000) that investigated the efficacy of FEES against VFSS in determining appropriate interventions for patients with dysphagia. The conclusion was that both were equally good at diagnosing dysphagia and in providing recommendations for treatment.

If no investigative procedure may be regarded as a gold standard, what should clinicians and researchers in the field do? Where there is no gold standard Sackett et al. (1991) recommend that one or more logical consequences (or constructs) of the disorder (dysphagia) are selected and made the gold standard. In dysphagia the consequences might be aspiration pneumonia or malnutrition. Alternatively, Sackett et al. (1991) also propose that clinicians could ask whether patients were better off as a result of undergoing the examination. There is moderate to strong evidence that individuals with dysphagia are better off as a result of VFSS examination. However, does it matter which examination they receive (FEES or VFSS)? Is one safer or more cost-effective than another? These questions have not yet been answered.

VFSS has been used in numerous studies as the independent, reference standard for comparison across studies. A reference standard should represent the truth and put patients into 'disease' and 'non-disease groups'. Sackett et al. (1991) outline eight steps for evaluating tests. It is clear, when applying these steps, that neither VFSS nor other commonly used diagnostic dysphagia tests, such as FEES, have undergone such rigorous scientific evaluation.

What is the relationship between the results obtained from instrumental and non-instrumental examinations?

Several well-designed, recently published studies have attempted, in different ways, to address the relationship between the clinical signs and symptoms gathered from the non-instrumental examination and the results obtained from instrumental (namely VFSS) investigation. The results from a number of studies are summarized in Table 7.3. All provide moderate evidence regarding the signs and symptoms predictive of moderate to severe dysphagia, as demonstrated on VFSS, and the detection of aspiration on VFSS. The evidence is also at a higher level (for example, a prospective clinical cohort study comparing VFSS and FEES (Mann et al., 1999)) than previously reported (clinical opinion). However, much is population-specific to stroke (Daniels et al., 1997), although the samples from Logemann et al. (1999)

Table 7.3 Studies that address the relationship between clinical signs, symptoms and characteristics of individuals with dysphagia with results from VFSS

Source	Sample	Population(s)	Methodology	Key findings
Daniels et al. (2000)	56	Acute stroke	Prospective CBE and VFSS	No single clinical feature a sufficiently sensitive indicator of dysphagia. When two or more features combined the sensitivity increased markedly.
Smith et al. (1999)	1100 aged 3–98 years	Neurological, head and neck, medical, gastrointestinal, unknown other	Retrospective record examination	36% aspirated (43% non-silent, 57% silently) Males more likely to aspirate silently. Aspiration more common in youngest and oldest age groups Aetiology of aspiration – disorder in pharyngeal motor response.
Logemann et al. (1999)	200 aged 14–97 years	Stroke (69) Head and neck cancer (26) Spinal cord injuries (21) Other (84)	Prospective CBE and VFSS	Single variables associated with aspiration: abnormal pharyngeal contraction, on trial swallows coughing, throat clearing, reduced laryngeal elevation, gurgly voice and multiple swallows per bolus. Combined variables associated with aspiration: coughing throat clearing, reduced laryngeal aspiration, history of recurrent pneumonia.
Mann et al. (1999)	128	Stroke (acute first stroke)	Prospective CBE and VFSS and outcome at six months	No clinical indicator of dysphagia or aspiration was independently predictive of swallowing outcome Delayed or absent swallow reflex single independent predictor of chest infection at six months (identified on VFSS) Delayed oral transit time single independent predictor of failure to return to normal diet (identified on VFSS) CBE not predictive of swallowing outcome.

(contd)

Table 7.3 (contd)

Source	Sample	Population(s)	Methodology	Key findings
Mann et al. (2000)	128	Stroke (acute first stroke)	Prospective CBE and VFSS and outcome at six months.	Compared to VFSS: CBE underestimated frequency of dysphagia CBE overestimated frequency of aspiration Costs of false positive and false negative diagnoses discussed.
Garon et al. (1995)	1000 (over a 10-year period)	Neurologic aetiologies (mainly stroke)	Retrospective outcome study CBE and VFSS.	57% aspirated Of these 52% aspirated silently, without clinical indication Results from CBE not sufficiently accurate to detect patients at risk of apsiration.
Garon et al. (1996)	102	Neurologic aetiology – 50% stroke	Retrospective outcome study comparing 3 oz water test (coughing) with aspiration on VFSS.	54 patients aspirated. Of these only 35% coughed. 65% did not cough on CBE but aspirated on VFSS. The 3 oz water test not an accurate sole indicator of aspiration.
Taniguchi and Moyer (1994)	142 (1–132 months)	Mixed paediatric diagnoses, including cerebral palsy, acquired brain injury, peripheral nervous system disorders, failure to thrive, genetic syndromes.	Retrospective study to examine the relationship between aspiration and (on VFSS) pneumonia. Notes reviewed retrospectively and VFSS scored.	44% aspirated on VFSS. History of pneumonia within one year of VFSS found in 35%. Significant risk factors for pneumonia: presence of any aspiration, gastro-oesophageal reflux, presence of a tracheostomy tube and age <1 year. Children with TBI less at risk for pneumonia than other diagnostic groups. Relationship between aspiration and pneumonia mediated by food consistency. Children who aspirated: Puree had a nine-fold greater risk for pneumonia. Thickened liquids were at intermediate risk (2.6 times > chance of developing pneumonia). Thin liquids did not have a statistically significant increase in pneumonia risk.

Reynolds et al. (1998)	102	Ischemic stroke patients with dysphagia	Prospective comparison of CBE and VFSS	20.6% of patients developed pneumonia. Pneumonia more common in those who aspirated on VFSS. Patients with pneumonia had longer length of stay, higher total stay costs, higher mortality and worse 24-hour stroke severity scores. Higher correction between VFSS and development of pneumonia than CBE and development pneumonia, but combined use yielded highest sensitivity (0.86) and negative predictive value (0.91).
Warms and Richards (2000)	23	Neurologic dysphagic patients	Prospective comparison of voice samples and VFSS – wet voice vs aspiration on VFSDS	In 57% of patients ingested barium remained in cervical region. Only 6.6% of the time was voice wetness judged to be present in those patients with residue in the cervical region. No association between wet voice and penetration/ aspiration on VFSS. Wet voice not useful as 'sole' indicator of aspiration/ penetration. Wet voice may be useful indicator of laryngeal dysfunction.
Schurr et al. (1999)	47	Acquired brain injury	Retrospective case series	Clinical examination normal in 14 subjects; two overtly abnormal and referred for gastrostomy; 31 referred for VFSS. Of those referred for VFSS 22 (71%) had abnormal studies. Of those with abnormal VFSS ($n = 22$) four received gastrostomy, 13 had penetration or minor aspiration responsive to therapy and were orally fed. Five had silent aspiration, nine received n/g tube) but responded to therapy and resumed oral feeding.

included some patients who had undergone treatment for head and neck cancer and other aetiologies. Until recently there were few paediatric studies. The first was a retrospective study of the records and outcomes for 142 children (Tanaguchi and Moyer, 1994). The study did not directly address signs and symptoms but focused more on co-morbidities as predictors and risk factors for the development of aspiration pneumonia.

In a more recent study, Schwartz et al. (2001) set out to determine the results of diagnostic evaluation and the effects of nutritional intervention on energy consumption, weight gain, growth and clinical status of children with neuro-developmental disability. These authors studied outcomes in 79 children who underwent a thorough diagnostic dysphagia work-up. They concluded that diagnosis-specific treatment results in significantly improved energy consumption (as measured by calorie intake) and weight gain (z scores for both weight and height and improved subcutaneous tissue stores). In addition, decreased morbidity (lower acute care hospitalization rates after treatment as compared to two-year pre-treatment baseline rates) was said to be related to diagnostic-specific treatment. The majority of children in the study (49 of 79) required a high level of intervention: 23% received a gastrostomy and fundoplication; 13% a gastrostomy tube only; and 22% required oral supplementation. This is one of the few studies to report on the results of a wide variety of outcomes in such children, in particular the lower rate of acute care hospitalization following diagnosis and treatment.

Is there any evidence that screening for dysphagia is effective?

Screening, as defined by the UK National Screening Committee is,

> the systematic application of a test, or inquiry, to identify individuals at sufficient risk of a specific disorder to warrant further investigation or direct preventative action, amongst persons who have not sought medical attention on account of symptoms of that disorder. UK National Screening Committee (1998, p. 6)

To date, two systematic reviews have evaluated the accuracy of different screening tests to detect dysphagia in stroke (Martino et al., 2000; Perry and Love, 2001). The reviews also examined the health-related outcomes reported and asked if screening altered these outcomes. Both reviews uncovered numerous articles (Martino and colleagues (2000) reviewed 154 sources) and found that the heterogeneity of the material made comparison and interpretation difficult and, at times, impossible. Martino et al. (2000) concluded that:

- Evidence for screening accuracy was limited by poor methodology and the predominant use of aspiration as the diagnostic reference.
- There was some (but limited) evidence to suggest that screening results in a reduction in pneumonia, hospital stay, personnel costs and patient charges.

The conclusion from both systematic reviews was that large, well-designed, controlled studies are needed before it may be stated conclusively that there are benefits to dysphagia screening. These studies should be undertaken in a variety of populations, including cerebral palsy. Recently, the need for screening in the severely disabled population was highlighted in a report published by the Community Services Commission (CSC) in New South Wales, Australia. The report (CSC, 2001) reviewed the characteristics and circumstances of 211 people with disabilities who died in care over a seven-year period. A significant number of the people who died were affected by dysphagia. Forty-two per cent of deaths were related to respiratory causes and pneumonia and 23% of these were directly attributed to aspiration pneumonia. The main cause of death in young people in the sample (aged 0–24 years) was respiratory disease, especially in those with dysphagia and identified aspiration. The report recommended several service improvement initiatives. People in care, in particular the disabled, would benefit from health screening (including a screen for dysphagia) to reduce morbidity (for example, the development of respiratory complications as a result of recurrent aspiration), to minimize harm (choking) and to prevent dysphagia-related deaths (for example, aspiration pneumonia) (CSC, 2001).

What is current best practice in the treatment of dysphagia?

Dysphagia treatment is not a 'package' that may be applied readily to all individuals. Given the considerable heterogeneity within the dysphagia population, it is not surprising that treatment is often prescribed individually and is dependent on the aetiology and the exact nature of individuals' problems. A common theme that emerges from the literature is 'team management' and the evidence underpinning this will be examined briefly here. Specific management approaches will be discussed and the evidence for each approach will be appraised for the relevant diagnostic groups.

Team management

Almost every textbook and publication espouses the view that a team approach should be adopted to the assessment and management of dysphagia. The rationales given include the following.

- Dysphagia is complex and cannot be managed adequately by any one profession.
- Dysphagia involves the whole digestive tract and therefore intersects a number of disciplines.
- The diagnostic investigations often require expertise from numerous different professionals.
- Advice given independently by various health professionals may be conflicting and confusing for carers and parents as well as the patients themselves.
- Team management is more efficient.

Although the reasons cited above appear sound, there is little evidence to support them. Few would argue against the need for multidisciplinary input into the evaluation and management of dysphagia. A variety of models has been proposed; however, no particular model has been evaluated. Furthermore, there is little empirical evidence to indicate that evaluation and management via multidisciplinary teams improves patient outcomes in dysphagia.

Twenty-eight papers concerned with team management were retrieved (resulting from a search of the following key terms: *dysphagia, swallowing disorder* and/or *team management, multidisciplinary team*). Twelve papers focused on paediatric dysphagia and 16 were concerned with adults with dysphagia; however, almost all the recommendations concerning team management arose from opinion and clinical experience. Only one article contained 'data' and attributed beneficial outcomes to the multidisciplinary team management of dysphagia. In a prospective study, Martens et al. (1990) compared multidisciplinary dysphagia team management ($n = 16$) with current 'best practice' according to a pre-existing ward routine ($n = 15$). Individual treatment programmes were devised by the team after bedside and VFSS examinations. A time series study design was used and the results demonstrated that multidisciplinary dysphagia team management resulted in a significant weight gain and increase in caloric intake in the group that underwent team management. There was no difference in the incidence of aspiration pneumonia in either group, which the authors attributed to the meticulousness of the best practice care adopted on the ward.

Curley et al. (1998) showed that providers of interdisciplinary care (albeit not in managing dysphagia) had a greater understanding of patient care, were more effective communicators and better team workers than providers of traditional (that is, non-team management) care models. Interdisciplinary care was also shown to be more efficient and of a higher quality with decreased costs associated with the hospital stay. To date there is moderate evidence (Level III.2) in support of team management (Martens et al. 1990). There has been no study of the effect of interdisciplinary care on a wide range of outcomes in patients with dysphagia, nor has there been study to ascertain if a particular model of care results in more efficient and more cost-effective care and results in positive patient satisfaction.

Management approaches

As highlighted previously, a variety of treatment options exists and some are population-specific. Logemann et al. (1983, 1992, 1994) and Logemann and Kahrilas (1990) categorized dysphagia treatment regimes into invasive and non-invasive therapies. Non-invasive therapies included compensatory techniques, indirect therapy and direct therapy, whereas invasive therapies included surgical interventions, pharmaceutical therapy and enteral feeding. (In this chapter only non-invasive therapies are considered.)

Tables 7.4, 7.5, 7.6, 7.7, 7.8 and 7.9 present the available evidence for the most commonly used non-invasive dysphagia treatments. Information on the dysphagia population(s) studied, the study design, main study outcomes and the strength of the evidence is displayed. Studies were included if they contained data on treated patients and if quantitative results were reported. Much of the evidence for the efficacy of specific treatment techniques and approaches in dysphagia is reported for specific diagnostic groups. In stroke, a number of systematic reviews (for example, Bath et al., 2001; Perry and Love, 2001) have been undertaken and this information is also summarized in tables 7.4, 7.5, 7.6, 7.7, 7.8 and 7.9. In Parkinson's disease a systematic review was undertaken to compare the efficacy and effectiveness of non-pharmacological swallowing therapy verses placebo or no interventions (Deane et al., 2001). An amendment was made to this review in November 2000 (Deane et al., 2002). No randomized controlled trials or controlled trials were found. However, the authors note that they know of one large randomized controlled trial in progress – comparing 'chin-down' posture with thickened liquids in the treatment of dysphagia. The reviewers concluded that there is currently no evidence to support or reject the efficacy of swallowing therapy for dysphagia in Parkinson's disease. The review made a number of recommendations about the need for large, well-designed trials and the inclusion of suitable outcome measures. In the following discussion the evidence underpinning each of the main approaches will be summarized.

Postural strategies

Evidence for the use of postural strategies ranges from low–moderate evidence (within-subject study design (Rasely et al., 1993; Table 7.4)) to high evidence (randomized controlled trial (Ohmae et al., 1998; Table 7.4)) that postural strategies, such as the chin tuck (the most effective postural strategy), reduce aspiration in adult head and neck surgical patients and in

Table 7.4 Evidence for postural modification in people with dysphagia*

Population	Source	Study design	Sample size	Outcome(s)	Results	Evidence level
Preterm infants	Hill et al. (2000)	Cross-over, repeated-measures design	20 preterm infants (duration of 40 bottle feeding sessions)	Oral support (cheek and jaw) influences on cardiopulmonary function and nutritive sucking	Infants not receiving support paused longer and more frequently than supported infants. Oxygen saturation and heart rate did not differ between groups. Post-feed saturation levels were lower for non-supported infants.	III.1
Cerebral Palsy	Lanert and Eckberg (1995)	Within-subject – comparative study	5 (mean age 6.6 years)	Aspiration Food/liquid retention	No aspiration with neck flexion and 30° recline Oral retention decrease 2/5. Posterior drooling decreased 3/5.	III.3
Mixed diagnoses	Ohmae et al. (1998)	Randomized conrolled trial, four postures: chin-down, head rotation chin-down + head rotation, head back to chin-down	95	Aspiration	Postural strategies effective in eliminating aspiration in 68 (72%) patients. Chin-down effective for majority	II
Lateral Mudullary Syndrome	Logemann et al. (1989)	Examined the effect of head rotation on swallowing.	5	Pharyngeal residue, pooling, upper oesophageal sphincter opening.	Head rotation decreased residue. Greater fraction of the bolus swallowed. Upper oesophageal sphincter opening increased.	IV

Population	Author	Study design	Sample size	Major outcomes	Results	Level of evidence
Head and neck and surgical	Logemann et al. (1994)	Within subject, head and/or body position modified.	32	Aspiration	Aspiration eliminated in 81%.	III.3
Oropharyngeal dysphagia – mixed	Rasley et al. (1993)	Within subject, five postures tested for each patient.	165	Aspiration	Aspiration eliminated with changes in head and/or body position in 77%.	III.3
Neurological	Bulow et al. (2001)	Case series: comparison study of three different techniques, supraglottic vs effortful vs chin tuck.	eight subjects (aged 46-81 years)	Aspiration, penetration, pharyngeal retention	Number of misdirected swallows not affected by any technique. Effortful swallow and chin tuck reduced depth of contrast penetration.	III.3
Neurogenic	Ertekin et al. (2001)	Experimental with control group of normal subjects and neurogenic subjects. Compared neutral chin position, chin up, chin tucked, head rotated right and head rotated left.	75 Control group (24) and Neurogenic patients (51)	EMG of laryngeal movements.	Changes in head and neck position did not alter dysphagia significantly.	III.2

*The populations studied, study design, sample size and major outcomes of interest are reviewed and level of evidence is provided for each.

Table 7.5 Evidence for diet modification in people with dysphagia*

Population	Source	Design	Sample size	Outcome(s)	Results	Evidence level
Pseudobulbar dysphagia (history of aspiration pneumonia)	Groher (1987)	RCT	46, Group 1 – pureed diet, thin liquids Group 2 – soft diet, thickened liquids	Pneumonia	Higher incidence of aspiration in group 1 (28) than in group 2 (5)	II
Stroke (previous aspiration detected on thin liquids)	Garon et al. (1997)	RCT – prospective design	20, two groups: 1 thickened liquids 2 thickened liquids but with free access to water	Aspiration pneumonia Dehydration	No pneumonia developed in either group. No major group differences in overall fluid intake.	II
Stoke	Goulding et al. (2000)	RCT	19: 10 cases 9 control subject	Aspiration	Higher viscosity did not protect against aspiration and may lead to reduced fluid intake.	II

*The populations studied, study design, sample size and major outcomes of interest are reviewed and level of evidence is provided for each.

Table 7.6 Evidence for oral motor exercises in people with dysphagia*

Population	Source	Design	Sample size	Outcome(s)	Results	Evidence level
Cerebral palsy (moderate impairment)	Gisel (1994)	Case series: no control 20 weeks of sensorimotor treatment, 5–7 min/day, 5 days/week	35 (aged 4.3–13.3 years)	Growth	No change in OM skills. Weight maintained. No catch up growth.	III.3
Cerebral palsy	Gisel and Alphonce (1995)	Case series: no control and 20 weeks of oral sensorimotor therapy	27 (mean age 5.1 years)	Growth (weight and skinfolds) OM skills (eating efficiency)	No change in OM skills. Weight maintained. No catch up growth. Concluded that eating efficiency may not be a good estimator of treatment outcome, but instead a diagnostic indicator re the severity of dysphagia.	III.3
Cerebral palsy (moderate impairment)	Gisel et al. (1996)	Case series with control period. 10 weeks of control followed by 10 weeks treatment. Stratified according to aspiration status.	27 (2.5–10 years), 7 aspirators, 20 non-aspirators	Growth (weight) OM skills (eating efficiency)	Children who aspirated had significantly poorer oral-motor skills. Significant changes in OM skills (spoon feeding, chewing and swallowing but not drinking). Weight maintained but no catch-up growth.	III.2

(contd)

Table 7.6 (contd)

Population	Source	Design	Sample	Outcome(s)	Results	Evidence level
Cerebral palsy (moderate impairment)	Gisel (1996)	Comparison of 2 treatments: controlled trial non-randomized to test the effect of oral sensori-motor treatment on eating efficiency and growth.	35 2 groups: 1. OM therapy (*n* = 11) 2. Chewing exercises (*n*=24)	Growth (weight) OM skills (eating efficiency)	Children who received oral motor therapy exceeded their expected centile line by 1.7 percentile points. Chewing exercises alone had no effect on weight gain. No significant group differences in eating efficiency.	II

*The populations studied, study design, sample size and major outcomes of interest are reviewed and level of evidence is provided for each.

Table 7.7 Evidence for modification of equipment in people with dysphagia*

Population	Source	Design	Sample size	Outcome(s)	Results	Evidence level
Cleft palate	Shaw et al. (1999)	RCT	101: two groups: 1. Compressible bottle 2. Rigid bottle	Weight	Compressible bottle preferable – improved weight gain.	II
Cleft palate	Brine et al. (1994)	RCT Both groups also received nutritional guidance and counselling	31: two groups: 1. Compressible bottle with x-cut nipple 2. Compressible bottle with long x-cut nipple	Weight	No significant differences between both groups on main outcome – weight gain.	II

*The populations studied, study design, sample size and major outcomes of interest are reviewed and level of evidence is provided for each.

Table 7.8 Evidence for the use of prostheses in people with dysphagia*

Population	Source	Design	Sample size	Outcome(s)	Results	Evidence level
Cerebral palsy	Gisel et al. (2000)	Case series	20 (4–13 years)	Sitting skills, ambulatory status, oral posture.	50% of subjects showed marked improvement in oral posture (e.g., closed mouth), ambulatory status (greater than expected via maturation) and sitting skills (head–trunk–foot control).	III.2
Cerebral palsy	Haberfellner et al. (2001)	Case series: multiple baseline design Phase 1. Control period. Phase 2. ISMAR treatment Phase 3. Facilitation ingestive skills	20 (4–13 years)	Oral skills Growth (after 1 year)	Weight gain and improved oral skills during intervention phase. But weight gain also occurred during control phase. Given cost and time commitment involved in use of ISMARs the cost-benefit would need to be carefully evaluated.	III.2
Cerebral palsy	Gisel et al. (2001)	Controlled trial non-randomized comparing treatment and non-treatment with ISMAR devices.	17 (6–15 years)	Seven domains of functional feeding and weight	No significant differences in weight changes between groups at 18 and 24 month follow-up. Maturation was equally effective as ISMAR therapy.	III.3

Population	Author	Study design	Sample size	Outcome	Results	Level of evidence
Post-surgical oral and oropharyngeal cancer patients	Pauloski et al. (1996)	Single-case design with control period	13	Swallowing function	Mixed: majority of patients had unchanged swallowing function or mixed results (i.e., some improvement but not for all bolus consistencies).	III.3
Stroke	Freed et al. (2001)	Controlled study: non-randomized comparing tactile thermal stimulation with electrical stimulation		Swallowing scale – 0 = aspirates own saliva and 6 = normal swallow. Daily treatments of 1 hour – average 5.5 treatments	Both groups showed improvement but higher gains in electrical treatment group.	III.1

*The populations studied, study design, sample size and major outcomes of interest are reviewed and level of evidence is provided for each.

Table 7.9 Evidence for the use of combined therapy approaches in people with dysphagia*

Population	Source	Design	Sample size	Outcome(s)	Results	Evidence level
Diet modification and exercises						
Stroke rehabilitation centre	DiPippo et al. (1994a)	RCT	115, three groups: 1. diet + exercises 2. diet + exercises and FU 3. diet + exercises and daily monitoring	Pneumonia	Pneumonia incidence, group results: 1. 2.6 % 2. 13.2 % 3. 5.1 % Group differences NS Pneumonia incidence did not correlate with intervention level.	II
	DiPippo et al. (1994b)	RCT	Compared therapist vs carer instruction	Hydration Recurrent upper airway obstruction Death	Patient and family instruction is as effective during inpatient stay as daily therapist rehearsal of treatment techniques.	
Swallow therapy (thermal stimulation, supraglottic swallow, bolus propulsion exercises)						
Neurologic and non-neurologic patients (+/- history of aspiration pneumonia)	Kasprisin et al. (1989)	Retrospective pseudo-controlled trial	69 three groups: 1. Treated (no aspiration pneumonia, n = 48) 2. Treated (aspiration pneumonia, n = 13) 3. No treatment (n = 8)	Pneumonia	Pneumonia incidence, group results: 1. 6.3% 2. 15.4% 3. 100% Group differences: 1 and 3, and 2 and 3 significant.	III.1

Diet, modification, exercises, counselling (individual treatment)

Neurologic and non-neurologic patients	Martens et al. (1990)	Historical prospective case series	Two groups: 1 Acute care patients (n = 16) - treated 2 Historical control subjects (n = 15)	Pneumonia	No reported cases in either group.	III.2

Diet modification, oral motor exercises, swallowing techniques, positioning

Stroke	Elmstahl et al. (1999)	Survey with follow-up treatment of a clinical case series.	38 patients, aged (53–89 years) Baseline recordings using VFSS followed by treatment and repeat VFSS	Nutritional status and anthropometry	Improved swallowing function (as measured by OM status and VFSS examination) was associated with improved nutritional parameters (e.g., improved levels of albumin and iron binding capacity). Body weight reduced in those with unchanged or decreased VFSS outcome.	III.3

Diet, modification, exercises, counselling (individual treatment)

Neurologic and non-neurologic patients	Martens et al. (1990)	Historical, prospective case series	Two groups, 1 Acute care patients (n = 16) - treated 2 Historical control subjects (n = 15)	Weight gain Intake	Treated group fared better on both variables – group differences: significant.	III.3

(contd)

Table 7.9 (contd)

Diagnostic specific treatment programmes – eclectic approach

Population	Source	Design	Sample size	Outcome(s)	Results	Evidence level
Children with neurodevelop-mental problems	Schwartz et al. (2001)	Follow-up study of outcomes following diagnosis specific treatment in a clinically referred population – case series.	79 children	Energy consumption, weight gain, growth, clinical status, acute care hospital use.	Improved energy consumption, nutritional status, growth, and decreased morbidity.	III.2

*The populations studied, study design, sample size and major outcomes of interest are reviewed and level of evidence is provided for each.

patients with dysphagia of mixed origin (structural and neurological aetiologies (Logemann et al., 1994; Table 7.4)). However, in children, despite its widespread use, the evidence that postural modification (chin-tuck combined with 30° postural recline) reduces aspiration is very low (from a small, single-case series of just six subjects (Lanert and Ekberg, 1995)).

Diet modification

The evidence for diet modification (thickened liquids) reducing aspiration and pneumonia is also conflicting. The three reported studies all focus on stroke patients: one used pneumonia as the main outcome and two used aspiration (demonstrated on VFSS) as the main outcome (Table 7.5). Two out of three randomized controlled trials (Garon et al., 1996; Goulding and Bakheit, 2000) demonstrated that there was no significant difference in aspiration rates or aspiration pneumonia rates according to whether or not fluids were thickened. The remaining randomized controlled trial demonstrated significantly lower pneumonia rates in the group receiving thickened liquids. In one trial (Garon et al., 1996) no group differences in the overall fluid intake were identified, whereas in the other (Goulding and Bakheit, 2000) there was a trend for reduced fluid intake in the group receiving thickened fluids. No such intervention studies were identified involving children.

Oral motor treatment

Throughout the literature numerous terms are used to describe variations on oral motor treatment (for example, oral sensory motor treatment, oro-motor exercises). For clarity, the term 'oral motor treatment' will be used throughout this section. Oral motor treatment and exercises were for many years the speech pathologist's (in particular paediatric speech pathologists') tools of the trade. But what of the evidence for their use? The literature concerned focuses mainly on children with cerebral palsy. The use of exercises in the adult population has been reported in combination with other treatment approaches (see Table 7.6). Pilot data are also emerging to suggest that a range of motion exercises (jaw, lip, tongue and larynx) result in improved global speech and swallowing measures in adult patients who have undergone oral or oropharyngeal ablative surgery (Logemann et al., 1997).

The majority of studies on children have been published by Dr Erika Gisel's research team in Canada. The studies have all been of a similar design: a series of cases with a baseline observation and control period followed by a treatment period. Common to all studies were the two outcome measures: growth (weight and skinfold thickness) and eating efficiency (expressed as oral motor control for spoon feeding, biting, chewing, etc.). Only one of the four studies conducted demonstrated a significant change in eating efficiency (two studies demonstrated limited but non-significant improvement). There was no significant change in weight outcomes as a result of oral motor treatment in any of the studies. There was also no change in drinking efficiency. In a summary to one of the studies, Gisel and Alphonce (1995) suggested that eating efficiency (as measured by oral motor control) was probably 'not a good estimator of treatment outcome, but rather a diagnostic indicator of the severity of eating impairment'.

Despite widely accepted clinical practice and views, there is currently weak evidence to suggest that oral motor treatment results in improved oral motor control and more efficient eating. Furthermore, there is no evidence that growth (weight gain and skinfold thickness) is enhanced by improved oral motor control in children. The largest treatment effects have been observed in children with moderately impaired oral motor skills – the same changes were not observed in those with severely impaired skills.

Pinelli et al. (2002) conducted a systematic review to determine whether non-nutritive sucking in pre-term infants influenced a range of variables, including weight gain, energy intake, heart rate, oxygen saturation, length of hospital stay, intestinal transit time, age when full oral feeds were instituted and any other clinically relevant outcomes. These authors reviewed 20 studies, of which 14 were randomized controlled trials. The results indicated that non-nutritive sucking:

- significantly reduced the length of hospital stay
- eased transition from tube to bottle feeds
- improved bottle feeding performance
- improved feeding behaviour.

There were no negative outcomes reported and there were no benefits identified for weight gain, energy intake, heart rate, oxygen saturation, intestinal transit time and age at full oral feeding. Pinelli et al. (2002) concluded that although were some methodological limitations (for example, variable outcomes, no longitudinal data, design issues) in some of the studies reviewed, non-nutritive sucking does appear to have benefits. The authors state in their implications for practice that non-nutritive sucking also appeared to facilitate the transition to full oral or bottle feeding as well as feeding performance and behavioural state. They went on to state that non-nutritive sucking appeared to reduce defensive behaviours during feeding and infants demonstrated less fussy and active states during and after feeds. They also settled more quickly into deep states.

Modified equipment

The use of modified feeding equipment (for example, modified cups, bottles and eating utensils) is discussed widely in the literature. However, apart from the two studies presented in Table 7.7 there is limited empirical evidence to support or refute their use. Modified equipment is used most commonly in particular paediatric populations, for example, children with cleft lip and palate and craniofacial anomalies. Two randomized controlled trials have examined the use of different types of bottles and teats for feeding babies with cleft lip and palate. In the largest study ($n = 101$) a significant difference was found in favour of the use of a soft, compressible bottle rather than a rigid one. The main outcome used in this study was weight gain. In the second study (Brine et al., 1994) a smaller number of infants were studied ($n = 31$). Both were fed by use of a compressible bottle, but different teats were tried: a cross-cut nipple versus a long cross-cut nipple. Both groups gained weight regardless of the nipple used. This is strong evidence (Level II) from randomized controlled trials, to support the use of compressible bottles with either a cross-cut or long cross-cut nipple for feeding babies with cleft lip and palate.

Prostheses

The use of prostheses is another area where a large body of literature exists, although most are descriptive papers, case studies or small series of cases without control (see Table 7.8). Three studies were published recently by Gisel and colleagues. The studies involved 20 children (11 girls and 9 boys) ranging in age from 4.2 years to 13.1 years (details available in Table 7.8). The children were randomized to treatment with an intra-oral device or to a control group (ongoing standard rehabilitation at school). Children in the control group were also offered the intra-oral device treatment after the six-month control period had ended. Treatment lasted for 12 months.

Each study used the same group of patients, but the aims of each study differed. In Study 1 (Gisel et al., 2000) the aim was to determine if the use of an intra-oral appliance resulted in improved functional feeding skills and growth outcomes in children with cerebral palsy after one year of treatment. Study 2 (Gisel et al., 2001) aimed to document the relationship between oral-motor, postural and ambulatory control, and in Study 3, functional feeding and growth outcomes were examined one year after treatment had ceased (Haberfellner et al., 2001).

These studies (in particular, the results from Study 3) demonstrate the importance of a longer term follow-up. Although initially a significant improvement in functional feeding skills was reported in the group treated with the intra-oral device, at follow-up no such difference was observed. Both the treatment and the control groups gained weight and at follow-up (one year post-treatment) there were no significant differences. However, an improvement in 'whole-body mobility' was reported (improvement in sitting, ambulatory status and oral posture) after one year of treatment, which the authors claim supports the hypothesis of interaction between oral structures and postural control.

It is important to note that treatment via the intra-oral devices used in these studies is time-consuming and requires a commitment to treatment for at least one year. Presumably in most countries there is also a cost involved in making the device, and repeated visits are required for adjustment. The benefit of improved whole body motility reported from this series of studies would need to be balanced against the cost effectiveness and compared to other treatments.

Numerous examples of the use of prostheses with dysphagic patients are reported in the literature. These have not been included in this review because the majority are case reports or case series and contain limited data with no baseline or outcome data reported.

Combined strategies

A number of studies have included and evaluated more than one intervention strategy (for example, diet modification and exercises). These are illustrated in Table 7.9. Di Pippo et al. (1994a) conducted a randomized controlled trial to evaluate the effects of intervention (diet modification and exercises) in three conditions:

- Group 1 received intervention only.
- Group 2, intervention plus follow-up.
- Group 3, intervention plus daily monitoring.

The main outcome was the development of pneumonia. The results demonstrated that pneumonia incidence did not correlate with the intervention type. Although the incidence of pneumonia was higher in Group 2 (13.2%) than in Group 1 (2.6 %) and Group 3 (5.1%), there were no significant group differences. Kasprisin et al. (1989) conducted a retrospective pseudo-controlled trial evaluating outcome (pneumonia) in three groups of patients with both neurologic and non-neurologic conditions:

- Group 1 (n = 48) consisted of patients with no demonstrated aspiration pneumonia who received treatment.
- Group 2 (n = 13) comprised patients with demonstrated aspiration receiving treatment.

- Group 3 (n = 8) was made up of patients who did not receive treatment and were considered control subjects.

The treatment included thermal stimulation, supraglottic swallow and bolus propulsion exercises. In Group 3 all patients developed pneumonia, whereas in Group 1 only 6.3% did and in Group 2 some 15.4% developed the condition. The differences between groups 1 and 3 and groups 2 and 3 were statistically significant.

In contrast to these findings, the prospective case series (weaker evidence) studied by Martens et al. (1990) did not demonstrate any difference in outcome (development of pneumonia) in a treated versus a non-treated group. However, Martens et al. (1990) did show increases in weight gain and intake in the treated group versus a set of 'historical' control subjects.

The studies that used combined treatment approaches provide beginning but conflicting evidence that these interventions reduce the development of aspiration-related pneumonia and result in increased oral intake and weight gain. However, the strength of the evidence is variable and the results of a well-designed randomized controlled trial are necessary to provide conclusive evidence (ACHPR, 1999).

Bath et al. (2001) concluded from their systematic review that there were too few studies with too few patients to draw definitive conclusions concerning many management strategies in common use with dysphagic stroke patients. These authors noted that further research was needed to assess how and when patients are fed and to evaluate the effect of swallowing or drug therapy on outcomes.

Conclusion: the way forward

This chapter aimed to summarize and guide readers to the best available evidence concerning the evaluation and management of dysphagia. It began by addressing some issues that are considered fundamental to the evolution of current best practice in dysphagia before moving on to evaluate best practice and the evidence for management of individuals with dysphagia.

Because the specialty developed primarily to meet clinical needs, there has been a notable lack of description and measurement of normal swallowing. It is clear from the material reviewed that the field of dysphagia lacks clear definitions of what is 'normal'. This has resulted in the lack of a reference standard against which clinicians can judge dysphagia. However, the problems of measurement are more widespread than this. Many of the studies reviewed for this chapter are affected by methodological issues, including small sample sizes and the lack of a properly constituted control group.

When reviewing the non-instrumental evaluation of dysphagia it was evident that many of the items routinely included in clinical practice have not undergone rigorous scrutiny to ascertain if they are predictive of, or associated with, dysphagia. It is becoming increasingly clear from a series of studies that have set out to examine the relationship between the clinical signs and symptoms and the results obtained from diagnostic investigations (for example, VFSS) that no single clinical feature is a sufficiently sensitive indicator, but when two or more features are combined the sensitivity increases markedly. Much research has focused on the detection of aspiration and some individual symptoms have been found to be predictive. However, the significance of identifying aspiration is unknown; not all individuals will go on to develop pneumonia. To date there is little reliable data from the non-instrumental examination to suggest which patients from which diagnostic groups will develop pneumonia. The majority of studies on the non-instrumental examination have focused on adults and single dysphagic populations, such as stroke victims. Studies in paediatrics were rare.

To date, no one diagnostic investigation has been found to be superior (ACHPR, 1999) and despite the fact that VFSS has been referred to as a 'gold standard' for some time, it does not meet the requirements of a gold standard (Sackett et al., 1997). As highlighted throughout this chapter, the lack of agreement regarding definitions and terminology is highly problematic and at times makes comparison impossible.

Clinicians should be able to rely on data that inform them about which clinical signs and symptoms (test thresholds for dysphagia populations) determine the need for investigation (what investigation is superior and for whom). Given the heterogeneity in the dysphagia population, the clinical signs and symptoms, test thresholds and need for investigation may vary from population to population. Furthermore, clinicians should know how sensitive, specific and reliable the tests are.

In summary, although the worthiness of the instrumental and non-instrumental examinations would not be questioned by clinicians, the scientific validity and psychometric properties of procedures in common use are some way from being established. The cost-benefit of instrumental diagnostic studies and the predictive validity of diagnostic tests (both instrumental and non-instrumental) are unknown for many populations (in particular, paediatrics). Furthermore, for many populations we do not know if the evaluation method chosen (for example, non-instrumentation alone versus instrumentation, or a combination of both) affects the treatment techniques or strategies adopted, the short and long-term patient outcomes or patient morbidity and mortality. There is no doubt that numerous questions about the evaluation of dysphagia remain unanswered (and until recently were unasked). These provide the research direction for the future.

Some challenging questions are summarized below.

Questions concerning the evaluation of dysphagia

- What evaluation result (for example, clinical evaluation and/or VFSS) determines an action or intervention threshold (such as safe versus unsafe to feed)?
- What is the relationship between the information collected on case history, patient observation, clinical examination and the results obtained from diagnostic investigations?
- Do the results obtained from diagnostic tests change management regimes?
- Do the results obtained from diagnostic tests provide clinically important information about prognosis?
- Do the results from diagnostic tests alter patient outcomes?

The evidence for evaluating interventions for dysphagia is highly variable and in many instances is population-specific (most information available refers directly to the adult stroke population). However, clinical practice probably reflects a generalization of this evidence to different diagnostic groups and from adults to children. Perhaps the biggest challenge in interpreting the dysphagia literature on treatment efficacy is the variability and poor quality of much of the research. This ranges from randomized controlled trials (for example, evidence for feeding babies with cleft palate) to areas where there is limited or no evidence (evidence for postural modification in cerebral palsy) available. For an excellent summary and discussion of methodological issues in dysphagia research, readers are directed to the AHCPR report (AHCPR, 1999, pp 10–12 and pp 135–45).

Unlike areas of medicine where treatment is aimed at 'curing' or reversing conditions, in dysphagia clinicians are primarily concerned with reducing morbidity and preventing mortality. Unfortunately, until recently, much of the dysphagia research was orientated towards the measurement of changes in levels of impairment rather than reduction in the disability, handicap or distress associated with dysphagia. In Tables 7.4–7.9 the main outcome measures used in each of the cited studies are reported.

In the ACHPR report (ACHPR, 1999) three main groups of outcomes were reported, including: short-term outcomes (changes in swallow function, food intake, feeding method, weight, and aspiration); morbidity (pneumonia, malnutrition, dehydration, tube complications); and long-term outcomes (quality of life, mortality, mortality resulting from morbidity, mortality resulting from treatment). The majority of studies (reported in Tables 7.4–7.9) were concerned primarily with short-term outcomes. Those involving adults focused primarily on aspiration and/or aspiration pneumonia as the main outcome, whereas there appeared to be a trend for the paediatric studies to concentrate on outcomes related to nutritional status and/or changes in oral motor function. The variations in the outcome measures used makes comparison and generalization difficult. Evidence about the morbidity and longer-term outcomes for patients with dysphagia is vital if clinicians are to prove that what they do with them and their families works.

Acknowledgement

Thanks are due to Professor Alison Perry for the many thoughtful discussions and helpful comments that helped to form this chapter.

References

Agency for Health Care Policy and Research (AHCPR). Diagnosis and Treatment of Swallowing Disorders (Dysphagia) in Acute-Care Stroke Patients. AHCPR publication no. 99-E024. Rockville, MD: US Department of Health and Human Resources, 1999.

American Speech and Hearing Association (ASHA) Omnibus Survey. American Speech and Hearing Association, 2001a. (http://www.asha.org)

American Speech and Hearing Association (ASHA). Clinical Indicators for Instrumental Assessment of Dysphagia. ASHA Special Interest report, 2001b. (http://dysphagia.com/asha_SID_12.htm)

Arvedson J, Rogers B, Buck G, Smart P, Msall M. Silent aspiration prominent in children with dysphagia. International Journal of Pediatric Otorhinolaryngology 1994; 28: 173-181.

Aviv JE. Prospective, randomized outcome study of endoscopy versus modified barium swallow in patients with dysphagia. Laryngoscope 2000; 110: 563-574.

Axelsson K, Asplund K, Norberg A, Eriksson S. Eating problems and nutritional status during hospital stay of patients with severe stroke. Journal of the American Dietetics Association 1989; 89: 1092-1096.

Barer DH. The natural history and functional consequences of dysphagia after hemispheric stroke. Journal of Neurology, Neurosurgery and Psychiatry 1989; 52: 236-241.

Bath PMW, Bath FJ, Smithard DJ. Interventions for dysphagia in acute stroke. The Cochrane Library, Issue 1, 2001.

Baum BJ, Bodner L. Ageing and oral motor function: evidence for altered performance among older persons. Journal of Dental Research 1983; 62: 2-6.

Bax M. Eating is important. Developmental Medicine and Child Neurology 1989; 31: 285-286.

Bower C. Assessing baseline risk: prevalence and prognosis. In: Moyer VA, Elliott EJ, Davis RL, Gilbert R, Klassen T, Logan S et al. (eds) Evidence Based Paediatrics and Child Health. London: BMJ Books, 2000.

Brine EA, Rickard KA, Brady MS, Liechty EA, Manatunga A, Sadove M, Bull MJ. Effectiveness of two feeding methods in improving energy intake and growth of infants with cleft palate: a randomized study. Journal of the American Dietetic Association 1994; 94: 732-738.

Bulow M, Olsson R, Ekberg O. Videomanometric analysis of supraglottic swallow, effortful swallow, and chin tuck in patients with pharyngeal dysfunction. Dysphagia 2001; 16: 190-195.

Bushman M, Dobmeyer SM, Leeker L, Perlmetter JS. Swallowing abnormalities and their response to treatment in Parkinson's disease. Neurology 1989; 39: 1309-14.

Cherney LR, Halper AS. Swallowing problems in adults with traumatic brain injury. Seminars in Neurology 1996; 16: 349-53.

Coates C, Bakheit AM. Dysphagia in Parkinson's disease. European Neurology 1997; 38: 49-52.

Coelho CA, Ferranti R. Incidence and nature of dysphagia in polio survivors. Archives of Physical Medicine and Rehabilitation 1991; 72: 1071-5.

Community Service Commission. Disability, Death and the Responsibility of Care. NSW Government: Sydney, 2001.

Cosgrove JL, Alexander MA, Kitts EL, Swan BE, Klein MJ, Bauer RE. Late effects of poliomyelitis. Archives of Physical and Medical Rehabilitation 1987; 68: 4-7.

Curley C, McEachern JE, Speroff T. A firm trial of interdisciplinary rounds on the inpatient medical wards. An intervention designed using continuous quality improvement. Medical Care 1998; 36: AS4-12.

Dahl M, Thommessen M, Rasmussen M, Selberg T. Feeding and nutritional characteristics in children with moderate or severe cerebral palsy. Acta Paediatrica 1996; 85: 697-701.

Daniels SK, McAdam CP, Brailey K, Foundas AL. Clinical assessment of swallowing and prediction of dysphagia severity. American Journal of Speech and Language Pathology 1997; 6: 17-24.

Daniels SK, Ballo LA, Mahoney MC, Foundas AL. Clinical predictors of dysphagia and aspiration risk: outcome measures in acute stroke. Archives of Physical Medicine and Rehabilitation 2000; 81: 1030-3.

Daniels SK, Brailey K, Priestly DH, Herrington LR, Weisberg LA, Foundas AL. Aspiration in patients with acute stroke. Archives of Physical Medicine and Rehabilitation 1998; 79: 14-19.

Deane KH, Ellis-Hill C, Jones D, Whurr R, Ben-Schlomo Y, Playford ED, Clarke CE. Non-pharmacological therapies for dysphagia in Parkinson's disease. Cochrane Database System Review 2001; 1.

Deane KH, Ellis-Hill C, Jones D, Whurr R, Ben-Schlomo T, Playford ED, Clarke CE. Systematic review of paramedical therapies for Parkinson's disease. Movement Disorders 2002; 17: 984-91.

DePippo KL, Holas MA, Reding MJ, Mandel FS, Lesser ML. Dysphagia therapy following stroke: a controlled trial. Neurology 1994a; 44: 1655-60.

DePippo KL, Holas MA, Reding MJ. The Burke Dysphagia Screening Test: validation of its use in patients with stroke. Archives of Physical Medical Rehabilitation 1994b; 75: 1284-6.

Edwards LL, Quigley EM, Harned RK, Hofman R, Pfeiffer RF. Characterization of swallowing and defecation in Parkinson's Disease. American Journal of Gastro-enterology 1994; 89: 15-25.

Elmstahl S, Bulow M, Ekberg O, Petersson M, Tenger H. Treatment of dysphagia improves nutritional conditions in stroke patients. Dysphagia 1999; 14: 61-6.

Ertekin C, Keskin A, Kiylioglu N, Kirazli Y, On AY, Tarlaci S, Aydogdu I. The effect of head and neck positions on oropharyngeal swallowing: a clinical and electrophysiologic study. Archives of Physical Medicine and Rehabilitation 2001; 82: 1255–60.

Evans-Morris S, Dunn Klein M. A Comprehensive Resource for Feeding Development. Arizona: Therapy Skill Builders, 1987.

Frazier JB, Friedman B. Swallow function in children with Down syndrome: a retrospective study. Developmental Medicine and Child Neurology 1996; 38: 695–703.

Freed ML, Freed L, Chatburn RL, Christian M. Electrical stimulation for swallowing disorders caused by stroke. Respiratory Care 2001; 46: 466–74.

Fuh JL, Lee RC, Wang SJ, Lin CH, Wang PN, Chiang JH et al. Swallowing difficulty in Parkinson's disease. Clinical Neurology and Neurosurgery 1997; 99: 106–112.

Garon BR, Engle M, Ormiston C. Reliability of the Three Ounce Water Swallow Test utilising cough reflex as sole indicator of aspiration. Journal of Neurologic Rehabilitation 1995; 9: 139–43.

Garon BR, Engle M, Ormiston C. Silent aspiration: results of 1000 videofluoroscopic swallow evaluations. Journal of Neurologic Rehabilitation 1996; 10: 121–6.

Garon BR, Engle M, Ormiston C. A randomised control study to determine the effects of unlimited oral intake of water in patients with identified aspiration. Journal of Neurologic Rehabilitation 1997; 11: 139–48.

Gisel EG. Oral motor skills following sensorimotor intervention in the moderately eating impaired child with cerebral palsy. Dysphagia 1994; 9: 180–92.

Gisel EG, Alphonce E. Classification of eating impairments based on eating efficiency in children with cerebral palsy. Dysphagia 1995; 10: 268–74.

Gisel EG, Applegate-Ferrante T, Benson J, Bosma JF. Oral-motor skills following sensorimotor therapy in two groups of moderately dysphagic children with cerebral palsy: aspiration vs nonaspiration. Dysphagia 1996; 11: 59–71.

Gisel EG, Haberfellner H, Schwartz S. Impact of oral appliance therapy: are oral skills and growth maintained one year after termination of therapy? Dysphagia 2001; 16: 296–307.

Gisel EG, Schwartz S, Petryk A, Clarke D, Haberfellner H. 'Whole body' mobility after one year of intraoral appliance therapy in children with cerebral palsy and moderate eating impairment. Dysphagia 2000; 15: 226–35.

Gordon C, Hewer RL, Wade DT. Dysphagia in acute stroke, British Medical Journal (Clinical Research Edition) 1987; 15: 295 (6595): 411–14.

Gottlieb D, Kipnis M, Sister E, Vardi Y, Brill S. Validation of the 50 ml^3 drinking test for evaluation of post-stroke dysphagia. Disability and Rehabilitation 1996; 18: 529–532.

Goulding R, Bakheit AM. Evaluation of the benefits of monitoring fluid thickness in the dietary management of dysphagic stroke patients. Clinical Rehabilitation 2000; 14: 119–24.

Groher ME. Bolus management and aspiration pneumonia in patients with pseudobulbar dysphagia. Dysphagia 1987; 1: 215–16.

Groher ME, Bukatman R. The prevalence of swallowing disorders in two hospitals. Dysphagia 1986; 1: 3–6.

Haberfellner H, Schwartz S, Gisel EG. Feeding skills and growth after one year of intraoral appliance therapy in moderately dysphagic children with cerebral palsy. Dysphagia 2001; 16: 83–96.

Hartelius L, Svensson P. Speech and swallowing symptoms associated with Parkinson's disease and multiple sclerosis: a survey. Folia Phoniatrica Logopedia 1994; 46: 9–17.

Hill AS, Kurkowski TB, Garcia J. Oral support measures used in feeding the preterm infant. Nursing Research 2000; 49: 2-10.

Hinds NP, Wiles CM. Assessment of swallowing and referral to speech and language therapists in acute stroke. QJM 1998; 91: 829-35.

Jones WB. Weight gain and feeding in the neonate with cleft: a three-center study. Cleft Palate Journal 1988; 25: 379-84.

Kagel MC, Leopold NA. Dysphagia in Huntington's disease: a 16 year retrospective. Dysphagia 1992; 7: 106-14.

Kasprisin AT, Clumeck H, Nino-Marcia M. The efficacy of rehabilitative management of dysphagia. Dysphagia 1989; 4: 48-52.

Kidd D, Lawson J, Nesbitt R, MacMahon J. Aspiration in acute stroke; a clinical study with videofluoroscopy. Quarterly Journal of Medicine 1993; 86: 825-9.

Larnert G, Ekberg O. Positioning improves the oral and pharyngeal swallowing function in children with cerebral palsy. Acta Paediatrica 1995; 84: 689-92.

Leder SB, Karas DE. Fiberoptic endoscopic evaluation of swallowing in the pediatric population. Laryngoscope 2000; 110: 1132-6.

Leighton SE, Burton MJ, Lund WS, Cochrane GM. Swallowing in motor neurone disease. Journal of the Royal Society of Medicine 1994; 87: 801-5.

List MA, Siston A, Haraf D, Schumm P, Kies M, Stenson K et al. Quality of life and performance in advanced head and neck cancer patients on concomitant chemoradiotherapy: a prospective examination. Journal of Clinical Oncology 1999; 17: 1020-1028.

Litvan I, Sastry N, Sonies BC. Characterising swallowing abnormalities in progressive supranuclear palsy. Neurology 1997; 48: 1654-62.

Logemann JA. Evaluation and Treatment of Swallowing Disorders. San Diego, CA: College Hill Press, 1983.

Logemann JA. Dysphagia: evaluation and treatment. Folia Phoniatrica et Logopedica 1995; 47: 140-64.

Logemann JA. Role of the modified barium swallow in management of patients with dysphagia. Otolaryngology, Head and Neck Surgery 1997; 116: 335-8.

Logemann JA. Evaluation and Treatment of Swallowing Disorders. Austin, TX: Pro-Ed, 1998.

Logemann JA. Do we know what is normal and abnormal airway protection? Dysphagia 1999; 14: 233-4.

Logemann JA, Kahrilias PJ. Relearning to swallow after stroke - application of maneuvers and indirect biofeedback: a case study. Neurology 1990; 40: 1136-1138.

Logemann JA, Kahrilas PJ, Kobara M, Vakil NB. The benefit of head rotation on pharyngoesophageal dysphagia. Archives of Physical Medicine and Rehabilitation 1989; 70: 767-71.

Logemann JA, Pauloski B, Rademaker A, Colangelo LA. Speech and swallowing rehabilitation for head and neck cancer patients. Oncology 1997; 11: 651-9.

Logemann JA, Rademaker A, Pauloski B, Kahrilas P. Effects of postural change on aspiration in head and neck surgical patients. Otolaryngology, Head and Neck Surgery 1994; 110: 222-27.

Logemann JA, Roa Pauloski B, Rademaker A, Cook B, Graner D, Milianti F, Beery Q, Stein D, Bowman J, Lazarus C. Impact of the diagnostic procedure on outcome measures of swallowing rehabilitation in head and neck cancer patients. Dysphagia 1992; 4: 179-86.

Logemann J, Veis S, Colangelo L. A screening procedure for oropharyngeal dysphagia. Dysphagia 1999; 14: 44-51.

McCullough GH, Wertz RT, Rosenbek JC, Dinneen C. Clinicians preferences and practices in conducting clinical/bedside and videofluorscopic swallowing examinations in an adult, neurogenic population. American Journal of Speech and Language Pathology 1999; 8: 149-63.

McCullough GH, Wertz RT, Rosenbek JC, Mills RH, Webb WG, Ross KB. Inter- and intrajudge reliability for videofluoroscopic swallowing evaluation measures. Dysphagia 2001; 16: 110-18.

Mann G, Hankey GJ, Cameron D. Swallowing function after stroke: prognosis and prognostic factors at six months. Stroke 1999; 4: 744-8.

Mann G, Hankey GJ, Cameron D. Swallowing disorders following acute stroke: prevalence and diagnostic accuracy. Cerebro-vascular diseases 2000; 5: 380-6.

Martens L, Cameron T, Simonsen M. Effects of a multidisciplinary management program on neurologically impaired patients with dysphagia. Dysphagia 1990; 5: 147-51.

Martino R, Pron G, Diamant N. Screening for oropharyngeal dysphagia in stroke: insufficient evidence for guidelines. Dysphagia 2000; 15: 19-30.

Martin-Harris B. The evolution of the evaluation and treatment of dysphagia across the Health Care continuum: a historical perspective - inception to proliferation. Nutrition in Clinical Practice 1999; 14 (Suppl.): S13-S19.

Martin-Harris B, Logemann JA, McMahon S, Scheicher M, Sandidge J. Clinical utility of the modified barium swallow. Dysphagia 2000; 15: 136-41.

Mayberry JF, Atkinson M. Swallowing problems in patients with motor neurone disease, Journal of Clinical Gastro-enterology 1986; 8: 233-4.

Morgan A, Ward E, Murdoch B. Incidence, characteristics and predictive factors for dysphagia following paediatric traumatic brain injury. Journal of Head Trauma Rehabilitation (in press).

Morton RE, Bonas R, Minford J, Kerr A, Ellis RE. Feeding ability in Rett syndrome. Developmental Medicine and Child Neurology 1997; 39: 331-5.

National Institute of Deafness and Other Communication Disorders (NIDOCD). National Strategic Research Plan for Language and Language Impairments, Balance and Balance Disorders, and Voice and Voice Disorders (NIH Publication No. 97-3217). Bethesda, MD, 1995.

Nilsson H, Ekberg O, Olsson R, Hindfelt B. Dysphagia in stroke: a prospective study of quantitative aspects of swallowing in dysphagia patients. Dysphagia 1998; 13: 32-8.

Ohmae Y, Ogura M, Kitahara S, Karaho T, Inouye T. Effects of head rotation on pharyngeal function during normal swallow. Annals of Otology, Rhinology and Laryngology 1998; 107: 344-8.

Pauloski BP, Logemann JA, Colangelo LA, Stein D, Beery Q, Heiser MA et al. Effective intra-oral prostheses on swallowing function in post-surgical oral and oropharyngeal cancer patients. American Journal of Speech Language Pathology 1996; 5: 31-46.

Perry L, Love CP. Screening for dysphagia and aspiration in acute stroke: a systematic review. Dysphagia 2001; 16: 7-18.

Pinelli J, Symington A, Ciliska D. Non-nutritive sucking in high-risk infants: benign intervention or legitimate therapy. Journal of Obstetric and Gynaecological Neonatal Nursing 2002; 31: 582-91.

Ramritu P, Finlayson K, Mitchell A, Croft G. Identification and Nursing Management of Dysphagia in Individuals with Neurological Impairment No 8. Adelaide: The Joanna Briggs Institute for Evidence Based Nursing & Midwifery, 2000.

Rasley A, Logemann JA, Kahrilas PJ, Rademaker AW, Pauloski BR, Dodds WJ. Prevention of barium aspiration during videofluoroscopic swallowing studies: value of change in posture. American Journal of Roentgenology 1993; 160: 1005-9.

Reilly S, Cass H. Growth and nutrition in Rett syndrome. Journal of Disability and Rehabilitation 2001; 23: 118-28.

Reilly S, Perry A. Is there an evidence base to the management of paediatric dysphagia? Asia Pacific Journal of Speech, Language and Hearing 2001; 6: 1-8.

Reilly S, Skuse D, Poblete X. Prevalence of feeding problems and oral motor dysfunction in children with cerebral palsy: a community survey. Journal of Paediatrics 1996; 129: 877-82.

Reilly S, Skuse DH, Wolke D. SOMA: The Schedule of Oral Motor Assessment. London: Whurr Publishers, 2000.

Reynolds PS, Gilbert L, Good DC, Knappertz VA, Crenshaw C, Wane SL, Pillbury D, Teqeler CH. Pneumonia in dysphagic stroke patients: effect on outcomes and identification of high-risk patients. Journal of Neurologic Rehabilitation 1998; 12: 15-21.

Sackett DL, Haynes RB, Guyatt GH, Tugwell P. Clinical Epidemiology – A Basic Science for Clinical Medicine. London: Little, Brown, 1991; 305-33.

Sackett DL, Richardson WS, Rosenberg WMC, Haynes RB. Evidence Based Medicine. London: Churchill-Livingstone, 1997.

Scott A, Perry A, Bench J. A study of inter-scorer reliability when using videofluoroscopy as an assessment of swallowing. Dysphagia 1998; 13: 223-7.

Schwartz SM, Corredor J, Fisher-Medina J, Cohen J, Rabinowitz S. Diagnosis and treatment of feeding disorders in children with developmental disabilities. Pediatrics 2001; 108: 671-6.

Schmidt J, Holas M, Halvorson K, Reding M. Videofluoroscopic evidence of aspiration predicts pneumonia and death but not hydration following stroke. Dysphagia 1994; 9: 7-11.

Schurr MJ, Ebner KA, Maser AL, Sperling KB, Helgerson RB, Harms B. Formal swallowing evaluation and therapy after traumatic brain injury improves dysphagia outcomes. Journal of Trauma 1999; 46: 817-23.

Shaw WC, Bannister RP, Roberts CT. Assisted feeding is more reliable for infants with clefts – a randomised trial. Cleft Palate and Craniofacial Journal 1999; 36: 262-8.

Siebens H, Trupe E, Seibens A, Cook F, Anschen S, Hanauer R, Oster G. Correlates and consequences of eating dependency in institutionalised elderly. Journal of American Geriatrics Society 1986; 34: 192-8.

Singer C, Weiner WJ, Sanchez-Ramos JR. Autonomic dysfucntion in men with Parkinson's disease. European Neurology 1992; 32: 134-40.

Smith CH, Logemann JA, Colangelo LA, Rademaker AW, Pauloski BR. Incidence and patient characteristics associated with silent aspiration in the acute care setting. Dysphagia 1999; 14: 1-7.

Smithard DG, O'Neill PA, Parks C, Morris J. Complications and outcomes after stroke. Does dysphagia matter? Stroke 1996; 27: 1200-04.

Spender Q, Stein A, Dennis J, Reilly S, Percy E, Cave D. An exploration of feeding difficulties in children with Down syndrome. Developmental Medicine and Child Neurology 1996; 38: 681-94.

Sullivan PB, Lambert B, Rose M, Ford-Adams M, Johnson A, Griffiths P. Prevalence and severity of feeding and nutritional problems in children with neurological impairment:

Oxford Feeding Study. Developmental Medicine and Child Neurology 2000; 42: 674-80.

Thommesen M, Heiberg A, Kase BF, Larsson S, Riis G. Feeding problems, height and weight in different groups of disabled children. Acta Paediatrica Scandinavia 1991; 80: 527-33.

Taniguchi MH, Moyer RS. Assessment of risk factors for pneumonia in dysphagic children. Significance of videofluroscopy swallowing evaluation. Developmental Medicine and Child Neurology 1994; 36(6): 495-502.

Trenouth MJ, Campbell AN. Questionnaire evaluation of feeding methods for cleft lip and palate neonates. International Journal of Pediatric Dentistry 1996; 6: 241-4.

UK Screening Committee. Second report of the UK National Screening Committee 1998, April: http://www.nsc.nhs.uk/pdfs/second report.pdf.

Volicer L, Seltzer B, Rheaume Y, Karner J, Glennon M, Riley ME, Crino P. Eating difficulties in patients with probable dementia of the Alzheimer type. Journal of Geriatric Psychiatry Neurology 1989; 2: 188-95.

Wade DT, Hewer RL. Motor loss and swallowing difficulty after stroke: frequency, recovery, and prognosis. Acta Neurologica Scandinavica 1987; 76: 50-4.

Warms T, Richards K. 'Wet voice' as a predictor of penetration and aspiration in oropharyngeal dysphagia. Dysphagia 2000; 15: 84-88.

Willig TN, Paulus J, Lacau Saint Guily J, Beon C, Navarro J. Swallowing problems in neuromuscular disorders. Archives of Physical Medicine and Rehabilitation 1994; 75: 1175-81.

Wintzen AR, Badrising UA, Roos RA, Vielvoye J, Liauw L, Pouwels EK. Dysphagia in ambulant patients with Parkinson's disease: common, not dangerous. Canadian Journal of Neurological Science 1994; 21: 53-6.

Williams K, Mellis C. Putting evidence into practice. In: Moyer VA, Elliott EJ, Davis RL, Gilbert R, Klassen T, Logan S et al. (eds) Evidence Based Paediatrics and Child Health. London: BMJ Books, 2000.

CHAPTER **8**

The evidence base for the diagnosis of developmental language disorders: research to clinical practice

PATRICIA EADIE

Introduction: developmental language disorders in context

This chapter discusses the emergence of evidence from the research literature regarding the diagnosis of developmental language disorders. Evidence is defined as 'the best available external clinical evidence from systematic research' (Sackett et al., 1996, p. 1). However, this chapter is particularly concerned with how recent research evidence may enable speech pathologists to incorporate more effective and efficient procedures into clinical assessment practice.

The chapter begins with a discussion of definitions of developmental language disorders and the diagnostic criteria that accompany them. Diagnostic criteria are then presented for specific language impairment, a subgroup of the larger group of children with developmental language disorders. Diagnosis in specific language impairment is based primarily on a set of exclusionary criteria and, as a consequence, little has been known about the underlying nature of the impairment. It has become apparent that however useful the exclusionary criteria have been in delineating children with specific language impairment, the criteria have not enabled the linking of cause with the consequence of language impairment. In addition, well-controlled cohort studies have suggested that some of these exclusionary criteria (for example, cognitive-language performance gaps) should not be used for diagnostic purposes. On a more positive note, recent research has revealed inclusionary criteria and ways to assess them, which, it will be argued, are more suitable for diagnostic purposes. The evidence for using these inclusionary criteria in clinical practice will be reviewed and discussed.

Defining developmental language disorder

Developmental language impairment occurs when there is a disruption in the normally accepted sequence and timing of the onset of language in the first years of life. Prevalence figures for developmental language impairment vary between 3% and 12% of the general population (Beitchman et al., 1986; Harasty and Reed, 1994). Children with developmental language disorders present with different aetiologies and very different skills across language parameters. Known causes of developmental language disorders include hearing loss, motor and intellectual disability, and neurological disorders.

Historical context

Inadequate language development has been given many different names over the last 100 years. Terms reflect the underlying theories and postulated causes of the language impairment at a particular point in time (for example, 'developmental dysphasia' versus 'specific language impairment'). Differences in terminology also reflect the different professional groups involved in investigating and diagnosing the impairment (for example, linguists, psychologists and speech pathologists). Lastly, as the symptoms of the impairment change over time, so can the label used to describe them. For example, the pre-school child with a language delay may become an 'adolescent with a learning disability'. In the 1990s alone, the following terms were used to define children who were not developing language normally:

- language-delayed (Cole et al., 1990)
- language-impaired (Curtiss, 1991; Rice et al., 1991; Fletcher, 1992)
- developmental language disorder (Tallal, 1991; Aram et al., 1992; Kamhi, 1998)
- language-disordered (Miller, 1991; Friel-Patti, 1992)
- specific language impairment (Aram et al., 1993; Fey, Long and Cleave, 1994; Rice and Wexler, 1996; Leonard et al., 1997).

Johnston (1988) points out that terminology is more likely to reflect the theoretical orientation of the author than a change in the population being referred to. However, the lack of agreement amongst researchers on what this group of children with language impairment should be called reflects a deeper problem with the absence of explicit criteria (Fazio et al., 1996) and arbitrary measures by which the impairment is to be diagnosed.

Definitions and diagnostic criteria

Definitions of language disorders are plentiful in the literature; for example, the American Speech–Language–Hearing Association (ASHA) has defined a language disorder as an impairment in:

> Comprehension and/or use of a spoken, written, and/or other symbol system. The disorder may involve (1) the form of language (phonologic, morphologic, and syntactic systems), (2) the content of language (semantic system), and/or (3) the function of language in communication (pragmatic system), in any combination. (ASHA, 1993, p. 40)

This definition describes language symptoms but provides no criteria on which to diagnose the disorder or discriminate children with different aetiologies. Consequently, as comprehensive as the definition is, it does not provide speech pathologists with criteria upon which to decide whether or not a language disorder is present.

Alternatively, both the World Health Organization (WHO) and the American Psychiatric Association (APA) have attempted to provide definitions of expressive and receptive language disorders with diagnostic criteria. Both the *Diagnostic and Statistical Manual of the Mental Disorders* (DSM-IV) (APA, 1994) and the *ICD-10* (WHO, 1992) separate specific language impairments from the language disorders where mental retardation, a speech-motor or sensory deficit, or environmental deprivation is present. In so doing they delineate the group of children with specific language impairment. The clinical utility of the term 'specific language impairment' has been much discussed (for example, see Kamhi, 1998); however, it is clear that there exists a group of children, who in the absence of any other problems find learning language considerably difficult.

Consequently, *ICD-10* (WHO, 1992, p. 265) provides a definition of specific expressive language disorder where 'the child's ability to use expressive spoken language is markedly below the appropriate level for its mental age, but in which language comprehension is within normal limits'. The accompanying diagnostic criteria include:

- Expressive language performance on standardized tests being below two standard deviations for the child's age.
- Expressive language skills that are at least one standard deviation below non-verbal IQ as assessed on standardized tests.
- Receptive language performance on standardized tests being within two standard deviations for the child's age.
- Normal use and understanding of non-verbal communication and imaginative language.

- No neurological, sensory, or physical impairment that affects language and no pervasive developmental disorder.

Similarly, a definition and diagnostic criteria are included for receptive language disorder. In comparison, the *DSM-IV* (APA, 1994) delineates the following diagnostic criteria for expressive language disorder:

- Scores obtained from standardized measures of expressive language are substantially below those obtained on standardized measures of non-verbal IQ and receptive language (the criterion continues by describing limited vocabulary, tense errors, recalling words, and producing sentences of appropriate complexity as possible clinical symptoms).
- Expressive language difficulties interfere with academic or occupational achievement or with social communication.
- Criteria not met for mixed receptive–expressive language disorder, pervasive developmental disorder.
- No mental retardation, speech-motor or sensory deficit, or environmental deprivation is present.

The difference in the *ICD-10* (WHO, 1992) approach, which is also mirrored in the definitions and diagnostic criteria of the *DSM-IV* (APA, 1994), is the explicit nature of the assessment required and the nature of the cognitive-language performance gap. In the speech pathology literature this method of diagnosing a specific language impairment has become known as 'cognitive referencing'. The use of cognitive referencing has been the subject of much research and clinical debate and there is now a body of research evidence attesting to problems in the use of this particular diagnostic criterion. This evidence has been primarily of a controlled cohort nature without randomization. The detailed cognitive and language assessments required for a diagnosis of language impairment based on cognitive referencing principles constrains the participants to those children requiring full diagnostic assessments, that is, clinical populations.

Research practice: diagnostic criteria of specific language impairment

Before reviewing the research literature with regard to cognitive referencing it is important to determine the basis upon which children are determined to have specific language impairment for research purposes. With few exceptions, research conducted to date has not used the prescribed criteria of the *ICD-10* (WHO, 1992) or the *DSM-IV* (APA, 1994). The majority of research conducted with children with specific language impairment in the past 15 years has used the work of Stark and Tallal (1981) to identify the language skills component of the diagnosis. Stark and Tallal (1981, p. 117) suggested a criterion that required the child 'to have an overall language age (LA) at least 12 months lower than their chronological age (CA) or their performance mental age (MAP) whichever was lower'. The language age was an average of the child's receptive and expressive language ages, as defined on a specific set of language assessment instruments, including the *Test of Auditory Comprehension of Language* (Carrow, 1972) and *The Token Test* (DiSimoni, 1978). Stark and Tallal (1981, p. 121) were forthright in their conclusion that 'a representative set of language tests is needed for selection purposes, not one alone'.

Most research, although retaining the general premise of a language gap when compared to chronological age or performance mental age, has been flexible in deriving its own definition of language impairment and the assessment tools used to confirm it. The result of this flexibility has been significant variability across studies in the criterion used to define the language impairment. Given current knowledge about the psychometric problems of the use of age scores, most language scores are now determined by and reported as standard scores. Recent studies involving children with specific language impairment consistently use the quantitative definition of at least one standard deviation below the mean, but vary considerably on whether they use one or more standardized measures and whether the impairment needs to be across both receptive and expressive language domains. In addition, the ecological validity of language sampling (Dunn et al., 1996), has meant that this less formal procedure is now also used in establishing the severity of the language impairment and the eventual diagnosis of specific language impairment.

What is clear, is that inherent within the definition of specific language impairment, is the acceptance that a cognitive age–language age gap will be present. There is some research evidence emerging to question this assumption, from both an assessment (Eadie, 1999) and therapeutic (Fey, Long, et al., 1994) perspective. However, regardless of the specific criterion used (for example, Stark and Tallal, 1981; APA, 1994) researchers consistently look for the discrepancy in IQ and language performance, that is cognitive referencing.

Cognitive referencing: what the study of children with developmental language disorders and specific language impairment has revealed

'Cognitive referencing' refers to the requirement that in order to qualify for speech and language services, children's cognitive performance must be higher than their language performance. If the two are equal the child is considered to be a poor candidate to improve during language intervention. Cognitive referencing as a model used to determine who receives intervention has been widely criticized (*see* Cole and Fey, 1996 for a complete review) not least because of weaknesses in the psychometric methods on which it is based.

In a series of studies investigating the stability of the relation between measures of cognition and language, Cole and colleagues have consistently reported unstable assessment results and significant problems with the theoretical model of cognitive referencing *per se* (Cole et al., 1990; Cole et al., 1992; Cole et al., 1994; Cole and Mills, 1997). For example, Cole et al. (1994) measured IQ by use of the *Columbia Mental Maturity Scale* (CMMS) (Burgmeister et al., 1972) and the *McCarthy Scales of Children's Abilities* (MSCA) (McCarthy, 1972) in 26 children who were developmentally delayed, diagnosed by a delay in two or more developmental areas, one of which was language. Despite these IQ tests purporting to measure the same general construct significant differences occurred in the results obtained (for example, CMMS mean IQ of 79.4; MSCA mean IQ of 61.2). In addition, the tests did not result in a consistent relative ranking of the individual participants by IQ.

Cole et al. (1994) also examined the likelihood of these same children qualifying for speech pathology services, based on a cognitive referencing model, where language testing results were poorer than measured IQ. Of concern was the lack of stability in the relation when different tests were used. Eligibility for speech and language pathology services varied from 11% to 84% of the participants. Such variability is concerning not only because of the service implications but because of the ramifications with regard to the reliability and validity of measures of language and cognition in children with language impairments. Cole and Mills (1997) continued by examining the stability of assessment profiles when different pairs of IQ and language tests were used. IQ measures included the *Leiter International Performance Scale* (LIPS) (Leiter, 1969), the MSCA (McCarthy, 1972) and the *Wechsler Preschool and Primary Scale of Intelligence* (WPPSI) (Wechsler, 1967), whereas the *Peabody Picture Vocabulary Test - Revised* (PPVT-R) (Dunn and Dunn, 1981), the *Test of Auditory Comprehension of Language - Revised* (TACL-R) (Carrow-Woolfolk, 1985) and the *Test of Early Language Development* (TELD) (Hresko et al., 1981) were the language measures administered.

The results demonstrated eligibility classifications, based on the different pairings of tests, ranged from 0% to 41%, with the MSCA–TACL profile identifying none of the children as eligible for intervention services. It is important to note that all participants in this study were part of a special education preschool programme and all had qualified under state guidelines as language-impaired with a minimum 1.5 standard deviation delay on at least one standardized language measure. As the authors concluded, the critical problem with cognitive referencing is demonstrated in the number of children with language impairment being denied services 'on the basis of an IQ/LQ profile that will change substantially with the use of different, but equally acceptable, assessment tools' (Cole and Mills, 1997, p. 128).

In one of the few studies to examine the stability of different definitions of the IQ criterion in diagnosing specific language impairment, Cole et al. (1995) found that significant differences between percentage IQs of children with specific language impairment over time altered the classification of them as having specific language impairment or not. Two methods of diagnosing specific language impairment by use of the *DSM III-R* (APA, 1987) criterion were compared, with one group adhering strictly to the *DSM III-R* criteria and the other requiring an absolute cut-off score but a difference between the overall cognitive and language performances. Twenty-two children with specific language impairment and 26 children with developmental lag language impairment participated in the study and were assessed on three occasions over a two-year period. The MSCA (McCarthy, 1972) was used as the IQ measure and significant decreases in the test results were found for the specific language impairment group without cognitive referencing between testing at times two and three, and times one and three. Results for the stability of the diagnosis of specific language impairment were quite remarkable. Over the three test periods only 23% of children originally diagnosed as having specific language impairment remained so. For the groups of children where the definition included a cognitive referencing component of at least one standard deviation difference between IQ and LQ scores, a significant decrease in MSCA was detected between time one and three for the children with specific language impairment. Again, the stability of the specific language impairment diagnosis was concerning with no child remaining in the specific language impairment group across all three assessment times; however, eight of the children, or 44% of the specific language impairment group, received a category of 'not delayed' by test time three. As Cole et al. (1995) pointed out, these results indicated instability in measurement more than real changes in the children's diagnostic classifications. Additional research that examines Performance IQ measurement both across tests and over time is needed to determine which standardized intelligence measures are likely to optimize performance and stability.

Consequently, if intelligence is to be a useful factor in describing language impairment then research must be able to demonstrate both its validity as an exclusionary criterion and the reliability of its measurement for children with language impairments. Although much is made of the difference between children with normal IQ and low language achievement and those children with below-average performance in both IQ and language, particularly in the specific language impairment literature, this difference is still largely assumed rather than proven. As Cole and Fey (1996, p.147) comment, 'it is remarkable that there has been so little experimental attention devoted to the assumption's verification'. What research has been conducted questions both the validity and the stability of intelligence quotients with this population (Cole and Harris, 1992; Cole et al., 1994; Fey, Cleave, et al., 1994). Discrepancy criteria have been shown to under-identify children with specific language impairment (Aram et al., 1993; Cole et al., 1995). Discrepancy models assume first, that language and non-verbal intelligence scores should be at the same level in normal children, and second, that if differences do exist in normal children then they are no larger than one standard deviation. There is little empirical evidence currently available that validates either assumption (Dunn et al., 1996). Further investigations exploring the relation between intelligence and specific language impairment are required to resolve these issues.

The search for inclusionary criteria in the diagnosis of specific language impairment

Despite the growing evidence questioning the validity of some of the diagnostic criteria, the primary definition of specific language impairment has relied on exclusion, and as a consequence, for many years little has been known about the underlying nature of the impairment (Lahey and Edwards, 1995). Current research trends have focused on addressing causation as well as the surface linguistic features of the language impairment. Research has been motivated to find inclusionary criteria that link the hypothesized causal factors to the linguistic output of children with specific language impairment. This research has attempted to validate the diagnostic category of specific language impairment by establishing inclusionary criteria, such as linguistic clinical markers.

To this end, the surface characteristics of the language of children with specific language impairment have been the focus of much research attention. No one area of the language skills of children with specific language impairment has been studied as extensively as grammatical morphology, particularly in the 1990s. It should be noted at the outset that differences between children with specific language impairment and children developing normally have been found to be far more significant in grammatical morphology than the differences noted in any of the other language parameters (Leonard, 1989; Fletcher, 1992). Dissociations between morphology and other language skill areas have also been documented in a generational study of an English-speaking family with specific language impairment (Gopnik and Crago, 1991) and by Moore and Johnston (1993). There is now a large body of literature that attests to the marked problems in grammatical morphology experienced by children with specific language impairment (Leonard, 1992; Rice and Oetting, 1993; Rice and Wexler, 1996; Leonard et al., 1997).

The verb system of children with specific language impairment has been the particular focus of much research. Early studies investigated the lexical nature of the verb system before investigating the morphosyntactic characteristics of children with specific language impairment. Investigations have demonstrated a deficit in the verb learning abilities of children with specific language impairment compared to their normally developing language-matched peers (Fletcher and Peters, 1984; Rice and Bode, 1993; Watkins et al., 1993; Oetting et al., 1995). Watkins et al. (1993) found that children with specific language impairment had a less diverse main verb lexicon when compared to both age- and language-matched peers. This study suggested that 5-year-old children with specific language impairment demonstrated less verb diversity than that expected of 3-year-old children at the same language level. Rice and Bode (1993) followed up this study with a detailed investigation of the verb lexicons of three pre-school boys with specific language impairment and found a small set of general all-purpose (GAP) verbs accounted for up to 50% of all verb use. These verbs corresponded to some of the earliest developing and most frequently used verbs in adult speech (for example, *want*, *go*, *get*, *do*, *put*, *need*, *come*, *did*, *look*, *make* and *work*). Verb errors frequently involved overuse of this set of GAP verbs.

Jones and Conti-Ramsden (1997) studied the verb use of three children with specific language impairment over a two-year period using their language matched younger siblings for comparison. Results indicated that, by the end of the two-year period, the size of the verb lexicons for the children in both groups were similar. However, during the latter part of the study there was a point where the younger siblings started using the verbs they knew more often and in a greater variety of forms than the children with specific language impairment. Jones and Conti-Ramsden (1997) suggest that the children with specific language impairment were deficient when compared to their younger siblings in generalizing knowledge of verb forms across different numbers of verbs. Certainly this pattern of verb use would influence the later morphological difficulties of children with specific language impairment. Conti-Ramsden and Jones (1997) then went on to compare the verb use of children with specific language impairment with a non-related language-matched control group. Again, sampling took place over a two-year period. The data revealed that children with specific language impairment used fewer verbs and fewer different verbs than their language-matched peers. The children with specific language impairment in this study did not rely more heavily on GAP verbs, as was suggested in the findings of Rice and Bode (1993), with usage of GAP verbs being similar across the two groups.

Studies investigating the grammatical morphology of children with specific language impairment have demonstrated a similar order of acquisition to normally developing children (Johnston and Schery, 1976; Leonard, 1979; Curtiss et al., 1992; Lahey et al., 1992), but differences in the time taken to achieve consistent use and in the overall error rates when compared to language-matched younger normally developing children (Johnston and Schery, 1976; Johnston and Kamhi, 1984; Curtiss et al., 1992; Lahey et al., 1992).

Not all grammatical morphemes appear equally affected in the language of children with specific language impairment. Although grammatical morphemes that mark tense and agreement have been widely and consistently demonstrated to be most problematic for children with specific language impairment (Khan and James, 1983; Johnston and Kamhi, 1984; Frome Loeb and Leonard, 1991; Rice and Wexler, 1996; Cleave and Rice, 1997), conflicting evidence characterizes the performance of children with specific language impairment on non-tense grammatical morphemes (Johnston and Schery, 1976; Khan and James, 1983; Lahey et al., 1992; Rice and Wexler, 1996; Leonard et al., 1997). Performance is generally characterized by omission of the obligatory markers of tense and agreement. The errors noted in the grammatical morphology of children with specific language impairment have been demonstrated to be rare but similar to those of younger children developing normally (Leonard, 1992; Rice et al., 1995).

In summary, most research detailing the linguistic characteristics of children with specific language impairment has been of a controlled cohort nature, using children with specific language impairment from clinical populations along with both age- and language-matched control subjects. This type of evidence lacks the strength of a well-controlled randomized trial, but pragmatically, provides good guidance for clinical practice. What has emerged throughout the 1990s is a set of inclusionary diagnostic criteria that can be adopted into clinical practice for preschool and early school-age children with language impairments. These studies were all controlled trials without randomization and are summarized in Table 8.1. Inclusionary criteria are more informative from both a diagnostic and intervention planning perspective. Ensuring they are readily assessable in everyday clinical practice is a remaining challenge.

Table 8.1 Description of the studies and level of evidence for the diagnostic criterion for specific language impairment

Diagnostic criterion for specific language impairment	Reference	Participants	Outcomes	Level of evidence Study type	Level
Weak use of grammatical morphology	Bedore and Leonard (1998)	SLI and age control subjects	Age>SLI	Controlled trial without randomization	III.1
	Goffman and Leonard (2000)	SLI, age and MLU control subjects	Age>MLU>SLI	Cohort study	III.2
	Rice and Wexler (1996)	SLI, age and MLU control subjects	Age> MLU>SLI	Controlled trial without randomization	III.1
	Eadie (1999)	SLI, DS and MLU control subjects	MLU>SLI=DS	Controlled trial without randomization	III.1
Verb elicitation task	Frome, Loeb et al, (1996)	SLI, age and MLU control subjects	Age>SLI>MLU	Controlled trial without randomization	III.2
	Klimacka and Brunger (1999)	SLI	Probe data = transcription data	Opinion based on research experience	IV
	Rice, Wexler and Hershberger (1998)	SLI and age controls	Probe data = transcription data	Controlled trial without randomization	III.2

(contd)

Table 8.1 (contd)

Diagnostic criterion for specific language impairment	Reference	Participants	Outcomes	Level of evidence Study type	Level
Processing skills (performance on non-word repetition)	Dollaghan and Campbell (1998)	SLI and age controls	Age > SLI	Controlled trial without randomization	III.2
	Montgomery and Leonard (1998)	SLI, age and receptive language controls	Age = RL > SLI	Controlled trial without randomization	III.2
	Adams and Gathercole (2000)	ND children with relatively good or poor language skills	Good language > Poor language	Controlled trial without randomization	III.2

MLU = minimum length of utterance; SLI = specific language impairment; ND = normally developing.

Clinical practice: diagnostic criteria of specific language impairment

Weak use of grammatical morphology as a clinical marker

It is clear that there is now a great deal of evidence that suggests that an inclusionary diagnostic criterion of specific language impairment lies in these children's production of grammatical morphology, at least for children acquiring English. Their use of morphemes associated with tense (for example, past tense [-ed], third person singular [3s], copular and auxiliary [BE]) has been shown to be even more consistently poor and more resistant to remedial efforts than has the use of other morphemes, such as plural and possessive, -s, or progressive, -ing (Rice and Wexler, 1996; Bedore and Leonard, 1998; Goffman and Leonard, 2000). Thus, Bedore and Leonard (1998) and Rice and Wexler (1996) have suggested that especially weak use of tense-related morphology is a phenotypic marker of specific language impairment.

What is the importance of a clinical marker for specific language impairment to evidence-based assessment practices? Primarily, the answer lies in the uncovering through this line of research of two highly robust inclusionary diagnostic criteria. First, the research that has identified the clinical marker has demonstrated that the elicitation of verb morphology is a reliable and valid procedure to assess this language component (Frome Loeb et al., 1996; Rice, Wexler and Hershberger, 1998; Klimacka and Brunger, 1999). Second, research attempts to account for the grammatical morphology deficits of children with specific language impairment have uncovered processing deficits, such as those proposed in deficits of phonological memory (Gathercole and Baddeley, 1990). Moreover, there is preliminary evidence available that tasks such as non-word repetition may prove to be good screening measures and predictive of language impairment in children (Bishop et al., 1995; Dollaghan and Campbell, 1998; Laws, 1998).

Research evidence advocating the use of verb elicitation tasks in the diagnosis of specific language impairment

There is now no doubt about the vulnerability of the verb system in children with specific language impairment. Both the range of verbs the children have to use and their ability to encode morphosyntactic information with them is affected. Clearly, then, the use of efficient and proven measures of the verb lexicon and morphosyntax are now acknowledged as critical to the diagnostic process.

The use of elicitation procedures is not new to the field of speech pathology. Elicitation can take many forms. The use of story books, games, picture presentation are all variations that can be used to elicit language. In this discussion, it will be argued that research has demonstrated elicitation tasks to be sensitive and efficient measures of the verb system in children with specific language impairment. Spontaneous language sampling and analysis can also be used for assessing the verb system, as can standardized assessments. The former measure has been demonstrated to be more sensitive than the latter in a study by Dunn et al. (1996). However, it needs to be acknowledged that language sampling and analysis is a time-consuming procedure that can often not lead to enough tokens of a particular language structure being observed. In turn, this makes it difficult for clinicians to conclude with certainty whether or not the structure in question is within the child's repertoire. Alternatively, standardized assessments generally offer insufficient items per language structure from which to make generalizations about productive use. Frome Loeb et al. (1996), Rice, Wexler and Hershberger (1998) and Klimacka and Brunger (1999) have advocated the use of elicitation probes. The authors argue that the research probes have been an accurate and, in the case of Rice (1998), sensitive measure of the verb system in children with specific language impairment. In our own research (Eadie, 1999), morphology probes were used from the *Wiig Criterion Referenced Inventory of Language* (Wiig, 1990) in conjunction with spontaneous language measures, and found to be effective.

What information we have available on verb elicitation is encouraging. The challenge for clinical practice is to provide more evidence from more diverse groups of children that verb elicitation probes are indeed as valid as initial limited controlled studies have suggested. The recent publication of the *Rice-Wexler Test of Early Grammatical Impairment* (TEGI) (Rice and Wexler, 2001) which yields criterion-referenced diagnostic information indicates that this avenue is promising.

Research evidence of processing skills affecting the language skills of children with specific language impairment

Research evidence attesting to subtle deficits in the non-linguistic skills of children with specific language impairment are 'now so commonplace that no theory of specific language impairment can be truly comprehensive without taking them into account' (Leonard, 1998, p. 237). Research has demonstrated that in the areas of lexical learning (Ellis Weismer and Hesketh, 1993; Ellis Weismer and Hesketh, 1996), comprehension (Bishop and Adams, 1992; Stark and Montgomery, 1995) and production (Leonard et al., 1983; McGregor and Leonard, 1994; Bortolini and Leonard, 1996) evidence exists for the relationship between processing capacity limitations and language differences between children with specific language impairment and their normally developing peers. It has now been consistently demonstrated that children with specific language impairment have significant difficulties with the manipulation of auditory–verbal information (Dollaghan, 1987; Bishop et al., 1996; Edwards and Lahey, 1996; Dollaghan and Campbell, 1998; Montgomery and Leonard, 1998; Bishop et al., 1999; Ellis Weismer et al., 1999; Ellis Weismer et al., 2000).

Such research allows diagnosis to move beyond surface characteristics and focus on the underlying deficit in the language learning process. Kamhi (1998, p. 41) has already suggested a 'basic-processing deficit' as one possible way to redefine specific language impairment. This would reduce the reliance on some of the more unreliable exclusionary criteria (for example, 85 or above performance IQ). Hence the interest in non-word repetition tasks as measures of the 'basic-processing deficit'; i.e. phonological working memory. Dollaghan and Campbell (1998) replicated previous research and demonstrated that school-aged children with language impairments had poorer non-word repetition performance than their age-matched peers. More critical to the present discussion, however, was their finding that the non-word repetition task distinguished between children with and without language impairments to a higher degree of accuracy than a traditional standardized language test. Ellis Weismer et al. (2000) found that second-grade children with specific language impairment were nearly three times more likely to fail a non-word repetition task than were same-age peers with normal language. The research groups of Bishop, Ellis Weismer and Tager-Flusberg have all suggested that non-word repetition performance may provide a phenotypic marker for developmental language impairment, irrespective of performance intelligence.

It is important to note that similar relationships between non-word repetition and language impairment have been demonstrated in other groups of children with developmental language disorders. Laws (1998) demonstrated similar findings for children with Down syndrome. Non-word repetition was significantly related to receptive vocabulary, language comprehension and reading when age and non-verbal ability were controlled for. Laws' (1998) results suggest that non-word repetition is a predictor of language comprehension and reading ability in children with Down syndrome and lends some support to the argument of Fowler (1995) that language impairments in children with Down syndrome are directly related to difficulties encoding acoustic information. Kjelgaard and Tager-Flusberg (2001) also reported a pattern of poor performance on phonological tasks similar to non-word repetition in a group of children with autism.

Last, the sensitivity of non-word repetition tasks in the identification of language impairment has been demonstrated in two other related studies. Bishop et al. (1999) conducted a twin study investigating the heritability of speech and language disorder. One interest of the study was to find a clinical marker of heritability of speech and language disorder that was sensitive regardless of whether the manifestation of the disorder was current or 'resolved'. One measure used in the study was *The Children's Test of Nonword Repetition* (Gathercole and Baddeley, 1996). Analysis of the performance of the twin pairs on this task demonstrated that it was indeed sensitive to both current and resolved language disorder. DeFries-Fulker analysis of heritability on this data yielded a factor in excess of one. More recently, Adams and Gathercole (2000) used the non-word repetition task to demonstrate language differences in normally developing 4-year-olds. Two groups of children were selected: one with relatively good performance on the non-word repetition task and one with relatively poor performance. The children with better non-word repetition skills produced a wider repertoire of words, generally longer utterances and greater variety in syntactic constructions. Findings that reveal non-word repetition performance can discriminate between two groups of normal language users confirm how sensitive and robust the task may prove to be in the diagnosis of language disorder.

Conclusions: putting research into practice

Currently, it is almost impossible to keep abreast of the sheer volume of new literature dealing with the processing skills of children with language impairments of many different aetiologies. This is indeed encouraging for building a strong evidence base for the use of non-word repetition tasks, reaction time tasks and sentence imitation tasks in the diagnosis of language impairments. The research discussed above argues persuasively for the use of measures of verb morphology performance and non-word repetition tasks being incorporated into the assessment practices of speech pathologists diagnosing developmental language disorders. Goffman and Leonard (2000, p. 159) concluded that 'to improve decision making during the assessment process, an analysis of grammatical features associated with verbs is highly diagnostic'.

There are a number of challenges remaining. First, there is a need for a systematic review of the processing skills literature to inform the clinical diagnostic practice of speech pathologists in a way that provides the strongest evidence possible. Second, current and future research should be aimed at elucidating the exact nature of the processing deficits of children with developmental language disorders. Finally, this will lead to well-designed (that is, controlled) studies of interventions targeted at processing deficits (for example, FastForword and Earobics) and grammatical morphology deficits (for example, Priming strategies). The research presented in this chapter will empower clinicians to continue to argue against the use of cognitive referencing and to incorporate both non-word repetition tasks and verb elicitation tasks as robust diagnostic indicators when assessing children for developmental language disorders.

References

Adams A, Gathercole SE. Limitations in working memory: implications for language development. International Journal of Language and Communication Disorders 2000; 35: 95–116.

American Psychiatric Association (APA). Diagnostic and Statistical Manual of the Mental Disorders (DSM-III-R) (third edition). Washington, DC: American Psychiatric Association, 1987.

American Psychiatric Association (APA). Diagnostic and Statistical Manual of the Mental Disorders (DSM-IV) (fourth edition. Washington, DC: American Psychiatric Association, 1994.

American Speech-Language-Hearing Association (ASHA). Guidelines for caseload size and speech-language service delivery in the schools. ASHA 1993; 35: 33–9.

Aram DM, Morris R, Hall NE. The validity of discrepancy criteria for identifying children with developmental language disorders. Journal of Learning Disabilities 1992; 25: 549–54.

Aram DM, Morris R, Hall NE. Clinical and research congruence in identifying children with specific language impairment. Journal of Speech and Hearing Research 1993; 36: 580–91.

Bedore LM, Leonard LB. Specific language impairment and grammatical morphology: a discriminant function analysis. Journal of Speech, Language, and Hearing Research 1998; 41: 1185–92.

Beitchman JH, Nair R, Clegg M, Patel PG. Prevalence of speech and language disorders in 5 year old kindergarten children in the Ottawa-Carleton region. Journal of Speech and Hearing Disorders 1986; 51: 98–110.

Bishop D, Adams C. Comprehension problems in children with specific language impairment: literal and inferential meaning. Journal of Speech and Hearing Research 1992; 35: 119–29.

Bishop D, Bishop S, Bright P, James C, Delaney T, Tallal P. Different origin of auditory and phonological processing problems in children with language impairment: evidence from a twin study. Journal of Speech, Language and Hearing Research 1999; 36: 155–68.

Bishop DVM, North T, Donlan C. Genetic basis of specific language impairment: evidence from a twin study. Developmental Medicine and Child Neurology 1995; 37: 56–71.

Bishop DVM, North T, Donlan C. Nonword repetition as a behavioural marker for inherited language impairment: evidence from a twin study. Journal of Child Psychology and Psychiatry 1996; 36: 1–13.

Bortolini U, Leonard L. Phonology and grammatical morphology in specific language impairment: accounting for individual variation in English and Italian. Applied Psycholinguistics 1996; 17: 85–104.

Burgmeister BB, Blum LH, Lorge F. Columbia Mental Maturity Scale (third edition). San Antonio TX: The Psychological Corporation, 1972.

Carrow E. Test of Auditory Comprehension of Language. Chicago, IL: Riverside Publishing Company, 1972.

Carrow-Woolfolk E. Test for Auditory Comprehension of Language - Revised Edition. Chicago, IL: Riverside Publishing Company, 1985.

Cleave PL, Rice ML. An examination of the morpheme BE in children with specific language impairment: the role of contractibility and grammatical form class. Journal of Speech, Language and Hearing Research 1997; 40: 480–492.

Cole KN, Harris SR. Instability of the intelligence quotient–motor quotient relationship. Developmental Medicine and Child Neuropsychology 1992; 34: 633-641.

Cole KN, Fey ME. Cognitive referencing in language assessment. In: Cole KN, Dale PS, Thal DJ (eds). Assessment of Communication and Language. Baltimore, MD: Paul Brookes Publishing Company, 1996.

Cole KN, Mills PE. Agreement of language intervention triage profiles. Topics in Early Childhood Special Education 1997; 17: 119-30.

Cole KN, Dale PS, Mills PE. Defining language delay in young children by cognitive referencing: are we saying more than we know? Applied Psycholinguistics 1990; 11: 291-302.

Cole KN, Dale PS, Mills PE. Stability of the intelligence quotient-language quotient relation: is discrepancy modelling based on a myth? American Journal of Mental Retardation 1992; 97: 131-43.

Cole KN, Mills PE, Kelley D. Agreement of assessment profiles used in cognitive referencing. Language, Speech and Hearing Services in Schools 1994; 25: 25-31.

Cole KN, Schwartz IS, Notari AR, Dale PS, Mills PE. Examination of the stability of two methods of defining specific language impairment. Applied Psycholinguistics 1995; 16: 103-23.

Conti-Ramsden G, Jones M. Verb use in specific language impairment. Journal of Speech, Language, and Hearing Research 1997; 40: 1298-313.

Curtiss S. On the nature of the impairment in language impaired children. In: Miller J (Ed.). Research on Child Language Disorders: A Decade of Progress. Austin, TX: Pro-Ed, 1991.

Curtiss S, Katz W, Tallal P. Delay versus deviance in the language acquisition of language-impaired children. Journal of Speech and Hearing Research 1992; 35: 373-83.

DiSimoni F. The Token Test. Texas: DLM, 1978.

Dollaghan C, Campbell TF. Nonword repetition and child language impairment. Journal of Speech, Hearing, and Language Research 1998; 41: 1136-46.

Dollaghan CA. Fast mapping in normal and language-impaired children. Journal of Speech and Hearing Disorders 1987; 52: 218-22.

Dunn L, Dunn L. Peabody Picture Vocabulary Test – Revised. Circle Pines, MN: American Guidance Service, 1981.

Dunn M, Flax J, Sliwinski M, Aram D. The use of spontaneous language measures as criteria for identifying children with specific language impairment: an attempt to reconcile clinical and research incongruence. Journal of Speech and Hearing Research 1996; 39: 643-54.

Eadie PA. The Clinical Construct of Specific Language Impairment: The Importance of Intelligence and Grammatical Morphology in Differential Diagnosis. Unpublished PhD thesis. La Trobe University, Melbourne, 1999.

Edwards J, Lahey M. Auditory lexical decisions of children with specific language impairment. Journal of Speech and Hearing Research 1996; 39: 1263-73.

Ellis Weismer S, Hesketh LJ. The influence of prosodic and gestural cues on novel word acquisition by children with specific language impairment. Journal of Speech and Hearing Research 1993 36: 1013-25.

Ellis Weismer S, Hesketh LJ. Lexical learning by children with specific language impairment: effects of linguistic input presented at varying speaking rates. Journal of Speech and Hearing Research 1996; 39: 177-90.

Ellis Weismer S, Evan J, Hesketh L. An examination of verbal working memory capacity in children with specific language impairment. Journal of Speech, Language, and Hearing Research 1999; 42: 1249-60.

Ellis Weismer S, Tomblin JB, Zhang X, Buckwalter P, Chynoweth JG, Jones M. Nonword repetition performance in school-age children with and without language impairment. Journal of Speech, Language, and Hearing Research 2000: 43: 865-78.

Fazio BB, Naremore RC, Connell PJ. Tracking children from poverty at risk of specific language impairment: a 3 year longitudinal study. Journal of Speech and Hearing Research 1996; 39: 611-24.

Fey ME, Cleave PL, Ravida AI, Long SH, Dejmal AE, Easton DL. Effects of grammar facilitation on the phonological performance of children with speech and language impairments. Journal of Speech and Hearing Research 1994; 37: 594-607.

Fey ME, Long SH, Cleave PL. Reconsideration of IQ criteria in the definition of specific language impairment. In: Watkins RV, Rice ML (eds). Specific Language Impairments in Children. Baltimore, MD: Brookes, 1994.

Fletcher JM. The validity of distinguishing children with language and learning disabilities according to discrepancies with IQ: introduction to the special series. Journal of Learning Disabilities 1992; 25: 546-8.

Fletcher P. Sub-groups in school-age language-impaired children. In: Fletcher P, Hall D (eds). Specific Speech and Language Disorders in Children. London: Whurr Publishers, 1992.

Fletcher P, Peters J. Characterizing language impairment in children: an exploratory study. Language Testing 1984; 1: 33-49.

Fowler AE. Linguistic variability in persons with Down syndrome. In: Nadel L, Rosenthal D (eds). Down Syndrome: Living and Learning in the Community. New York, NY: Wiley-Liss, 1995.

Friel-Patti S. Research in child language disorders: what do we know and where are we going? Folia Phoniatrica 1992; 44: 126-42.

Frome Loeb D, Leonard LB. Subject case marking and verb morphology in normally developing and specifically language-impaired children. Journal of Speech and Hearing Research 1991; 34: 340-6.

Frome Loeb D, Pye C, Redmond S, Zobel Richardson L. Eliciting verbs from children with specific language impairment. American Journal of Speech-Language Pathology 1996; 5: 17-30.

Gathercole S, Baddeley A. Phonological memory deficits in language disordered children: is there a causal connection. Journal of Memory and Language 1990; 29: 336-60.

Gathercole SE, Baddeley AD. The Children's Test of Nonword Repetition.: Psychological Corporation, 1996.

Goffman L, Leonard J. Growth of language skills in preschool children with specific language impairment: implications for assessment and intervention. American Journal of Speech-Language Pathology 2000; 9: 151-61.

Gopnik M, Crago M. Familial aggregation of a developmental language disorder. Cognition 1991; 39: 1-50.

Harasty J, Reed VA. The prevalence of speech and language impairment in two Sydney metropolitan schools. Australian Journal of Human Communication Disorders 1994; 22: 1-23.

Hresko W, Reid D, Hammill D. Test of Early Language Development. Austin, TX: Pro-Ed, 1981.

Johnston J, Schery T. The use of grammatical morphemes by children with communication disorders. In: Morehead D, Morehead A (eds). Normal and Deficient Child Language. Baltimore, MD: University Park Press, 1976.

Johnston JR. Specific language disorders in the child. In: Lass N, McReynolds L, Northern J, Yoder D (eds). Handbook of Speech-Language Pathology and Audiology. Toronto: BC Decker Inc., 1988.

Johnston JR, Kamhi AG. Syntactic and semantic aspects of the utterances of language-impaired children: the same can be less. Merrill-Palmer Quarterly 1984; 30: 65–86.

Jones M, Conti-Ramsden G. A comparison of verb use in children with specific language impairment and their younger siblings. First Language 1997; 17: 165–93.

Kamhi AG. Trying to make sense of developmental language disorders. Language, Speech and Hearing Services in Schools 1998; 29: 35–44.

Khan L, James S. Grammatical morpheme development in three language disordered children. Journal of Communication Disorders 1983; 6: 85–100.

Kjelgaard MM, Tager-Flusberg H. An investigation of language impairment in autism: Implications for genetic subgroups. Language and Cognitive Processes 2001; 16: 287–308.

Klimacka L, Brunger K. Elicitation in verb morphology. Child Language Teaching and Therapy 1999; 15: 247–59.

Lahey M, Edwards J. Specific language impairment: preliminary investigation of factors associated with family history and with patterns of language performance. Journal of Speech and Hearing Research 1995; 38: 643–57.

Lahey M, Liebergott J, Chesnick M, Menyuk P, Adams J. Variability in children's use of grammatical morphemes. Applied Psycholinguistics 1992; 13: 373–98.

Laws G. The use of nonword repetition as a test of phonological memory in children with Down syndrome. Journal of Child Psychology and Psychiatry 1998; 39: 1119–30.

Leiter RG. The Leiter International Performance Scale. Chicago, IL: Stoelting Company, 1969.

Leonard L. Language impairment in children. Merrill Palmer Quarterly 1979; 25:205–32.

Leonard L, Nippold M, Kail R, Hale C. Picture naming in language impaired children. Journal of Speech and Hearing Research 1983; 26: 609–15.

Leonard LB. Children with Specific Language Impairment. Cambridge, MA: MIT Press, 1998.

Leonard LB. Language learnability and specific language impairment in children. Applied Psycholinguistics 1989; 10: 179–202.

Leonard LB. The use of morphology by children with specific language impairment: Evidence from three languages. In: Chapman RS (Ed.). Processes in Language Acquisition and Disorders. St Louis, MI: Mosby-Year Book Inc., 1992.

Leonard LB, Eyer JA, Bedore LM, Grela BG. Three accounts of the grammatical morpheme difficulties of English-speaking children with specific language impairment. Journal of Speech, Language, and Hearing Research 1997; 40: 741–753.

McCarthy D. Manual for the McCarthy Scales of Children's Abilities. San Antonio, TX: The Psychological Corporation, 1972.

McGregor K, Leonard L. Subject pronoun and article omissions in the speech of children with specific language impairment: a phonological interpretation. Journal of Speech and Hearing Research 1994; 37: 171–81.

Miller J. Research on language disorders in children: a progress report. In: Miller J (Ed.). Research on Child Language Disorders: A Decade of Progress. Austin, TX: Pro-Ed, 1991.

Montgomery JW, Leonard LB. Real-time inflectional processing by children with specific language impairment: effects of phonetic substance. Journal of Speech, Language, and Hearing Research 1998; 41: 1432–43.

Moore M, Johnston JR. Expressions of past time by normal and language-impaired children. Applied Psycholinguistics 1993; 14: 515–34.

Oetting JB, Rice ML, Swank LK. Quick incidental learning (QUIL) of words by school-age children with and without specific language impairment. Journal of Speech and Hearing Research 1995; 38: 434–45.

Rice ML, Sell M, Hadley P. Social interactions of speech and language impaired children. Journal of Speech and Hearing Research 1991; 34: 1299–1307.

Rice ML, Wexler K. Rice–Wexler Test of Early Grammatical Impairment. San Antonio, TX: The Psychological Corporation, 2001.

Rice ML, Bode JV. GAPS in the verb lexicons of children with specific language impairment. First Language 1993; 13: 113–31.

Rice ML, Oetting JB. Morphological deficits of children with specific language impairment: evaluation of number marking and agreement. Journal of Speech and Hearing Research 1993; 36: 1249–58.

Rice ML, Wexler K. Toward tense as a clinical marker of specific language impairment in English-speaking children. Journal of Speech and Hearing Research 1996; 39: 1239–57.

Rice ML, Wexler K, Cleave PL. Specific language impairment as a period of extended optional infinitive. Journal of Speech and Hearing Research 1995; 38: 850–63.

Rice ML, Wexler K, Hershberger S. Tense over time: the longitudinal course of tense acquisition in children with specific language impairment. Journal of Speech, Language, and Hearing Research 1998, 41(6), 1412–31.

Sackett DL, Rosenberg WMC, Muir Gray JA, Haynes RB, Richardson WS. Evidence-based medicine: what it is and what it isn't. NHS Research and Development Centre for Evidence Based Medicine, 1996. (http:cebm.jr2.ox.ac.uk/ebmisisnt.html) (Accessed 13 February 2001.)

Stark R, Montgomery J. Sentence processing in language-impaired children under conditions of filtering and time compression. Applied Psycholinguistics 1995; 16: 137–54.

Stark RE, Tallal P. Selection of children with specific language deficits. Journal of Speech and Hearing Disorders 1981; 46: 114–22.

Tallal P. Back to the future: research on developmental disorders of language. In: Miller J (Ed.). Research on Child Language Disorders: A Decade of Progress. Austin, TX: Pro-Ed, 1991.

Watkins RV, Rice ML, Moltz CC. Verb use by language-impaired and normally developing children. First Language 1993; 13: 133–43.

Wechsler D. Wechsler Preschool and Primary Scale of Intelligence. New York, NY: Psychological Corporation, 1967.

World Health Organization. International Classification of Mental and Behavioural Disorders: Clinical Descriptions and Diagnostic Guidelines (ICD-10). Geneva: World Health Organization, 1992.

Wiig E. Wiig Criterion Referenced Inventory of Language. San Antonio, TX: The Psychological Corporation, 1990.

CHAPTER 9

The evidence base for the management of late talkers

PATRICIA EADIE

'If not now, when? If not me, who?'
(Ethics of the Fathers)

Introduction: late talking in context

For clinicians involved in the diagnosis and intervention of young children with language impairments (that is, 2–3-year-olds), the past two decades has produced an abundance of research. Those children with early language delays are now most commonly referred to as 'late talkers' in the research literature. The criteria on which to base a diagnosis of 'late talking' are clearly defined, as are the factors associated with better outcomes in the pre-school and school years. But what of the intervention for these late talkers? Is there evidence to suggest *when* we should intervene, *how* we should intervene, *who* should be the target of this intervention and *what* the outcomes of intervention might be?

The purpose of this chapter is to review the evidence that addresses these crucial questions about intervention with late talkers. The chapter begins with a brief overview of the research that has defined this group of children and the issues this research has raised concerning the provision of intervention services. The chapter then describes in more detail the types of intervention studies reported in the literature and the levels of evidence that each represents.

Defining the group of children who are late talkers

During the 1980s, two research groups began research programmes that followed cohorts of very young children in the beginning stages of developing language skills. The work of Rescorla (1989), Rescorla and Schwartz (1990) and Paul (1991) in describing the development of these children's skills over a number of years has led to a clear definition of late talking and its associated diagnostic criteria. Late talkers are characterized as having obvious delays in language acquisition in contrast to what appears to be normal development in other areas. The diagnostic criteria include children who, at 24 months of age, have fewer than 50 words in their expressive vocabulary and/or who demonstrate no word combinations. Rescorla (1989) and Rescorla et al. (1993) estimate that the prevalence rate of late talkers among the general population of 2-year-olds is between 10% and 15%.

Spontaneous improvement and risk factors of language change

Follow-up investigations of children who are late talkers have identified a number of positive predictors for spontaneous improvement of language skills and risk factors for on-going language difficulties. Law et al. (2000) found in their systematic review of the prevalence and natural history of primary speech and language delay that up to 60% of children identified with speech and/or language delay at age 2 years may resolve without treatment between the ages of 2 and 3 years. This conclusion is consistent with the work of Paul (1993, 1996) and Rescorla et al. (1997), who found that anywhere between 35% and 79% of children who were diagnosed as late talkers improved spontaneously, depending on the language measure chosen to determine progress (for example, expressive vocabulary versus mean length of utterance (MLU)). Whether or not the delay resolves, multiple educational and social difficulties are noted for children with earlier speech and language delay (for example, 41–75% demonstrate reading difficulties at age 8 years) (Law et al., 2000).

Risk factors associated with poorer outcomes of early language delay include:

* Hearing, in particular early fluctuating conductive hearing loss (Shriberg et al., 2001; Casby, 2001).
* Positive family history of speech and/or language delay (Bishop et al., 1995; Rice et al., 1998).
* Receptive and expressive language both delayed (Olswang and Bain, 1996).
* No use of sequenced gestures (Thal and Bates, 1988; Capirci et al., 1996).
* Low proportion of consonant to vowel babble and a small consonant inventory in babble (Mirak and Rescorla, 1998; Oller et al., 1998; Pharr et al., 2000).
* A small number of verbs in expressive vocabulary (Rice and Bode, 1993).

The evidence for the 'when' and 'how' to intervene with late talkers

Better understanding of the natural course of late talking necessitated the re-examination of intervention decisions for late talkers. (This information, along with intervention studies is summarized in Table 9.1.) Paul (1996) recommends the 'watch and see' approach for late talkers who were from 'functional families' with no additional risk factors (for example, poverty or serious medical problems). By use of this model, late-talking 2-year-olds were re-evaluated every three to six months between the ages of 2 and 3 years and re-evaluated every six to 12 months between the ages of 3 and 5 years. Paul's (1996) attempt to provide a guideline for service provision was met with mixed review (Olswang et al., 1998). What it did very successfully was create the impetus for discussion to occur.

Van Kleeck, Gillam, and Davis (1997) suggest that implementing a 'watch and see' approach demands being able to predict with certainty those children who will improve spontaneously and those who will continue to evidence language delay. Although predicting outcome is now a more informed process (Olswang et al., 1998), the multi-layered nature of language and communication development makes clinical decision-making an uncertain process at best. As an example, there is now a body of literature describing the parent–child relationship and family characteristics of a family when a child is language delayed. (In a later section of this chapter it is argued that research on this 'family factor' is one of a number of important pieces of evidence to consider when making decisions about intervention with late talkers.)

When searching the literature for intervention studies with late talkers, databases such as the Cumulative Index to Nursing and Allied Health (CINAHL) retrieve in excess of 30 published articles. However, a review of these articles reveals one-third to be related to predicting outcomes, not intervention, for late talkers and approximately another seven articles that deal with intervention issues, but not with late talkers. What remains are two core categories of articles: the first is best described as 'expert opinion'; the second (and the one that will be the focus of the rest of this chapter) deals with what are best described as 'case-control studies'. Such studies represent a level of evidence common in speech pathology, that is, on the middle rung of the possible methodologies ladder. They demonstrate controlled data collection but do not exhibit the strength of a randomized controlled trial in that they use clinical cohorts of participants.

The Hanen model of early language intervention

Most of the studies that will be reviewed focus on the therapeutic outcomes of the Hanen model of early language intervention (Manolson, 1992). Briefly,

Table 9.1 Description of the studies and level of evidence for the language intervention studies with late talkers

Language intervention with late talkers	Reference	Level of evidence
'Watch and see' approach	Law et al., (2000)	Systematic review
	Olswang and Bain (1996)	Expert opinion, based on clinical and research experience (level IV)
	Olswang et al., (1998)	Expert opinion, based on clinical and research experience (level IV)
	Paul (1996)	Expert opinion, based on clinical and research experience (level IV)
	Van Kleek et al. (1997)	Expert opinion, based on clinical and research experience (level IV)
Hanen model of early language intervention	Girolametto et al. (1997)	Cohort studies (Level III.2)
	Girolametto et al. (1999)	Cohort studies (Level III.2)
	Pearce et al. (1996)	Cohort studies (Level III.2)
Intervention studies	Glogowska et al. (2001)	Pragmatic randomized controlled trial (Level II)
	Pre-kindergarten NOMS (2001)	Cohort studies (Level III.2)
Parent–child relationship and intervention	Carson et al. (1998a)	Controlled trial without randomization (Level III.1)
	Carson et al. (1999)	Controlled trial without randomization (Level III.1)
	Robertson, and	Controlled trial without randomization (Level III.1)
	Ellis Weismer (1999)	

this model of intervention is based in social interactionist accounts of how children learn language from the adult input. The model encourages parents to use contingent and simplified linguistic input when communicating with their children. (For a full description of the Hanen programmes see the Hanen Centre website (www.hanen.org/).) Parents are the primary mediators of the intervention with their late-talking toddlers by use of this model. The series of studies has been jointly conducted by the Hanen Centre and the University of Ontario, Canada.

Evidence for parent-focused intervention with late talkers

Published research exploring the outcomes of parent-focused intervention with late talkers has, without exception, revealed positive changes in toddlers' language abilities (Girolametto et al., 1996, 1997; Pearce et al., 1996; Girolametto et al., 1999). The study by Girolametto et al. (1996) involved 25 mothers and their late-talking toddlers in an interactive focused stimulation targeting expressive vocabulary skills. The mothers and toddlers were randomly assigned to intervention or delayed intervention groups. Mothers participating in the intervention programme were taught how to use focused stimulation. The mothers were the mediators of the intervention to their toddlers. Individually selected vocabulary targets were based on parents' responses to their toddlers' vocabulary skills, based on the *MacArthur Communicative Development Inventories* (MacArthur CDI) (Fenson et al., 1993). The mothers who had participated in the intervention group demonstrated language input that was slower, less complex and more focused on their child's utterances after intervention when compared with the delayed intervention group. At the same time, the children of the participating mothers used more words and were reported to have larger vocabularies than the children in the delayed intervention group. They used more words in free-play interactions, used more multi-word combinations and demonstrated more early morphemes than the children in the delayed intervention group.

In a subsequent study, Girolametto and colleagues (Girolametto et al., 1999) further explored the relationship between maternal language change and language development in toddlers. In this study, mother–toddler dyads were compared before intervention and four months later, after involvement in the Hanen programme. Maternal language features of interest included four structural measures (that is, total number of utterances, rate of speech in words per minute, type-token ratio and MLU) and four measures of contingent responsiveness (imitations, interpretations, labelling and expansions). Measures of child language behaviour included talkativeness (that is, total number of utterances), vocabulary (number of different words used) and complexity (the number of multi-word combinations). The MacArthur CDI (Fenson et al., 1993) and the *Sequenced Inventory of Communicative Development* (SICD) (Hedrick et al., 1984) were used in gathering data along with videotaped free-play interactive sessions with mother–toddler dyads. Twelve toddlers with expressive vocabulary delays and their mothers participated. A robust relationship between maternal use of imitation and expansion with measures of child language after intervention was found. The authors conclude that the findings support stronger effects for responsive language input on the language abilities of this group of late-talking toddlers. This study is perhaps most significant in that it establishes a direct link between changing maternal language behaviours and the increase in language abilities of the late-talking toddlers. Although it cannot be assumed that other factors (for example, developmental progress) may not have influenced the intervention outcomes, the studies by Girolametto and colleagues provide strong evidence that parent-focused intervention is a viable treatment option for young children with language delays.

The parent–child relationship when the child is a late talker

The study of the interaction between language delay and behavioural and social difficulties has a long history (Richman and Stevenson, 1977). More recently, the association has been established in young children aged from 2 years (Caulfield et al., 1989). If evidence exists for the emergence of concomitant language and behavioural difficulties in very young children then early language intervention may serve the dual purpose of developing language abilities and preventing behavioural problems. In addition, the effect of behavioural and social difficulties along with language delay, on the parent–child relationship cannot be underestimated. As eluded to earlier in this chapter, one of the mediating factors in both spontaneous recovery for late-talking toddlers and in the success of intervention is the parent–child relationship. Consequently, it is important to know what evidence exists detailing the behavioural characteristics of late talking toddlers and the effect these difficulties may have on the parent–child relationship.

Research conducted by Carson and colleagues (Carson et al., 1998a; Carson et al., 1998b; Carson et al., 1999) has investigated whether behavioural difficulties, social development and family characteristics differentiate children with language delay and children developing language normally. Carson et al. (1998a) and Carson et al. (1998b) followed 36 and 64 children, respectively, with delayed expressive language development from age 2 years to 3 years. Measures included the language development survey (Rescorla, 1989), the *Infant Mullen Scales of Early Learning* (MSEL) (Mullen, 1989), the child behaviour checklist (CBCL) (Achenbach, 1992) and the *Developmental Profile II* (DPII) (Alpern et al., 1980). Although none of the children in the studies had behaviours in the clinical disturbance range there was an association between delays in expressive language and children's behavioural difficulties. More specifically, based on maternal report the children who were late talkers exhibited more symptoms of anxiety, depression, withdrawal and sleep problems. Measures of social development for the group of late talkers were significantly lower than for the normally developing children.

Subsequently, Carson et al. (1999) went on to examine differences in the family characteristics and parenting behaviours of families with toddlers who had language delay and toddlers developing normally. Sixty-four parents of children aged 2 years participated in this case control study. The language development survey (Rescorla, 1989) was used to categorize the participants into families with a toddler with language delay or developing normally. Seventeen toddlers were identified as language-delayed and 47 were identified as developing normally. The family characteristics and parenting behaviours were then compared across the two groups. Another comparison was conducted with 26 families who agreed to be re-evaluated when their children were between 5 and 6 years of age. The measures used included the *Colorado Self-Report Measure of Family Functioning - Revised* (CSMFF-R) (Bloom and Lipetz, 1987), the *Family Evaluation Form - Revised* (FEF-R) (Emery et al., 1984), the *Mother–Child Relationship Evaluation* (MCRE) (Roth, 1980) and the *Parent Behavior Checklist* (PBC) (Fox, 1994). Results indicated that parents were less nurturant and the families were less sociable and more enmeshed when there was a toddler with language delay. Less nurturant behaviour towards the child with language delay was found to be a consistent feature of parental perceptions, emerging again on re-assessment when the children were between 5 and 6 years of age.

The results of these studies consistently support the notion that early intervention is critical and that parent involvement and education is an important preventative component of any intervention. For those late talkers who do not improve spontaneously, the long-term risk for ongoing language difficulty (such as specific language impairment), as well as educational and social difficulties, is well documented. For example, the literature regarding the social skills of older pre-school children with a diagnosis of specific language impairment should make us cognisant of the long-term negative social outcomes for these children. Gertner, Rice and Hadley (1994) report on the negative effect of poor communication skills on peer acceptance for children with specific language impairment. Rice et al. (1993) discusses the long-term interplay of negative social consequences and language difficulties. Such evidence, taken in conjunction with behavioural and family characteristics of families with children with language delay, argues against a 'watch and see' approach with late-talking toddlers and advocates early intervention involving both parents and their toddlers.

Evidence for the positive effect on parent–child relationship from early language intervention

One study to date has attempted to examine the effect of early language intervention on the parent–child relationship. Robertson and Ellis Weismer (1999) investigated the effect of language intervention on a set of linguistic variables and parents' perceptions of the child's socialization and their own stress levels. Twenty-one parent–child dyads participated in the study and were randomly assigned to treatment or no treatment groups for comparison. The average age of the late-talking toddlers was 25 months. The intervention programme was of 12 weeks' duration. The parents received no formal training with this intervention and did not participate in sessions, although they were invited to observe. Speech pathologists implemented the treatment and utilized parallel talk, expansion, expatiations and recasts. Pre- and post-intervention language measures included MLU, total number of words used, number of different words used and percentage of intelligible utterances. Social skills were measured by use of the 'socialization' domain of the *Vineland Adaptive Behaviour Scales* (VABS) (Sparrow et al., 1984). Parental stress was measured by use of the 'child' domain of *The Parenting Stress Index* (PSI) (Abidin, 1995). Post-intervention measures were obtained immediately after the 12-week intervention programme was completed. Improvements were noted in two of the children's language measures from pre- to post-intervention: MLU, indicating increased use of multi-word combinations; and the lexical diversity measures. Parents' perceptions of their children also improved from pre- to post-intervention. This was the case for both scores on the socialization domain of the VABS and in measures of parent acceptance and use of reinforcing behaviours on the PSI. This study provides preliminary evidence that early language intervention, mediated by speech pathologists can have short-term effects on linguistic, social and parenting behaviours. Results such as these further reinforce the argument that intervention as early as possible is the preferred option to a 'watch and see' approach. It is highly probable that the positive communicative cycle established by intervention encourages further flow-on effects that affect both children's language abilities and parents' perceptions of their child and themselves.

Other sources of evidence regarding language intervention with young children

Since 1998 the American Speech–Language–Hearing Association (ASHA) has been encouraging speech and language pathologists to participate in the National Outcomes Measurement System (NOMS). A series of disorder-specific, seven-point rating scales allow speech and language pathologists to describe change in individuals' communication and swallowing ability over the course of intervention. Data are collected across multiple sites from large numbers of speech and language pathologists tracking the progress in intervention of their client populations. Collation of this type of data fits within the cohort studies level of evidence. One of the three components measured in the NOMS is the progress of pre-school children in intervention, categorized as 'pre-kindergarten health/schools'. In a recent ASHA publication (Pre-kindergarten NOMS, 2001) preliminary outcome data for the pre-kindergarten NOMS was disseminated. Details about the numbers of children and the nature of interventions was not provided. Although the data reported revealed a great deal of variance, better outcomes in language comprehension intervention appear strongly associated with the type of service delivery model. More specifically, better progress is obtained in group intervention (80% of participants showed progress) compared to individual intervention (52% of participants showed progress). This finding is consistent with social interaction accounts of language learning which predict development will occur in socially relevant and contextually meaningful environments (for example, group communication versus clinician–client dialogue). More data will need to be added before judgements can be made with regard to expressive language intervention and, more specifically, who receives the intervention (for example, parents or toddlers). However, large-scale outcome projects such as NOMS sit well alongside intervention research and will continue to provide valuable data that can inform future speech and language intervention practices.

Lastly, it is important to consider the first randomized controlled trial investigating speech and language intervention services across 16 different community clinics in Bristol. The study by Glogowska, Roulstone, Enderby and Peters (2001) compared routine speech and language therapy provided to pre-school children against a 12-month period of 'watchful waiting'. One hundred and fifty-nine children were included in the randomized controlled trial. Although outcome was measured across many different language parameters, the only measure to show significant improvement in favour of children who received therapy was auditory comprehension. This study concluded that there was little evidence for providing speech and language therapy over watchful waiting. However, this conclusion must be considered with the following points in mind. First, the study did not prove (or disprove) the efficacy of speech therapy, but rather it was an evaluation of the existing service provision. The mean of 6.2 hours of therapy across the period of the study can hardly be considered ideal or what the speech pathologists wanted to provide. In addition, the study tells us that children with speech and language delay in this sample did not spontaneously recover. In other words it should caution us against watchful waiting as a treatment option. The findings of the study may be initially disconcerting to speech pathologists, but they provide valuable evidence of *what does not* achieve positive outcomes for young children with speech and language delays (Reilly and Eadie, 2000).

Conclusions: future directions

A number of questions remain unanswered with respect to intervention with late talkers. There is a need for a large epidemiological study to provide stronger evidence of the concomitant risk factors (such as social–emotional development and parent–child relationship) associated with early language delay. Moderate evidence (Level III.2) exists to support parent-mediated interventions (within the Hanen model) for late talkers. However, future research is needed to determine if it is the 'whole' Hanen programme or specific components of it that contribute to its reported success (for example, instructional material, video feedback, home visiting). Lastly, because a significant number of children who have participated in parent-mediated intervention programmes go on to require individual therapy, medium to long-term outcome research is of vital importance (Girolametto et al., 2001).

This chapter has argued that speech pathologists can now confidently diagnose late-talking toddlers, based on diagnostic criteria established through rigorous research evidence. Although the evidence is still minimal and predominantly from case-control studies, the risk of concomitant linguistic, social and parenting difficulties requires intervention to occur as early as possible. Although spontaneous recovery from late talking will occur in a majority of cases of children aged between 2 and 3 years, the approach of watching and waiting is contraindicated. This conclusion is based on evidence that suggests that parent-mediated intervention (the 'who') is effective and when carried out as early as possible (the 'when') has positive outcomes on the parent–child relationship.

References

Abidin R. The Parenting Stress Index. Charlottesville, VA: Pediatric Psychological Press, 1995.

Achenbach TM. Manual for the Child Behaviour Checklist 2/3 and 1992 Profile. Burlington, VT: University of Vermont Department of Psychiatry, 1992.

Alpern G, Boll T, Shearer M. Developmental Profile II. Aspen, CO: Psychological Development Publications, 1980.

Bishop DVM, North T, Donlan C. Genetic basis of specific language impairment: evidence from a twin study. Developmental Medicine and Child Neurology 1995; 37: 56–71.

Bloom BL, Lipetz ME. Revisions on the Self-Report Measure of Family Functioning. Boulder, CO: University of Colarado, 1987.

Capirci O, Iverson JM, Pizzuto E, Volterra V. Gestures and words during the transition to two-word speech. Journal of Child Language 1996; 23: 645–73.

Carson DK, Klee TM, Lee S, Williams KC, Perry CK. Children's language proficiency at ages 2 and 3 as predictors of behaviour problems, social and cognitive development at age 3. Journal of Children's Communication Development 1988a; 19: 21–30.

Carson DK, Klee TM, Perry CK, Muskina G, Donaghy T. Comparisons of children with delayed and normal language at 24 months of age on measures of behavioural difficulties, social and cognitive development. Infant Mental Health Journal 1998b 19(1), 59-75.

Carson DK, Perry CK, Diefenderfer MS, Klee TM. Differences in family characteristics and parenting behaviour in families with language-delayed and language-normal toddlers. Transdisciplinary Journal of Infant–Toddler Intervention 1999; 9: 259–79.

Casby MW. Otitis media and language development: a meta-analysis. American Journal of Speech–Language Pathology 2001; 10: 65–80.

Caufield MB, Fischel JE, DeBaryshe BD, Whitehurst GJ. Behavioural correlates of developmental expressive language disorder. Journal of Abnormal Child Psychology 1989; 19: 187–201.

Emery RE, Weintraub S, Neale JM. Family Evaluation Form – Revised. Stony Brook, NY: SUNY, Department of Psychology, 1984.

Fenson L, Dale P, Reznick S, Bates E, Thal D, Pethick S. MacArthur Communicative Development Inventories. San Diego, CA: Singular Publishing Group Inc., 1993.

Fox RA. Parent Behaviour Checklist. Brandon, VT: Clinical Psychology Publishing Co., 1994.

Gertner BL, Rice ML, Hadley PA. Influence of communicative competence on peer preferences in a preschool classroom. Journal of Speech and Hearing Research 1994; 37: 913–23.

Girolametto L, Pearce P, Weitzman E. Interactive focussed stimulation for toddlers with expressive vocabulary delays. Journal of Speech and Hearing Research 1996; 39: 1274–83.

Girolametto L, Pearce P, Weitzman E. Effects of lexical intervention on the phonology of late talkers. Journal of Speech, Language and Hearing Research 1997; 40: 338–48.

Girolametto L, Weitzman E, Wiigs M, Pearce P. The relationship between maternal language mesures and language development in toddlers with expressive language delays. American Journal of Speech–Language Pathology 1999; 8: 364–74.

Girolametto L, Wiigs M, Smyth R, Weitzman E, Pearce P. Children with a history of excpressive vocabulary delay: outcomes at 5 years of age. American Journal of Speech Language Pathology 2001; 10: 358–69.

Glogowska M, Roulstone S, Enderby P, Peters TJ. Randomised controlled trial of community based speech and language therapy in preschool children. British Medical Journal 2001; 321: 1–5.

Hedrick DL, Prather EM, Tobin AR. Sequenced Inventory of Communicative Development Revised. Seattle, WA: University of Washington Press, 1984.

Law J, Boyle J, Harris F, Harkness A, Nye C. Prevalence and natural history of primary speech and language delay: findings from a systematic review of the literature. International Journal of Language and Communication Disorders 2000; 35: 165-88.

Manolson A. It Takes Two to Talk: A Parent's Guide to Helping Children Communicate. Toronto, Ontario, Canada: The Hanen Centre, 1992.

Mirak J, Rescorla L. Phonetic skills and vocabulary size in late talkers: concurrent and predictive relationships. Applied Psycholinguistics 1988; 19: 1-17.

Mullen E. Infant Mullen Scales of Early Learning. Cranston, RI: TOTAL Child Inc., 1989.

Oller D, Eilers RE, Neal AR, Cobo-Lewis AB. Late onset canonical babbling: a possible early marker of abnormal development. American Journal on Mental Retardation 1998; 103: 249-63.

Olswang L, Bain B. Assessment information for predicting upcoming change in language production. Journal of Speech and Hearing Research 1996; 39: 414-23.

Olswang LB, Rodriguez B, Timler G. Recommending intervention for toddlers with specific language learning difficulties: we may not have all the answers, but we know a lot. American Journal of Speech-Language Pathology 1998; 7: 23-32.

Paul R. Profiles of toddlers with slow expressive language development. Topics in Language Disorders 1991; 11: 1-13.

Paul R. Patterns of language development in late talkers. Journal of Children's Communication Development 1993; 15: 7-14.

Paul R. Clinical implications of the natural history of slow expressive language development. American Journal of Speech-Language Pathology 1996; 5: 5-21.

Pearce P, Girolametto L, Weitzman E. The effects of focussed stimulation intervention on mothers of late-talking toddlers. Transdisciplinary Journal of Infant-Toddler Intervention 1996; 6: 213-27.

Pharr A, Bernstein Ratner N, Rescorla L. Syllable structure development of toddlers with expressive specific language impairment. Applied Psycholinguistics 2000; 21: 429-49.

Pre-Kindergarten NOMS. Leader. ASHA 2001; 6: 25.

Reilly S, Eadie P. Speech therapy has its place [Letter to the editor]. Medical Observer 2000; 24.

Rescorla L. The language development survey: a screening tool for delayed language in toddlers. Journal of Speech and Hearing Disorders 1989; 54: 587-99.

Rescorla L, Schwartz E. Outcomes of toddlers with specific expressive language delay (SELD). Applied Psycholinguistics 1990; 11: 393-408.

Rescorla L, Hadicke-Wiley M, Escarce E. Epidemiological investigation of expressive language delay at age two. First Language 1993; 13: 5-22.

Rescorla L, Roberts J, Dahlsgaard K. Late-talkers at 2: outcome at age 3. Journal of Speech, Language, and Hearing Research 1997; 40: 556-66.

Rice ML, Bode JV. GAPS in the verb lexicons of children with specific language impairment. First Language 1993; 13: 113-31.

Rice ML, Hadley PA, Alexander AL. Social biases toward children with speech and language impairments: a correlative causal mode of language limitations. Applied Psycholinguistics 1993; 14: 445-71.

Rice ML, Haney KR, Wexler K. Family histories of children with SLI who show Extended Optional Infinitives. Journal of Speech, Language, and Hearing Research 1998; 41: 419-32.

Richman N, Stevenson J. Language delay in three-year-olds. Acta Pediatrica Belgica 1977; 30: 213-19.

Robertson S, Ellis Weismer S. Effects of treatment on linguistic and social skills in toddlers with delayed language development. Journal of Speech, Language, and Hearing Research 1999; 42: 1234-8.

Roth RH. The Mother–Child Relationship Evaluation Manual. Los Angeles, CA: Western Psychological Services, 1980.

Shriberg LD, Friel-Patti S, Flipsen P, Brown RL. Otitis media, fluctuant hearing loss, and speech–language outcomes: a preliminary structural equation model. Journal of Speech, Language, and Hearing Research 2000; 43: 100-20.

Sparrow SS, Balla DA, Ciccetti DV. Vineland Adaptive Behaviour Scales. Circle Pines, MN: American Guidance Services, 1984.

Thal D, Bates E. Language and gesture in late talkers. Journal of Speech and Hearing Research 1988; 31: 115-23.

van Kleeck A, Gillam RB, Davis B. When is 'watch and see' warranted? A response to Paul's 1996 article, 'Clinical implications of the natural history of slow expressive language development'. American Journal of Speech-Language Pathology 1997; 6: 34-9.

CHAPTER **10**

The evidence base for the evaluation and management of motor speech disorders in children

BEVERLY JOFFE AND SHEENA REILLY

Introduction: motor speech disorders in context

When defining paediatric motor speech disorders, Enderby and Emerson (1996) excluded speech disorders that arise as a result of structural problems (for example, cleft palate) or those that are of psychological origin. These will also be excluded from further discussion in this chapter. It is acknowledged from the outset that this chapter focuses more on dyspraxia than dysarthria; this reflects both the degree of controversy that exists about dyspraxia and to some extent the abundance of literature on the subject. This chapter is divided into two sections: the first section presents an overview of the historical aspects of paediatric motor speech disorders and the controversy that surrounds their diagnosis and classification; the second section presents the evidence and discusses the main factors that affect the types and levels of evidence available.

The features of adult and paediatric motor speech disorders have been described in a number of publications and some of the similarities and differences have been highlighted. (Table 10.1 summarizes the main features of paediatric motor speech disorders.)

Historical context

The neurological classification and differential diagnosis of paediatric motor speech disorders have mainly been based on conceptual frameworks from adult-acquired neurological disorders. There is increasing recognition that the situation in children is likely to be more complex and less predictable than acquired lesions in adults. This is particularly likely in paediatric motor speech disorders, because of the widespread effects of damage either during embryogenesis or post-natally, on the developing central nervous system.

Table 10.1 Characteristics of paediatric motor speech disorders

Source	Characteristics
Sheppard (1964)	Primitive oro-motor reflexes may persist in children contributing to lack of establishment of voluntary speech control.
Crary (1984)	In children the types of motor speech disorders (for example, dyspraxia and dysarthria) and phonological disorders can present superficially as very similar.
	Paediatric motor speech disorders may co-exist with deficits in phonology and grammar.
	The paediatric dyspraxia and dysarthria diagnostic groups may contain considerable heterogeneity – different subgroups may exist within each group.
Ozanne (1994)	The speech errors of adults with dyspraxia indicate a deficit at the phonemic rather than phonetic level of speech production.
Murdoch et al. (1995)	Motor impairment forms at least part of the basis for developmental dyspraxia in children and may be indicative of the presence of a concomitant dysarthria.
Morgan Barry (1995a, 1995b)	Child characteristics are subject to many influences during growth and maturation – different symptom clusters may be seen during stages of development.
	Children demonstrate greater impairment of involuntary and vegetative functions (for example, more drooling).
Clark et al. (2000)	Children are evolving through neurological maturational phases while acquiring developmental skills – expression of impairment may be highly variable or even silent.

Examination of the data in Table 10.1 reveals that motor speech disorders in children may differ from motor speech disorders in adults. Therefore, the direct transfer of the motor speech classification system used for acquired adult disorders to children (regardless of whether the condition is acquired or developmental) may not be appropriate.

The lack of a clear and empirically derived classification system, or the use of an inappropriate one (derived for the most part for use in adults), has influenced the development of the evidence base for the management of paediatric motor speech disorders.

Much has been published about the theoretical viewpoints on paediatric motor speech disorders. Although it is beyond the scope of the present chapter to review these, this literature is touched upon because the differing theoretical viewpoints affect and influence clinical treatments and research directions. This is particularly true of dyspraxia.

In the 1960s, children who exhibited features consistent with dyspraxia were said to experience problems with the voluntary motor aspects of speech articulation (Morley, 1967). During the late 1970s and onwards, the linguistic paradigm came to the fore within speech pathology and this exerted a considerable influence on the manner in which problems in communicating were construed (Ingram, 1976; Crystal, 1980). 'Distinctive features' and 'phonological processes' became common terms, used to describe speech problems as well as accounting for commonalities and patterns of speech errors. At the same time a tendency to refrain from the use of terminology relating to speech articulation or motor aspects also emerged. During this time the distinct entity of developmental verbal dyspraxia (DVD) was introduced (for example, Edwards, 1973). Disorders containing DVD-type features tended to be increasingly described using linguistic phenomena and managed using principles derived from a linguistic framework.

Debate emerged between proponents of linguistic frameworks and those who aligned with a motor framework. To an extent, these opposing views have persisted to the present time, although recently there has been a move towards viewpoints that are more encompassing and acknowledge the potential contribution of both linguistic and motor factors in DVD-type disorders.

The changing theoretical viewpoints over the past 50 years has had an effect on the accumulation of evidence underpinning paediatric motor speech disorders. This will be addressed later in this chapter when treatment approaches are reviewed and the evidence for each approach is evaluated.

Defining paediatric motor speech disorders

Because controversy surrounds the diagnosis of paediatric motor speech disorders it is necessary to define each disorder.

What is dysarthria?

Dysarthria comprises a group of speech disorders resulting from disturbances in muscular control owing to impairment of any of the basic motor processes involved in the execution of speech (Darley et al., 1975). It is generally accepted that this group of disorders occurs as a result of impairment of the central or peripheral nervous system. This impairment affects the motor and sensory activity of the speech mechanism resulting in weakness, slowness, incoordination and/or a reduction in the range of movement as well as altered muscle tone. Respiration, phonation, articulation and resonance may be affected to various degrees leaving speech sounding nasal, slurred and/or breathy. The exact nature of the dysarthria and the resulting speech characteristics are dependent on the type of impairment.

In children, dysarthria is classified as acquired (for example, post-natal acquired brain injury) or 'congenital or developmental' (for example, insult to the central nervous system during embryogenesis or perinatally, as in cerebral palsy). The bulk of the literature on paediatric dysarthria focuses primarily on acquired dysarthrias rather than developmental cases.

Communicating Quality (RCSLT, 2000, p. 167) described developmental dysarthria as 'a disorder manifest from infancy affecting voluntary movement of the oral and pharyngeal structures'. Acquired dysarthria was described as:

> a speech disorder resulting from the disturbance of neuromuscular control. This is caused by damage to the central or peripheral nervous system, which may result in weakness, slowing, incoordination or altered muscle tone, and changes the characteristics of speech produced. (RCSLT, 2000, p. 158)

Not included in this definition is any mention of when the disorder was acquired, but presumably this can occur anytime after birth. There are many different types of dysarthria and the speech characteristics vary according to the subtypes described. For a detailed discussion see Murdoch et al. (1990) and Murdoch and Horton (1998).

What is dyspraxia?

Dyspraxia remains one of the most controversial diagnoses in paediatric speech pathology practice. Various terms have been coined to denote the disorder, including 'developmental verbal dyspraxia', 'developmental articulatory dyspraxia' and 'developmental apraxia of speech'. Throughout this chapter the term 'dyspraxia' is used.

In 1981 Guyette and Diedrich wrote a highly critical review that concluded, 'no pathogonomic symptoms or necessary and sufficient conditions were found for the diagnosis ... the diagnosis 'developmental apraxia of speech' is neither appropriate nor useful'. These authors went on to state that dyspraxia was a 'label in search of a population'. Despite this, a plethora of literature on the subject of dyspraxia continues to emerge.

There has always been a strong suggestion that at least some forms of dyspraxia are familial and likely to be heritable. Recently, further light has been shed on possible genetic transmission and the somewhat mystifying aetiology surrounding dyspraxia. A mutation on the gene FOXP2 was found in an individual with severe speech and language disorder of which severe dyspraxia was the main characteristic (Lai et al., 2001). These authors hypothesized that FOXP2 haplo-insufficiency in the brain at key stages of embryogenesis leads to abnormal development of the neural structures important for speech and language development.

Regardless of the controversies that exist, it is generally agreed that dyspraxia is a motor programming disorder (Yorkston et al., 1999). Many also believe that underlying this condition is a disturbance of higher level functions responsible for the organization of movement related to speech. Perhaps it is for reasons such as this that researchers such as Ozanne (1994) view dyspraxia as a 'multi-deficit motor-speech disorder'. Problems include difficulties with pre-planning or programming the order and the duration of movement sequences (Blakely, 1983; Strand, 1995).

Traditionally, it has been accepted that there is no impairment of muscle function in dyspraxia, in contrast to dysarthria where the primary features involve problems with strength and speed of movement (Square, 1994). In dyspraxia, according to La Pointe and Katz (1998), features relate essentially to difficulties with timing and the direction of movements required for speech production.

Proponents of the existence of verbal dyspraxia in children (for example, Robin, 1992, p. 19) argue that because dyspraxia primarily involves a problem with movement, 'notions of linguistic bases for the disorder are misguided'. Such a view accentuates the necessity for consideration of multiple factors in assessment and treatment. In line with Robin's thinking are views that question the use of approaches that incorporate auditory discrimination and phonological approaches with children who manifest with dyspraxic problems (Rosenbek et al., 1974; Pannbacker, 1988). Conversely, others such as Marion et al. (1993) postulate an underlying poor phonological representation system in these children (based on signs such as an inferior ability to rhyme) and argue against the exclusion of auditory discrimination and other linguistic strategies in treatment.

A cursory examination of the literature reveals immediately, even to the inexperienced, that there are many opposing views among clinicians and researchers regarding motor speech disorders, in particular dyspraxia. Numerous questions arise as to the diagnosis and classification of paediatric motor speech disorders and it is necessary to examine these further before considering the evidence for treatment.

Is there evidence for a paediatric motor speech disorders continuum?

Numerous authors have identified that part of the controversy in paediatric motor speech disorders is the lack of diagnostic exclusivity (Crary, 1984; Morgan-Barry, 1995a, 1995b; Clark et al., 2000). For example, phonological processes of initial and final consonant deletion may be present in children considered to have dyspraxia, as well as in those not thought to exhibit dyspraxia. Similarly, difficulties in producing multi-syllabic words and in diadochokinesis may be evident in young children, irrespective of a diagnosis of dyspraxia. Moreover, features considered by some to be exclusionary criteria for the diagnosis of a motor speech disorder such as dyspraxia (for example, deficits in expressive semantics and syntax) may co-exist with what on first impression appears to be a primary motor speech problem (Crary and Towne, 1984). On the other hand, researchers such as Stackhouse (1992) suggest that syntax restrictions are part of the disorder; some children may reduce utterance length in an attempt to compensate for speech production problems.

Nonetheless, others believe that children with dyspraxia also manifest with idiosyncratic speech and praxis features, for example, inconsistency or variability of error patterns, deficient consonant inventories, transpositions of phonemes within words, sequencing difficulties, vowel errors, prosody disturbances, silent posturing and/or groping of the articulators, and believe that these distinguish them from other motor speech disorders (Rosenbek and Wertz 1972; Chappell, 1973; Ozanne, 1994).

The overlap, mentioned earlier, is not confined to dyspraxia as there is considerable symptom overlap between dyspraxia and dysarthria, and other speech disorders (not construed to involve any major motor planning deficit). This is most clearly illustrated by Rosemary Morgan Barry's (1995a) continuum (reproduced with permission in Figure 10.1). Morgan Barry formulated the continuum from her clinical experience, her own research data, and an appraisal of the literature on paediatric dysarthria and dyspraxia. Morgan Barry (1995a) proposed that dyspraxia and dysarthria overlap in children and that the overlap might be integral to the motor speech system. The fact that the two conditions might co-exist had also been proposed by others (Crary, 1984). Morgan Barry (1995a) stated that the combination of symptoms may be such that no clear diagnosis may be made and therefore the term 'motor speech disorder' might be best applied as a speech diagnosis in its own right. Diagnosis would, therefore, presumably be reliant on the presence of more symptoms from one end of the continuum than the other.

Other frameworks for understanding paediatric motor speech disorders have also been proposed by Shriberg et al. (1997), and Stackhouse (1992). Shriberg et al. (1997) developed the Speech Disorders Classification System, an aetiological-based classification system that can be used to classify an individual's speech production status through the lifespan. (It contains reference data on more than 800 subjects ranging in age from 3 to 40 years.) Stackhouse (1992) reviewed the literature to determine if children with dyspraxia exhibited distinctive features and attempted to address the question by devising broad categories that included the following.

• The clinical perspective, including clinical signs, oral motor skills and familial factors.

- The phonetic perspective, including sub-parameters such as history of speech difficulties, articulatory characteristics, prosodic features and co-ordination of the vocal tract.
- The linguistic perspective, including phonological and syntactic factors.
- The cognitive perspective, including intelligence, perceptual skills and reading and spelling.

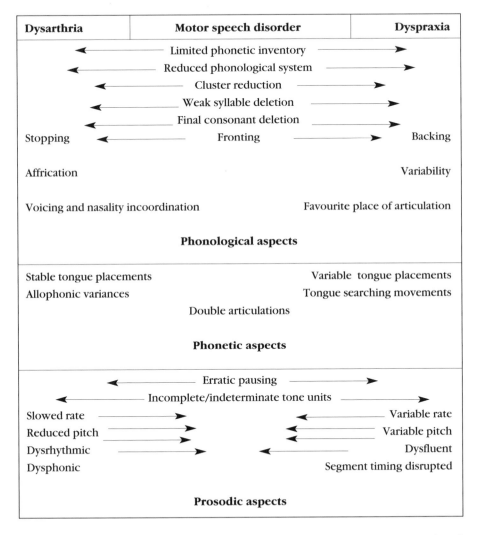

Figure 10.1 Paediatric motor speech continuum (Morgan Barry, 1995a). (Reproduced with permission.)

The review was comprehensive and Stackhouse (1992) concluded that difficulties within any of these areas may manifest, change or cease to exist at different stages in children with dyspraxia. She suggested that no one perspective was sufficient to characterize the disorder and that a combination should be present before contemplating the diagnosis. However, Stackhouse's observations highlight the confounding nature of dyspraxia and the challenges presented to researchers and clinicians alike in defining the clinical population for research purposes.

Reviewing the literature, we wanted to identify the main theoretical viewpoints regarding paediatric motor speech disorders. Two main or general theories regarding motor speech disorders were found:

- dyspraxia and dysarthia are distinct diagnostic paediatric motor speech disorders
- there is a motor speech disorders continuum – the extreme ends of this continuum represent the classic diagnostic entities of dyspraxia and dysarthria.

Four theories specific to dyspraxia were also identified:

- dyspraxia is a disorder of motor programming or planning
- dyspraxia is a disorder of motor impairment, programming and planning (in other words it also contains some features of dysarthria)
- dyspraxia is a severe, phonologically based linguistic disorder
- dyspraxia is a multi-system disorder.

Is there any evidence to support any one of these theoretical viewpoints over another? First, the theoretical literature was examined, then reviewed and the evidence underpinning each theory was evaluated. In so doing, a number of key issues were identified, which neither prove nor disprove each of these theories. Following this review there was no doubt that the methodological issues identified have a major effect on the validity and strength of the evidence for any of the theories listed above. The key issues identified are as follows:

1. Although the majority of studies were reasonably well conducted, many were contaminated by the manner in which the sample was recruited and the stated inclusion or exclusion criteria. Classic and oft-quoted studies have pre-selected subjects on the basis of speech-related tasks thought to characterize dyspraxia. For example, Crary (1984) selected subjects on the basis of their difficulty with volitional oral movements (it was one of the main inclusion criteria). Others pre-defined their samples by excluding children with any known co-existing language disorder. The problem with such

studies is best exemplified by the following quotation from Jaffe (1984, p. 171) who wrote, 'It is extremely circular to select studies on the basis of behavioural characteristics that the study itself is designed to discover.'

2. The majority of studies involved 'clinical' or 'referred samples', meaning that subjects had been pre-diagnosed as having dyspraxia or dysarthria by experienced clinicians. Given the lack of agreement as to what constitutes the condition, this would seem a major flaw and to date few comprehensive studies have been undertaken to ascertain if there is any agreement among clinicians regarding the diagnosis of dyspraxia. Unfortunately, even the subject samples used in recent and promising cross-validation studies originated from referred clinical samples. For example, Thoonen et al. (1997) conducted some cross-validation studies using maximum performance tasks. These authors demonstrated that it was possible to differentially diagnose or separate dyspraxia from dysarthria (normal speakers were included as control subjects) with high diagnostic accuracy: sensitivity was 95% and specificity 97%. These results were strong even when borderline or milder cases were included as part of the validation exercise. There have been a few notable studies that have attempted to address subject selection criteria (Morgan Barry, 1995a; Shriberg et al., 1997). Both did not include a 'referred' clinically diagnosed sample (instead children described as having 'persistent phonological disorders' were recruited). Morgan Barry (1995a) concluded from her study of just four children that although dyspraxia and dysarthria probably do exist as separate entities they are inter related and it is possible that a continuum may exist. Shriberg et al. (1997, p. 282) stated that the construct, 'otherwise inexplicable lack of progress' was one of the strongest features associated with dyspraxia.

3. To date the majority of studies have described small samples of pre-defined clinical series of cases and have not included a properly constituted comparison group of normal speakers, children with other motor speech disorders or children with other speech disorders (non-motor).

4. Attempts to establish if elements of dyspraxia and dysarthria co-exist have also been contaminated by the way in which the samples were ascertained and the results are not comparable because different assessment methods have been used. For example, Rosenbek and Wertz (1972) studied a clinical sample and found that 26% of children referred with dyspraxia also had characteristics of dysarthria (established via traditional methods). In contrast, Murdoch et al. (1995) used instrumentation to demonstrate that elements of dysarthria (impaired tongue strength and endurance) were present in six children with dyspraxia.

5. Much of the evidence for the theory that dyspraxia is a severe, phonologically based linguistic disorder comes from descriptive case studies and clinical case series of small samples of subjects (for example, 10–25

subjects). Descriptive profiles obtained from the individual participants in these studies (most do not include a comparison group) are used to support the theory. The exception is the series of studies carried out by Shriberg et al. (1997) who were able to statistically differentiate children with dyspraxia from those with speech delay and from normal speakers. One linguistic variable, a deficit in phrasal stress, was found to differentiate 52% of the dyspraxic children. However, these authors also proposed that at least one other subtype also exists and that it was marked by one or more segmental deficits.

6. A range of tools and assessment techniques have been used to establish the presence or absence of the condition and therefore comparison between studies is almost impossible. Few tools have been shown to have adequate psychometric properties (for example, validity and reliability). Analysis methods also lack sensitivity; for example, analysis is often only conducted at the segmental speech level and not at the suprasegmental level. There are exceptions, e.g. the study by Velleman and Shriberg (1999). The lexical stress errors these workers found did not differentiate children with suspected dyspraxia from those with speech delay. They did find, however, that such types of errors persisted longer in children with suspected dyspraxia.

7. The age range of subjects within some studies has been broad (for example, Crary and Towne, 1984). This is particularly problematic if, as suggested, the characteristics and/or communication profiles in dyspraxia change or cease to exist at different stages. Stackhouse (1992) raised reservations about the wide age span evident in the research for this clinical group and how this might affect the interpretation of results.

From the literature review it was evident that many of the above theoretical approaches arose primarily from expert opinion and were not underpinned by evidence. Together, the issues described above contaminate the evidence that underpins the theories regarding motor speech disorders, in particular dyspraxia. There appears to be a lack of recognizable, clear and distinct diagnostic entities and considerable heterogeneity among children with motor speech disorders. There is growing support for the idea of a paediatric motor speech disorders continuum and this certainly seems a sensible and attractive option. However, could the reason why this is an attractive option be because speech pathologists simply failed to adequately identify the key diagnostic components of the disorders? Do we still have labels looking for populations, as proposed by Guyette and Diedrich (1981)?

The epidemiological work carried out by Shriberg and colleagues (1997), although distinguishing distinct entities also suggests that a number of subtypes exist in children (especially in dyspraxia) and that this may contribute to heterogeneity within this population. A continuum of severity also appears to exist. As Morgan Barry proposed, diagnosis might well be reliant on the severity or presence of symptoms from different ends of a spectrum. To complicate things even further it appears that many different aetiologies give rise to similar symptoms. For example, dyspraxia in children has been described as a concomitant of conditions as diverse as galactaseamia (Nelson, 1995; Heidrich-Hansen et al., 1996), autosomal dominant rolandic epilepsy (Scheffer et al., 1995) and Fragile X syndrome (Spinelli et al., 1995). Although the aetiological pathway might in some cases be congenital (for example, Fragile X), in others it is acquired (for example, traumatic brain injury) and in many the aetiology remains unknown. Might clinicians then have a speech deficit that expresses itself in an identical or similar way, despite distinctly different aetiological pathways? Alternatively, perhaps this speech deficit clinicians label as dyspraxia is actually expressed differently in each of these conditions? Furthermore, it is important to keep in mind that in many congenital conditions, dyspraxia is just one of a number of multiple system deficits.

Prevalence of paediatric motor speech disorders

It is not surprising to discover that the reported prevalence data for paediatric motor speech disorders is variable. As already highlighted, the epidemiology and natural history of paediatric motor speech disorders is not adequately understood. The validity of the prevalence data was affected by deficient ascertainment methods, the variable diagnostic definitions adopted and the particular populations that have been studied. What is more, obtaining these data would seem a distant goal given the limits in our understanding of the diagnosis and classification of paediatric motor speech disorders. To complicate the situation even further, although paediatric motor speech disorder may be a speech diagnosis in its own right (as suggested by Morgan Barry (1995a)), in many cases motor speech disorders do not occur in isolation but as part of a cluster of symptoms of disorders or disease processes.

Nonetheless, some prevalence estimates for developmental dyspraxia do exist. They range from 0.125% (Shriberg et al., 1997) to 1–1.3% (Morley, 1967; Yoss and Darley, 1974). The prevalence estimates for dysarthria are condition-specific. For example, prevalence rates exist for dysarthria in cerebral palsy, ranging from 31% to 59% (Wolfe, 1950) to 88% (Achilles, 1955). Although dysarthria is a frequently reported consequence of acquired brain injury, in particular in the 15% of children who suffer severe brain injuries (for example, Bak et al., 1983; Costeff et al., 1985; Murdoch and Horton, 1998), there are no definite prevalence estimates.

In a recent survey of two London education authorities in the UK, 37% of children identified as having a primary speech and language problem were diagnosed as having developmental verbal dyspraxia (Dockrell and Lindsay, 1998). Presumably, the huge range that exists in the reported prevalence estimates is due in part to the lack of a clear diagnostic entity.

Diagnosis of and differentiation of paediatric motor speech disorders

The preceding discussion gives rise to numerous questions about the assessment and diagnosis of paediatric motor speech disorders. First, is there any agreement regarding diagnosis? Second, how do clinicians differentially diagnose a motor speech disorder from other speech disorders in children, and last, how do they decide if a child has dysarthria as opposed to dyspraxia or whether both disorders exist?

Guyette and Diedrich (1981) reviewed the diagnostic process in motor speech disorders, focusing primarily on dyspraxia. These authors argued and concluded that because the characterization of dyspraxia is vague, it makes it almost impossible to distinguish it from other types of paediatric speech disorders. In order to evaluate this further it is necessary to consider if there are symptoms or sets of symptoms that together distinguish, with certainty (and reliability), motor speech disorders from other paediatric speech disorders. Furthermore, can motor speech disorder subgroups (such as dyspraxia and dysarthria) be differentiated on the basis of symptomatology?

Diagnostic signs or symptoms may be divided into two main groups: non-speech and speech-related signs. Traditionally, non-speech signs include dimensions such as soft or hard signs, revealed on neurological examination, abnormal results from EEGs, abnormal results obtained from scans such as CAT, MRI or PET. For some time it has been accepted that one factor that differentiated motor speech disorders from other speech disorders was the presence of 'soft' neurological signs (Horwitz, 1984). Within the paediatric motor speech disorders group, dysarthria could also be differentiated from dyspraxia by the presence of soft neurological signs (for example, abnormalities on cranial nerve testing). However, this is now accepted to be a 'naïve' belief and the validity of soft neurological signs for the demonstration of brain damage has been questioned (Horwitz, 1984).

Table 10.2 summarizes the speech-related signs used to differentiate between and within paediatric motor speech disorder groups. The results are confusing and at first glance there seems to be little consensus. The studies that have engaged a comparison group of children with non-specific speech disorders yield interesting results. When children with dyspraxia were compared to children with non-specific speech disorders there do not appear to be major differences and the characteristics that make up dyspraxia also seem to be present in children with 'other' speech disorders. Children with dysarthria, on the other hand, do appear to be different on a number of features, including

Table 10.2 Speech-related tasks used to differentiate paediatric motor speech disorder groups from other speech disorders*

Task	Source	Type of study	Finding	Evidence
Volitional oral movements (VOM)	Rosenbek and Wertz (1972)	Case series: 36 subjects; included a neurological examination.	Often but not always present.	III.3
	Darley and Spreisterbach (1978)	Based on result from Yoss and Darley (1974). However the main inclusion criteria was difficulty with VOM.	Accompanying VOM problem usually present.	III.3
	Aram and Howritz (1983)	Case series: 7 subjects; used a standardized test but did not report cut-offs or scores.	5 subjects had VOM difficulties.	III.3
	Ferry et al. (1975)	Descriptive study: 60 subjects; no measures taken or described. Described also difficulties with vegetative functions for example, drooling, sucking, chewing.	36 subjects said to have VOM problems.	III.3
	Kools et al. (1971); Kools and Tweedie (1975)	Descriptive: 87 normal subjects	Weak correlation only between VOM and speech at 2 years none at 3, 4 and 5 years of age.	III.3
Diadochokinetic rates (DR)	Aram and Howritz (1983)	Case series: 7 subjects; repetition of /pa/ and /pataka/	All children had difficulty; limited number of repetitions and slow and arrythmic.	III.3
	Nicolosi et al. (1978)	Case series: functional articulation disorders	Normal diadokinetic rate in all children.	III.3
	Yoss and Darley (1974)	Case control study of three groups: (1) functional articulation disorders; (2) Dyspraxic; (3) Matched control subjects	No difference between groups 1 and 2 on diadchokinetic rate. Significant difference between matched control subjects and groups 1 and 2. 50% of subjects with dyspraxia could not produce diadchokinetic rate /pataka/, but results for /pa/ only slightly below age matched control subjects.	III.2

(contd)

Table 10.2 (contd)

Task	Source	Type of study	Finding	Evidence
	Thoonen et al. (1999)	72 subjects: four groups (1) clear cases of dyspraxia and dysarthria; (2) mixed disorders or mild cases; (3) non-specific articulation disorders; (4) normal speakers; aged 4–12 years	Diadokinetic rate discriminated between all groups but different aspects were important. Dysarthria diagnosed on basis of maximum diadchokinetic rate and maximum vowel prolongation. Dyspraxia diagnosed on basis of maximum rate of alternating diadchokinetic rate sequences and maximum fricative prolongation. Sensitivity and specificity ranged from 89% to 100%. Dysarthic and dyspraxic speech characteristics also observed in children with non-specific speech disorders.	III.2
Language deficits (LD)	Rosenbek and Wertz (1972)	Case series: 36 subjects; no effort made to exclude children with language disorders from sample	56% of dyspraxic children in the study had accompanying aphasia.	III.3
	Chappell (1973)	Case series of apraxic subjects only	Intact cognitive and receptive language skills.	III.3
	Aram and Howritz (1983)	Case series: 7 subjects	Delayed acquisition of language milestones, normal comprehension of vocabulary and syntax but increasing difficulty with longer utterance. Delayed expressive language and learning difficulties.	III.3

Muscular weakness, paralysis or inco-ordination (MW)	Yoss and Darley (1974)	Case control study of three groups	No language delay *but* subject inclusion criteria excluded language-delayed children.	III.2
	Finley et al. (1977)	Case series: 4 subjects aged 6–10 years with cerebral palsy	Oromotor examination revealed muscular weakness.	III.3
	Love et al. (1980)	Descriptive study of 60 subjects with cerebral palsy aged 3–20 years	Oromotor examination revealed muscular weakness.	III.3
	Bak et al. (1983)	Single-case study: 6-year-old – brainstem infarct	Oromotor examination revealed muscular weakness.	III.3
	Van Dongen et al. (1987)	Case series: 8 subjects – variety of aetiologies	Oromotor and neurological examination revealed muscular weakness.	III.3
	Robin and Eliason (1991)	Case series: 7 subjects with von Recklinghausen's disease	Oromotor and neurological examination revealed muscular weakness.	III.3
	Morgan Barry (1995a)	Comparison of two groups: (1) dysarthria – $n = 2$; (2) dyspraxia – $n = 2$	Overall incoordination of respiration, phonation, resonance and articulation found primarily in dysarthric children.	III.2
	Murdoch et al. (1995)	Case-control study: (1) Dyspraxia ($n = 6$); (2) Normally speaking children ($n = 6$), aged 5–11 years	Tongue strength and endurance was weaker and reduced in the dyspraxic children than control subjects. Concluded that a motor impairment forms at least part of the basis for dyapraxia.	III.2
Prosody	Morgan Barry (1995b)	Comparison of two groups: (1) dysarthria – $n = 2$; (2) dyspraxia – $n = 2$	Erratic pausing with uneven word stress found in both group but more pronounced in dysarthric children.	III.2

(contd)

Table 10.2 (contd)

Task	Source	Type of study	Finding	Evidence
	Shriberg et al. (1997)	Comparison of two groups: (1) dyspraxia ($n = 14$); (2) speech delay ($n = 73$)	Stress was the only linguistic domain that differentiates children with dyspraxia from delayed speech.	III.2
Speech characteristics	Thoonen et al. (1994)	Case control study: 11 children with dyspraxia; 11 age-matched normal speaking control subjects	Few qualitative differences found in error patterns between case and control subjects. Dyspraxic children produced higher substitution and omission rates, but the profiles were similar.	III.2
	Thoonen et al. (1997)	Case-control study: (1) dyspraxic subjects ($n = 11$); (2) matched control subjects ($n = 11$)	Children with dyspraxia produced a higher rate of singleton consonant errors and cluster errors than normally speaking children. Substitution rate yields an adequate measure of severity in dyspraxia.	III.2
	McCabe et al. (1998)	Retrospective examination of clinical records ($n = 50$), children aged 2–8 years	Characteristics regarded as diagnostic for dyspraxia also occurred in the general speech impaired population There was a relationship between the number of dyspraxic features and the severity of the speech production problem.	III.3

*Also distinguishes between subgroups of motor speech disorders; basic details regarding the type of study are provided as well as the main findings and evidence levels.

the fact that there is an overall lack of co-ordination of respiration, phonation, resonance and articulation, and muscular weakness. However, to a lesser extent, symptoms regarded as characteristic of dysarthria (reduced tongue strength and endurance) have also been found in children with dyspraxia (Murdoch et al., 1995). From the evidence reviewed it seems we are no closer to establishing a clinical phenotype for paediatric motor speech disorders.

Consequences of paediatric motor speech disorders

Motor speech disorders affect speech intelligibility. Although the characteristics may vary, there is accepted overlap between dyspraxia and dysarthria (as illustrated in Figure 10.1). In addition, difficulties with eating, swallowing and saliva control may also co-exist. The severity of the disorder may vary from being one that is so mild it is just noticeable during rapid speech or only apparent to those familiar with the speaker, to a disorder so severe that no intelligible or functional speech is present. In the most severe case a child may be unable to produce any vocal utterances.

Motor speech disorders disable children by reducing their ability to function in situations that require intelligible speech and efficient communication, and consequently individuals face considerable frustration when trying to communicate. Environmental factors (such as stimulation, expectations and mobility) may further impair children's speech and language processes. Slow progress in response to treatment has been documented (Hall et al., 1993) and this, coupled with ongoing breakdown in transmitting effective messages that listeners can understand, affects a child's confidence in communicating. Intractability of this problem can have profound consequences with respect to psychosocial as well as later academic functioning (Dockrill and Lindsay, 1998).

What are the aims of intervention in paediatric motor speech disorders?

In paediatric motor speech disorders the primary aim of intervention is to maximize communicative function. Implicit in this aim is the understanding that not all children will achieve fully intelligible speech and some may be reliant on other methods to augment communication (see Chapter 12). Part of the intervention process will also involve encouraging and enabling carers, parents, teachers and important others in a child's life to participate in the therapeutic process and thereby facilitate communication with the child. Because many motor speech disorders also involve a co-existing dysphagia, this may also form part of the intervention process. In this chapter the management of dysphagia is not addressed further (see Chapter 7), nor is the use of alternative or augmentative communication (see Chapter 12).

The considerable controversies surrounding whether dysarthria and particularly dyspraxia are distinct diagnostic conditions have already been highlighted earlier in this chapter. As indicated, some have proposed the idea of a motor speech continuum. However, a review of the intervention literature indicates that this has not been considered with regard to treatment. As far as intervention is concerned, the conditions appear to have been regarded as totally separate diagnostic entities. Therefore the evidence for intervention will be presented and reviewed separately for both conditions.

Dyspraxia

Treatment for dyspraxia (where oral speech is considered achievable) aims to teach children to programme their articulators to achieve accurate production of speech sounds as well as sequencing of speech sounds within words. Expansion of a child's phonetic inventory, elaboration of word and syllable shapes and extension of utterance length are further targets. The overall aim of these treatment strategies is to improve speech intelligibility thereby enabling a child to communicate more readily and easily. An often unstated aim is to reduce the likelihood of associated problems (such as poor self-esteem or learning difficulties).

Many treatment strategies for children with dyspraxia are drawn from those in common use for traditional articulation problems. Similarities include approaches that advocate use of multi-modal input, active and frequent motor practice and addressing of motor skill (Diedrich, 1981; Blakely, 1983; Hadders-Algra, 2000).

As well as approaches used to treat other articulation problems, linguistic and phonological approaches are also used. Many treatment strategies are eclectic in that other modalities are accessed and incorporated in an attempt to compensate for difficulties. These include cueing, use of repetition and drills and melodic intonation therapy. There has been some contention as to whether specialized strategies and/or approaches are indicated for children with dyspraxia (Love, 2000). Cueing (visual, tactile, kinaesthetic and auditory) is one example of a specialized strategy that has been developed for use in dyspraxia. Touch-cue, as the name suggests, incorporates tactile cues applied (usually by the clinician) to areas of the face and neck to depict particular speech sounds (Bashir et al., 1984). Cueing has been further extended into whole approaches such as the 'prompts for restructuring oral muscular phonetic targets' (PROMPT) (Chumpelick, 1984). PROMPT (Loucks and De-Nil, 2001) involves manipulation of speech structures through motor movements involved in the production of various speech sounds; it is a combination of tactile stimulation and cueing.

Whole programmes have also been developed based on drills and repetition, such as the Nuffield Centre Dyspraxia Programme (Nuffield

Hearing and Speech Centre, 1985). The Nuffield programme involves visual cues in the form of picture symbols to depict various sounds. In addition, approaches such as 'melodic intonation therapy', which involves altering and exaggerating prosody within utterances, have also been applied to children with dyspraxia (Helfrich-Miller, 1984).

Although much is written about these approaches and programmes there are very few published reports that have evaluated the efficacy of each approach. In the few studies identified, often a combination of approaches has been used. This was emphasized by Yorkston et al. (1999), who discussed how the uncertainty regarding diagnostic entity affects decisions as to whether to incorporate an exclusively motor approach to dyspraxia treatment, or to use such a strategy and combine it with a linguistic approach. The majority of treatment studies have adopted an 'all or nothing' approach to the treatment of developmental verbal dyspraxia. At best, the literature comprises single-case studies (Level III.3) or small-case series (Level III.3) that contain few subjects. For example, Velleman (1994), reporting on just two case studies, found that sequencing of syllables appeared to be assisted by targeting sentence level prosody. Relatively few studies have adopted a case-control approach or multiple-baseline design and there are no studies that have compared one treatment strategy to another. (Available data are summarized in Table 10.3.)

Some approaches, such as PROMPT, have been growing in popularity with clinicians as a treatment of choice. However, despite claims by the developers (Loucks and De-Nil, 2001) that PROMPT has the facility to enhance speech motor skills, to our knowledge there has been no scientific evaluation of this approach. Other approaches that have been in use for some years now (for example, Nuffield Dyspraxia Programme) have also not been the subject of scientific evaluation.

Dysarthria

The treatment aims for children with dysarthria (where oral speech is considered achievable) are similar to those for dyspraxia. That is, the therapist aims to teach the child to achieve more accurate production of speech sounds with perhaps less emphasis on programming the articulators. As for dyspraxia, many treatment strategies are drawn from those in common use for other articulation problems. The emphasis in treatment is to improve speech intelligibility so that children can function as effectively as possible as oral communicators and maximize oral communication opportunities.

To summarize the approaches in common use, the treatment classification system or framework proposed by Fukusako et al. (1989) and others (for example, Murdoch and Horton, 1998) for dysarthria was adapted. Five treatment types were identified:

Table 10.3 Treatment strategies and approaches used for children with dyspraxia*

Approach	Source (s)	Strategy	Study information	Level of evidence
Multi-modal**	Rosenbek et al. (1974)	Techniques such as slowing speech, using auditory and visual modality; emphasizing movement sequences in CV and VC syllables, selecting contexts to facilitate production (e.g., places of articulation in close proximity) Utilizing spaced drill and use of serial items (e.g., counting) Utilizing rhythm, intonation and gross motor movements to assist production 22 treatment sessions over a three-month period	Single-subject case study – 9 years Results: reported increase in speech intelligibility.	III.3
	Yoss and Darley (1974)	Altering stress and intonation patterns, discriminating between words with different initial consonants, cues such as clapping, arm swinging, whole-body movements to accentuate stress and intonation patterns Suggests principles of treatment such as mirror work imitating oral movements, exaggerated movements, range of movements, imitating	Single-subject case study – 6 years. Results not reported.	IV
	Powell (1996)	Series of brief modules within sessions: using sound play activities, for example sound associated with a toy motor car together with a movement to depict a feature of the consonant	Single-case study – 5 years Results: reported gains in size of phonetic inventory and increased complexity noted in child's sound system.	III.3

		Utilize visual, auditory and tactile cues and then fading cues. Advocates stimulation of all sounds that are missing from the child's phonetic inventory. Four sessions per week of one hour's duration over the summer months		
	Watson and Gillon, (1999)	'Traditional apraxia treatment' (Nuffield + carrier phrases + DDK task practice) versus adapted phonological awareness training	Case-series – two cases aged 5 years Results: phonological awareness training resulted in improved production of consonants.	III.3
Multi-modal	Hall (1989)	Described a variety of approaches	No evaluation – expert opinion.	IV
	Harlan (1984)	Eclectic – non-speech approach (signing) plus direct work on oral expression (for example, imitation of mouth positions for vowel production) plus tactile cues combined with visual and gross motor movements (arm movements)	Case study Results: reported progress (but qualitative only and little information provided).	IV
	Cumley and Swanson (1999)	Largely an augmentative and alternative communication approach combining speech, gestures, manual signs and AAC resources (for example, picture communication dictionary or voice output device)	Series of single-case studies – aged 3;7, 8 years and 12;9 years. Results: case one achieved an increase in MLU. In case two there was an increase in the number of successful instances of communication and in case three an increase in assertive communicative behaviours as well as a reported reduction in frustration. Little if any improvement in articulation was reported.	III.3

(contd)

Table 10.3 (contd)

Approach	Source (s)	Strategy	Study information	Level of evidence
	Tessel and Joffe (2000)	Adapted touch cueing combined with Nuffield programme (graphic + Nuffield) and AAC (Compic + Makaton) as well as adapted music and movement programme (Joffe, 1995, 2000)	Series of single-case studies; aged 4 years and 3 years 2 months. Multiple baseline design with pre- and post-treatment outcome measures. Results: gains in phonetic and syllabic structure inventories and in phonetic distribution of speech.	III.3
	Watson and Leahy (1995)	Signing; combined with finger spelling, visual cues, tactile cues, gross motor movement, orthographic cues and modelling. In addition, reading books and telling stories with continued use of signs. Written word to trigger production of some sounds. Modelling of CVC words containing stops. Gradual fading of signs Twice weekly (one hour individual plus one-hour group activities) for 12 weeks and daily for six weeks	Single-case study – 3.1 years. Results: increase in use of spontaneous signs and emergence of sign combinations after 12 weeks. Increased consonant inventory and use of reduplicated syllables at end of second semester. By age 5;8 only some vowel errors and some unusual prosody remained.	III.3
Prosody***	Velleman (1994)	Subject 1: approach included increasing variety of syllables; improving language skills; working on sentence level prosody; pacing board for syllables; oral motor activities; sequencing activities Subject 2: expanding word and syllable shapes; improving language skills; book	Two case studies: case 1 aged 3;11 years and case 2: aged 2;4 years. Results: subject 1: improved production and sequencing of syllables; increase in MLU. Subject 2: increased consonant harmony and reduplication.	IV

Cueing	Klick (1985)	reading and pretend play as contexts for syllable practice; repetitions of words instead of counting (for example, *fish*, *fish*... etc.); naming multiple similar objects Cueing; adapted cueing; visual cueing	Single-case study aged 5;6 Results: increased intelligibility reported.	IV
	Bashir et al. (1984)	Cueing; tactile	Single-case study: 5-year-old Results: improved intelligibility reported.	IV
PROMPT	Chumpelik (1984); Hayden (1998)	Prompts: restructuring oral muscular phonetic targets	No formal evaluation.	IV
Nuffield	Nuffield Hearing and Speech Centre (1985)	Visual cues and pictorial symbols used to depict various sounds	No formal evaluation.	IV
Melodic intonation therapy	Helfrich-Miller (1984)	Melodic intonation therapy programme	Single-case study: Results: improvement in speech articulation and sequencing.	III.3

*Each study is classified according to the approach adopted. The source and information about the treatment strategy is provided as well as information about the study and the level of evidence.

**'Multi-modal' is used here to describe the combined use of many different approaches to treat children with dyspraxia.

***Although described as prosodic approach the example given is, in fact, multi-modal and differs for both subjects.

- physiological
- motor speech
- instrumentation
- pharmacology
- combined approaches.

Physiological approaches include muscle strengthening exercises and approaches such as proprioceptive neuromuscular facilitation. Motor speech approaches include more traditional speech pathology techniques, such as work on articulation, prosody, resonance and phonation. The use of instrumentation can include intra-oral appliances, amplification or biofeedback and specific approaches, such as electropalatography. An increased use of pharmacology in treatment is to be expected. This might include the use of drug treatment or botox injections (as highlighted in Table 10.4). Lastly, a category was included to enable review of combined approaches, which may reflect how different approaches are adopted in clinical practice.

The majority of authoritative journal articles reviewed on the treatment of paediatric dysarthria contained no data. The treatments and intervention programmes espoused were, in the main, anecdotal and the opinion of respected authorities in the field. Many of the traditional approaches in common use had not been the subject of scientific evaluation. The evidence for the main treatment strategies and approaches are depicted in Table 10.4 where brief descriptions of studies, participants, study design and level of evidence are displayed. At best, the majority of studies reviewed offer low levels (III.3) of evidence to support the common speech pathology approaches used with dysarthric children. Evidence for effectiveness comes from single-case studies (III.3) or case-series (III.3). Studies involving control groups or comparison treatments were rare.

It is important to note that almost all the treatment approaches described in the literature address only speech impairment (see Enderby and Emerson, 1995). Most focus solely on improvement in speech intelligibility as the main outcome measure. Such studies fail to consider or measure the disability and the functional limitations that might result from motor speech disorder. It is possible that there are other benefits (apart from changes in impairment level) that result from the speech pathology interventions on offer. Intervention might, for example, alter the strategies used in communication to enable individuals with a motor speech disorder to become more active participants in conversation. For example, in a child's school environment this might focus on changing how the child interacts or initiates communication. To date, however, only changes in degree or severity of impairment (primarily speech intelligibility) have been explored in children with motor speech disorders.

Table 10.4 Treatment strategies/approaches used for children with dysarthria*

Approach	Source (s)	Strategy	Study information	Level of evidence
Physiological	Butler and Darrah (2001)	Neuro-developmental treatment; uses the study of motor control, motor learning and motor development as the basis for understanding motor dysfunction	Although said to be highly effective, efficacy studies are inconclusive and the effect on breathing and speech has not been studied. Efficacy not evaluated in children.	IV
	Netsell and Rosenbek (1985)	Use of instrumental and biofeedback techniques to monitor attempts	Theoretical discussion only. Efficacy not evaluated in children.	IV
	Jones et al. (1963)	Exercises to improve respiratory muscle weakness and inco-ordination – expiratory muscle strength	Studied children with speech impairments and respiratory hypotonia; non-speech expiratory muscle conditioning resulted in changes to speech intelligibility.	III.3–IV
	Rothman (1978)		Case series – no control subjects used in any of the studies; most did not take speech measures as a main outcome with the exception of Cerny et al. (1997) who reported changes in speech intelligibility when non-speech expiratory muscle exercises were implemented.	
	Cerny et al. (1997)			
	Nwaobi et al. (1983); Nwaobi (1986); Nwaobi and Smith (1986)	Postural adjustment in children with cerebral palsy. Postural muscular activity minimized in the upright position	In three studies (all case series – $n = 11$) the effects of improved posture on respiratory function was studied. Improvements in tidal volume and minute ventilation and vital capacity resulted but the benefits to speech not measured but claimed as an outcome. Efficacy not evaluated in children.	IV

(contd)

Table 10.4 (contd)

Approach	Source (s)	Strategy	Study information	Level of evidence
	Rood (1956); Haynes (1985)	Aimed at increasing orosensory awareness in children with neuromuscular dysfunction. Uses techniques such as brushing, icing, rubbing or touching oral structures. Involves use of different textures and applications (for example, deep pressure and resistance)	Efficacy not evaluated in children.	IV
Specific speech pathology techniques	Vaughn and Clark (1979)	Speech facilitation via extra-oral stimulation – involving manipulation, cueing and stimulation of placement of the articulators	Efficacy not evaluated in children.	IV
	Crary (1993); Netsell and Rosenbek (1986)	Oromotor drills and exercises with and without resistance	Case series: uncontrolled experiments.	III.3/IV
	Hayden (1998); Hayden and Square (1993, 1994)	PROMPT – based on neurological, anatomical and motor theory principles	Efficacy not evaluated in children.	IV
	Yorkston et al., (1988); Dworkin (1991); Love (1992)	Increasing speech intelligibility though effort, strength, precision and rate	Efficacy not evaluated in children.	III.3
	Dean and Howell (1986)	Non-speech activities	Efficacy not evaluated in children.	IV
	Dworkin (1991)	Prosody	Efficacy not evaluated in children.	

	Ansel et al. (1983)	Other: modification of speech behaviours when faced with communication failure	Efficacy not evaluated in children.	IV
	Tjaden and Liss (1995)	Utilization of breathing strategies	Efficacy not evaluated in children.	IV
Instrumentation	Tudor and Selley (1974) Shaugnessy et al. (1983)	Use of prostheses, for example, palatal lift to aid speech intelligibility and decrease hypernasality	Single-case studies.	III.3
	Thomas-Stonell et al. (2001)	Computer program to train speech (Stepping Stones)	12 children and young adults; three-phase repeated measures design; significant changes in speech rate noted achieved gains maintained for four week follow-up phase.	III.2
	Morgan Barry (1995a)	Electropalatography (EPG)	Single-case study (12-year-old) with congenital suprabulbar paresis. Results inconclusive. Multiple baseline measures	III.3
	Gibbon et al., (1999)		Single-case study – 8year-old boy. Normal articulatory placements achieved for /t/ and /d/.	
Pharmacology	Lapco et al. (1999)	Botox injection	Case study: one adolescent with cerebral palsy. Reported improvement included increased fluency, quieter voice and a reduction in the staccato vocal quality Intelligibility increased from 40% to 85% at single-word level and from 60% to 94% for connected speech with familiar listeners. Voice changes documented with instrumentation, including the endoscopic and aerodynamic records. Improved oral communication resulted and telephone usage became possible.	III.3

(contd)

Table 10.4 (contd)

Approach	Source (s)	Strategy	Study information	Level of evidence
Combined approaches	Light et al. (1988)	AAC and behavioural	Single case study – 13-year-old with Cerebral Palsy – Resulted in transition to reliance on natural speech. Uncontrolled experiment.	IV
	Love (1969)	Sensory modality stimulation – visual, aural and combined	22 subjects (age range 7.6 years to 19 years). Intensive stimulation for 22 consecutive days. Combined aural and visual produced fewer errors than aural alone; voicing improved with aural and visual stimulation.	IV

*Each study is classified according to the approach adopted. The source and information about the treatment strategy is provided as well as information about the study and the level of evidence.

More often than not single treatments (for example, physiological) are not offered in isolation. Instead, they have been combined with other treatments (for example, both physiological and traditional). Approaches that use physiological and motor speech techniques (displayed in Table 10.4) focus primarily on increasing or decreasing muscle tone or strength and articulatory placements to improve speech intelligibility and have usually been applied as components of a 'treatment package'.

Summary of treatment for motor speech disorders

There is limited evidence that treatment programmes developed specifically for children with motor speech disorders (either dyspraxia or dysarthria) are any more effective than other 'traditional' articulation or phonological programmes. Often, adult rehabilitation programmes have been applied to children with limited success. It must therefore be concluded that the evidence for improving speech intelligibility outcomes in children with motor speech disorders is weak. There are a few case studies (Level III.3) and even fewer studies that have used a control or comparison group. No studies were found that compared one treatment with another. The majority of studies were constrained by methodological limitations, including poor case definition, inadequately defined treatment regimes, questionable subject selection criteria and ill-defined outcomes that focused almost solely on the level of impairment.

Interestingly, although few clinicians would dispute the need for family education and training, to date there has been no evaluation of this important and often time-consuming component of 'therapy' for children with motor speech disorders (Strand, 1995).

What factors affect the type and quality of the evidence in paediatric motor speech disorders?

Given the paucity of evidence and that the existing evidence is weak, it is important to ask why this should be so? As already highlighted, numerous problems exist concerning the definition, classification and therefore our understanding of paediatric motor speech disorders. These limitations affect the type and quality of the evidence underpinning the treatment of motor speech disorders. Jaffe (1989) summarized the problems aptly in a discussion of dypraxia as follows:

> Apraxia is defined by a symptom cluster ... Not all symptoms must be present; no one characteristic or symptom must be present; and the typically reported symptoms are not exclusive to developmental apraxia of speech. Compounding the problem is the observation that children change over time. (Jaffe, 1989, pp 166, 170)

In the following discussion the three main factors identified to have a major affect on both the type and quality of the existing evidence are summarized:

- diagnostic issues
- theoretical issues
- methodological issues.

Each will be discussed in turn.

Diagnostic issues

The controversy as to whether discrete diagnostic motor speech entities exist has had a major impact on the type of studies that have been conducted. Apart from a few exceptions, this is unacknowledged in much of the literature. As far as the treatment literature is concerned, dyspraxia and dysarthria are distinct diagnostic entities that require different treatment approaches. However, considerable heterogeneity is reported to exist between and within the diagnostic groups or the proposed continuum. This heterogeneity, along with individual variation, is often proposed as the main reason why it is not possible to conduct well-designed treatment studies in paediatric motor speech disorders. Until there is further elucidation regarding the diagnosis and classification of paediatric motor speech disorders it is difficult to know how big a problem heterogeneity may be in the design of controlled trials. This is no excuse for the lack of robust evidence. In conditions such as aphasia and cerebral palsy heterogeneity is also a factor in the design of controlled trials and the interpretation of results. In aphasia, there has been a shift away from randomized controlled trials toward studies that employ single-subject methodology because of the recognized heterogeneity (*see* Chapter 3). However, in paediatric motor speech disorders it may be premature to consider such decisions until the condition is better defined.

A further confounding issue in motor speech research is the reported phenomenon that spontaneous changes occur over time; hence the recognition of dyspraxic signs and symptoms may vary according to the child's age (Miller, 1986; Ozanne, 1994).

Theoretical issues

There are numerous theoretical issues that warrant discussion. First, general theoretical issues are briefly considered, and second, we look at theoretical issues regarding motor learning theories.

General issues

To date, many of the treatment strategies used with children with motor speech disorders have been adopted directly from those developed for use with adults. However, we have already learned that there are significant differences in the manifestation of motor speech disorders in children as compared to adults (Strand, 1995). Adults and children have differing processing demands. Unlike adults, children are simultaneously and interactively developing their cognitive, semantic, phonologic and motor control skills. It is not therefore surprising that motor speech disorders in children cannot be considered in isolation of the development of other language skills. Activities such as strength exercises in children are influenced by the linguistic, cognitive and motor demands placed on them. Similarly, motor learning principles (for example, repetition, performance feedback, effects of rate on performance) will also interact with these other demands.

Beliefs about the theoretical underpinning of motor speech disorders affect intervention frameworks and strategies. For example, should a multi-focus or single-focus treatment approach be adopted? If, for example, a clinician believes that dyspraxia and dysarthria are separate entities, and that dyspraxia is a disorder of motor planning and programming, then particular treatment strategies will be chosen accordingly. In contrast, the belief that dyspraxia is a multi-system deficit disorder as proposed by Ozanne (1994) would presumably result in selection and application of a wider variety of treatment strategies and options. Treatment in such cases may be multi-focal and involve the use of simultaneous approaches as described by Murdoch and Horton (1998). Strand (1995), discussing paediatric dysarthria, pointed out that treatment should not be single-focus. Instead, treatment should take into account factors such as the stage of language development.

Motor learning theories

Theory about motor learning has advanced in recent years, and these advances are not necessarily reflected in the treatment approaches described in the literature. First, there has been acknowledgment that children evolve through different neurological maturational phases and as they do so they acquire developmental skills. Therefore, the expression of the motor speech impairment may vary, its characteristics may change and at some stages even be silent during this process (Clark et al., 2000).

Second, for many years traditional approaches have focused on non-speech exercises that aim to improve strength and control. In adults, speech and non-speech behaviours are regarded as distinct and separate (Moore et al., 1988), whereas in infants it has long been suggested that novel motor patterns may be assembled by adapting established movement dynamics (for example, oral motor movements for feeding) to achieve new movement goals (for example, oral motor movements for speech). Clinical treatments in infants and children therefore have built on this premise (Mueller, 1972) and have been designed to elicit vegetative activities to enhance speech (Netsell and Rosenbek, 1985). However, doubts about the relevance of this approach have been raised (Luschei, 1991) and recent evidence does not support the suggestion that speech coordination emerges from earlier oral motor behaviours (Moore and Ruark, 1996). Further, it has been demonstrated that different control mechanisms mediate speech and non-speech behaviours in young children (Ruark and Moore, 1992). These findings are critical as the conceptualization of developing speech, as a successor to earlier appearing oral motor behaviours, is an explicit part of some models of motor speech control. Understandably, treatment strategies have been chosen to incorporate such aspects of the motor speech control model but the evidence suggests that this is misplaced.

Third, recent theories of motor learning, such as the neuronal group selection theory (NGST), suggest that children with motor deficits not only have a limited repertoire of primary neuronal networks but also impairments in processing afferent information (Hadders-Algra, 2000). For example, studies of manipulative skills in children with cerebral palsy suggest that deficits in sensory processing contribute to the motor output of children with mild to moderate cerebral palsy (Hadders-Algra, 2000). The results from intervention studies showed that practice, repetition of self-generated sensory input and augmentation of movement-related afferent information resulted in a decrease in motor output and in better task-specific adaptation of motor behaviour. Could these findings be applied to children with motor speech disorders?

Methodological issues

Given the major controversies highlighted throughout this chapter, it initially seemed pointless to attempt to address and reiterate the major methodological problems in the existing treatment studies. Nonetheless, it is important to ensure that readers are aware of areas where limited evidence exists. Readers should also be cognisant of the current best evidence underpinning the management of paediatric dysarthria and dyspraxia.

The majority of papers reviewed that did contain data failed to adequately describe the treatment components, how the treatment was delivered (some exceptions can be found in the case studies included in Murdoch and Horton (1998) and Murdoch et al. (1990)) or the intensity of the therapy. Further, many reported case studies provide insufficient data on the subject(s) and how they were recruited. For example, the many studies that used 'clinical referred' samples failed to mention how clinicians identified suitable subjects and if they used a specific set of diagnostic criteria. No study has been undertaken to measure how reliably the clinical and diagnostic judgements of paediatric speech pathologists are with regard to motor speech disorders.

If clinical and diagnostic judgements were found to be unreliable between and within clinicians then the evidence from existing clinical studies would be weakened further.

Conclusions: future directions

There is as an urgent need to address the methodological issues that weaken the existing studies on the treatment of motor speech disorders. It is also critical that we develop valid and reliable diagnostic markers and an improved classification system for paediatric motor speech disorders. We need to design and conduct studies that address the needs of children rather than relying on the 'trickle-down' effect of the results of trials conducted solely in adults' (Slinger and Mogher, 2001, p. 43). Treatment studies should also ensure that new information regarding motor learning theories is incorporated into the design of new treatment regimes. Given the need to investigate multiple factors (for example, linguistic, articulatory and motor or praxis aspects in children), well-designed multiple-baseline, single-case or single-subject research designs may be more suitable than the randomized controlled trial.

This review of speech pathology treatment for paediatric motor speech disorders revealed low levels of evidence (Level III.3). In 1974, Yoss and Darley, concluded that the results from treatment studies were badly needed. Almost ten years later, in 1981, Guyette and Diedrich again stated that there were still no published empirical studies that compared treatment programmes across children. (They were referring specifically to dyspraxia.) Twenty years later the situation in motor speech disorders remains little changed.

The major challenge facing researchers and clinicians considering undertaking treatment studies is whether it is possible given the basis of our existing knowledge. There is currently no clearly established phenotype for dyspraxia and the phenotypic characteristics for developmental and acquired dysarthria originate from the adult classification system. Many have suggested that there is a continuum and that the disorders co-exist in some form. There remains no clear biological correlate (Guyette and Diedrich, 1981). How then can we begin to evaluate the evidence for treatment of a condition, such as dyspraxia, about which there is little agreement?

The research of the future must be directed towards identifying a clinical and behavioural phenotype. It is clear from a series of studies aimed at elucidating the genetic and neurological basis of developmental speech and language disorders, that in many cases what has traditionally been termed 'dyspraxia' may not occur in isolation but in fact in association with multiple speech, language and cognitive impairments (Watkins et al., 2002a; Watkins et al., 2002b). Flint (1999) highlighted that only through careful delineation of the clinical and behavioural phenotype will the pathway from genotype to phenotype be accessed.

References

Achilles R. Communicative anomalies of individuals with cerebral palsy. Cerebral Palsy Review 1955; Sep-Oct: 15-24.

Aram DM, Horwitz SJ. Sequential and non-speech praxic abilities in developmental verbal apraxia. Developmental Medicine and Child Neurology 1983; 25: 197-206.

Bak E, Van Dongen HR, Arts WFM. The analysis of acquired dysarthria in childhood. Developmental Medicine and Child Neurology 1983; 25: 81-94.

Bashir AS, Grahamjones F, Botswick RY. A touch-cue method of therapy for developmental verbal apraxia. In: Perkins WH, Northern JL (eds). Seminars in Speech and Language. New York, NY: Thième-Stratton, 1984.

Blakeley RW. Treatment of developmental apraxia of speech. In: Perkins WH (Ed.). Current Therapy of Communication Disorders: Dysarthria and Apraxia. New York, NY: Thième-Stratton, 1983.

Butler C, Darrah J. Effects of neurodevelopmental treatment (NDT) for cerebral palsy: an AACPDM evidence report. Developmental Medicine and Child Neurology 2001; 43: 778-90.

Cerny FJ, Panzarella KJ, Stathopoulos E. Expiratory muscle conditioning in hypotonic children with low vocal intensity levels. Journal of Medical Speech–Language Pathology 1997; 5: 141-52.

Chappell GE. Childhood verbal apraxia and its treatment. Journal of Speech and Hearing Disorders 1973; 38: 362-8.

Chumpelik D. The PROMPT system of therapy: theoretical framework and applications for developmental apraxia of speech. In: Perkins WH, Northern JL (eds). Seminars in Speech and Language. New York, NY: Thième-Stratton, 1984.

Clark M, Carr L, Reilly S, Neville BG. Worster-drought syndrome, a mild tetraplegic perisylvian cerebral palsy: review of 47 cases. Brain 2000; 123: 2160-70.

Costeff H, Groswasser Z, Landman Y, Brenner T. Survivors of severe traumatic brain injury in childhood. I. Late residual disability. Scandinavian Journal of Rehabilitation Medicine 1985; 12: 10-15.

Crary MA. Phonological characteristics of developmental verbal dyspraxia. Seminars in Speech and Language 1984; 5: 71-83.

Crary MA. Developmental Motor Speech Disorders. San Diego, CA: Singular Publishing, 1993.

Crary MA, Towne RC. The asynergistic nature of developmental verbal dyspraxia. Australian Journal of Human Communication Disorders 1984; 12: 27-37.

Crystal D. Introduction to Language Pathology. London: Edward Arnold, 1980.

Cumley GD, Swanson S. Augmentative and alternative communication options for children with developmental apraxia of speech: three case studies. Augmentative and Alternative Communication 1999; 15: 110-25.

Darley FL, Aronson AE, Brown JE. Motor Speech Disorders. London: WB Saunders Company, 1975.

Darley FL, Spriesterbach DC. Diagnostic Methods in Speech Pathology (second edition). New York, NY: Harper & Row, 1978.

Dean E, Howell J. Developing linguistic awareness: a theoretically based approach to phonological disorders. British Journal of Communication Disorders 1986; 21: 223–36.

Diedrich WM. Toward an understanding of communicative disorders. In: Lass N, Northern J, Yoder D, McReynolds L (eds). Speech, Language and Hearing. Philadelphia, PA: WB Saunders, 1981.

Dockrell J, Lindsay G. The ways in which speech and language difficulties impact on children's access to the curriculum. Child Language Teaching and Therapy 1998; 14(2): 117–133.

Dworkin PI. Motor Speech Disorders: A Treatment Guide. St Louis, MI: Mosby Yearbook, 1991.

Edwards M. Developmental verbal dyspraxia. British Journal of Disorders of Communication 1973; 8: 64–70.

Enderby P, Emerson J. Speech language and therapy: does it work? BMJ 1996; June 29: 312.

Ferry PC, Hall SM, Hicks JL. Dilapidated speech: developmental verbal dyspraxia. Developmental Medicine and Child Neurology 1975; 17: 749–56.

Finley WW, Niman C, Standley J, Wansley RA. Electrophysiologic behaviour modification of frontal EMG in cerebral palsied children. Biofeedback and Self-Regulation 1977; 2: 59–79.

Flint J. The genetic basis of cognition. Brain 1999; 122: 2015–32.

Fukusako Y, Endo K, Konno K, Hasegawa K, Talsumi, Masaki S, Kawamura M, Shiola J, Hirose H. Changes in speech of spastic dysarthric patients after treatment based on perceptual analysis. Annual Bulletin RILP 1989; 23: 119–40.

Gibbon F, Stewart F, Hardcastle WJ, Crampin L. Widening access to electropalatography for children with persistent sound system disorders. American Journal of Speech–Language Pathology 1999; 8: 319–34.

Guyette TW, Diedrich WM. A critical review of developmental apraxia of speech. In: Lass NJ (Ed.). Speech and Language: Advances in Basic Research and Practice. New York, NY: Academic Press, 1981.

Hadders-Algra M. The neuronal group selection theory: promising principles for understanding and treating developmental motor disorders. Developmental Medicine and Child Neurology 2000; 42: 707–15.

Hall PK. The occurrence of developmental apraxia of speech in a mild articulation disorder: a case study Journal of Communication Disorders 1989; 22(4): 265–76.

Hall PK, Jordan LS, Robin DA. Developmental Apraxia of Speech: Theory and Clinical Practice. Austin, TX: Pro-Ed., 1993.

Hansen TW, Henrichsen B, Rasmussen RK, Carling A, Andressen AB, Skjeldal O. Neuropsychological and linguistic follow-up studies of children with galactosaemia from an unscreened population. Acta Paediatric 1996; 85(10): 1197–201.

Harlan NT. Treatment approach for a young child evidencing developmental verbal apraxia. Australian Journal of Human Communication Disorders 1984; 12: 121–7.

Hayden D. Motor disorders of speech and the PROMPT system. (www.apraxia-kids.org/slps/hayden.html) 1998.

Hayden DA, Square PA. A systems approach for the differential diagnosis of developmental apraxia. Paper presented at the Annual Convention of the American Speech-Language-Hearing Association, Anaheim, CA, 1993.

Hayden DA, Square PA. Motor speech treatment hierarchy: a systems approach. Clinical Communication Disorders 1994; 4(3): 162–74.

Haynes S. Developmental apraxia of speech: symptoms and treatment. In: John D (Ed.). Clinical Management of Neurogenic Communication Disorders. Boston, MA: Little, Brown & Co., 1985.

Helfrich-Miller KR. Melodic intonation therapy with developmentally apraxic children. Seminars in Speech and Language 1984; 5: 119–26.

Horwitz SJ. Neurological findings in developmental verbal apraxia. Seminars in Speech and Language 1984; 5: 111–18.

Ingram D. Phonological Disability in Children. New York, NY: Elsevier, 1976.

Jaffe MB. Childhood articulatory disorders of neurological origin. In: Leahy MM (Ed.). Disorders of Communication: The Science of Intervention. New York, NY: Taylor & Francis, 1989.

Jones EI, Hardy JC, Shipton HW. Development of electrical stimulation in modifying respiratory patterns of children with cerebral palsy. Journal of Speech and Hearing Disorders 1963; 28: 230–238.

Klick SL. Adapted cueing technique for use in treatment of dyspraxia. Language, Speech and Hearing Services in Schools 1985; 15: 256–9.

Kools JA, Williams AF, Vickers MJ, Caell A. Oral and limb apraxia in mentally retarded children with deviant articulation. Cortex 1971; 7: 387–400.

Kools JA, Tweedie D. Development of praxis in children. Perceptual and Motor Skills 1975; 40: 11–19.

Lapco PE, Forbes MM, Murry T, Rosen CA. Laryngeal botulinum toxin A for spastic dysarthria associated with cerebral palsy: a case study. Journal of Medical Speech–Language Pathology 1999; 7: 63–8.

Lai CSL, Fisher SE, Hurst JA, Vargha-Khadem F, Monaco AP. A forkhead-domain gene is mutated in a severe speech and language disorder. Nature 2001; 413: 519–22.

La Pointe LL, Katz RC. Neurogenic disorders of speech. In: Shames G, Wiig E, Secord WA (eds). Human Communication Disorders. Boston, MA: Allyn & Bacon, 1998.

Light J, Beesley M, Collier B. Transition through multiple augmentative and alternative communication systems: a three-year case study of a head injury adolescent. Augmentative and Alternative Communication 1988; 4: 2–14.

Loucks TMJ, De-Nil LF. Assessing the physiological and behavioural evidence for the role of kinesthesia in speech production. Journal of Speech Language Pathology and Audiology 2001; 25: 152–69.

Love RJ. Effects of Sensory Modality Stimulation on the Dysarthria of Cerebral Palsy. Vanderbilt University, Nashville, TN, Division of Hearing and Speech Science, 1969.

Love R. Childhood Motor Speech Disability. New York, NY: Macmillan, 1992.

Love RJ. Childhood Motor Speech Disability. Boston, MA: Allyn & Bacon, 2000.

Love RJ, Erman EL, Taimi EG. Speech performance, dysphagia and oral reflexes in cerebral palsy. Journal of Speech and Hearing Disorders 1980; 45: 59–75.

Luschei E. Development of objective standards of non-speech oral strength and performance: an advocate's view. In: Moore C, Yorkston K, Beukelman D (eds). Dysarthria and Apraxia of Speech: Perspectives on Management. Baltimore, MD: Paul H Brooks, 1991.

McCabe P, Rosenthal JB, McLeod S. Features of developmental dyspraxia in the general speech-impaired population. Clinical Linguistics and Phonetics 1998; 12: 105–26.

Miller N. Dyspraxia and its Management. London: Croom Helm, 1986.

Moore CA, Smith A, Ringel R. Task-specific organization of activity in human jaw muscles. Journal of Speech and Hearing Research 1988; 31: 670-80.

Moore CA, Ruark JL. Does speech emerge from early developing oral motor behaviours? Journal of Speech and Hearing Research 1996; 39: 1034-47.

Morgan Barry R. The relationship between dysarthria and verbal dyspraxia in children: a comparative study using profiling and instrumental analyses. Clinical Linguistics and Phonetics 1995a; 9: 277-309.

Morgan Barry R. A comparative study of the relationship between dysarthria and verbal dyspraxia in adults and children. Clinical Linguistics and Phonetics 1995b; 9: 311-32.

Morley ME. Development and Disorders of Speech in Childhood (second edition). Baltimore, MD: Williams & Williams, 1967.

Mueller H. Facilitating feeding and prespeech. In: Pearson P, Williams C (eds). Physical Therapy Services in the Developmental Disabilities. Springfield, IL: Thomas, 1972; 283-308.

Murdoch BE, Ozanne AE, Cross JA. Acquired childhood speech disorders: dysarthria and dyspraxia. In: Murdoch BE. Acquired Neurological Speech/Language Disorders in Childhood. London: Taylor & Francis, 1990.

Murdoch BE, Attard MD, Ozanne A, Stokes PD. Impaired tongue strength and endurance in developmental verbal dyspraxia: a physiological analysis. European Journal of Disorders of Communication 1995; 30: 51-64.

Murdoch BE, Horton SK. Acquired and developmental dysarthria in childhood. In: Murdoch BE. Dysarthria: A Physiological Approach to Assessment and Management. London: Stanley Thornes, 1998.

Nelson D. Verbal dyspraxia in children with galactosemia. European Journal of Pediatrics 1995; 154(7 Suppl 2): 56-7.

Netsell R, Rosenbek JC. Treating the dysarthrias. In: Darby J (Ed.). Speech and Language Evaluation in Neurology: Adult Disorders. New York, NY: Grune & Stratton, 1985.

Nicolosi L, Harryman E, Kresheck J. Terminology of Communicative Disorders: Speech, Language, Hearing. Baltimore, MD: Williams & Wilkins, 1978.

Nuffield Hearing and Speech Centre. Nuffield Centre Dyspraxia Programme. London: Nuffield Hearing and Speech Centre, 1985.

Nwaobi OM. Effects of body orientation in space on tonic muscle activity of patients with cerebral palsy. Developmental Medicine and Child Neurology 1986; 28: 41-4.

Nwaobi OM, Smith PD. Effect of adaptive seating on pulmonary function of children with cerebral palsy. Developmental Medicine and Child Neurology 1986; 28: 351-4.

Nwaobi OM, Brubaker CE, Cusick B, Sussman MD. Electromyographic investigation of extensor activity in cerebral-palsied children in different seating positions. Developmental Medicine and Child Neurology 1983; 25: 175-83.

Ozanne A. The search for developmental verbal dyspraxia. In: Dodd B. Differential Diagnosis and Treatment of Speech-disordered Children. London: Whurr Publishers, 1994.

Pannbacker M. Management strategies for developmental apraxia of speech: a review of literature. Journal of Communication Disorders 1988; 21(5): 363-71.

Powell T. Stimulability considerations in the phonological treatment of a child with a persistent disorder of speech-sound production. Journal of Communication Disorders 1996; 29: 315-33.

Robin DA, Eliason MJ. Speech and prosodic problems in children with neurofibromatosis. In: Moore CA, Yorkston KM, Beukelman DR (eds). Dysarthria and Apraxia of Speech: Perspectives on Management. Baltimore, MD: Paul H Brooks, 1991.

Rood MS. Neurophysiological mechanisms utilized in the treatment of neuromuscular dysfunction. American Journal of Occupational Therapy 1956; 10: 220.

Rosenbek J, Wertz RT. A review of 50 cases of developmental verbal dyspraxia of speech. Journal of Speech and Hearing Disorders 1972; 3: 23-33.

Rosenbek J, Hansen R, Baughman C, Lemme M. Treatment of developmental apraxia of speech: a case study. Language, Speech and Hearing Services in Schools 1974; 5: 13-22.

Rothman JG. Effects of respiratory exercises on the vital capacity and forced expiratory volume in children with cerebral palsy. Physical Therapy 1978; 58: 421-425.

Royal College of Speech and Language Therapists (RCSLT). Communicating Quality. London: Royal College of Speech and Language Therapists, 2000.

Ruark J, Moore CA. Coordination of Orofacial Muscles during Sucking by Human Infants. Paper presented at the 25th Annual ASHA Convention, San Antonio, TX, 1992.

Scheffer IE, Jones L, Pozzebon M, Howell RA, Saling MM, Berkovic SF. Autosomal dominant rolandic epilepsy and speech dyspraxia: a new syndrome with anticipation. Annals of Neurology 1995; 38: 633-642.

Shaugnessy A, Netsell R, Farrage J. Treatment of a four-year-old with a palatal lift prosthesis. In: Berry W (Ed.) Clinical Dysarthria. Boston, MA: College-Hill Press, 1983.

Sheppard JJ. Cranio-oropharyngeal motor patterns in dysarthria associated with cerebral palsy. Journal of Speech and Hearing Research 1964; 7: 373-80.

Shriberg LD, Aram DM, Kwiatkowski J. Developmental apraxia of speech: III. A subtype marked by inappropriate stress. Journal of Speech, Language and Hearing Research 1997; 40: 313-37.

Slinger R, Moher D. Assessing therapy. In: Moyer VA, Elliott EJ, Davis RL, Gilbert R, Klassen T, Logan S, Mellis C, Williams K. Evidence Based Paediatrics and Child Health. London: BMJ Books, 2001.

Spinelli M, Rocha AC, Giacheti CM, Richieri-Costa A. Word-finding difficulties, verbal paraphasias, and verbal dyspraxia in ten individuals with Fragile X syndrome. American Journal of Medical Genetics 1995; 60: 39-43.

Square PA. Treatment approaches for developmental apraxia of speech. Clinics in Communication Disorders 1994; 4: 151-61.

Stackhouse J. Developmental verbal dyspraxia I: a review and critique. European Journal of Disorders of Communication 1992; 27: 19-34.

Strand EA. Treatment of motor speech disorders. Seminars in Speech and Language 1995; 16: 126-139.

Tessel L, Joffe B. Evidence-based Practice: An Intensive Eclectic Multimodal Treatment Program for DAS. Paper presented at the Speech Pathology Association of Australia National Conference, Melbourne, 2001.

Thomas-Stonell N, Leeper HA, Young P. Evaluation of a computer-based program for training speech rate with children and adolescents with dysarthria. Journal of Medical Speech Language Pathology 2001; 9: 17-29.

Thoonan G, Maassen B, Gabreels F, Schreuder R. Feature analysis of singleton consonant errors in developmental verbal dyspraxia (DVD). Journal of Speech and Hearing Research 1994 Dec; 37(6): 1424-60.

Thoonen G, Maassen B, Gabreels F, Schreuder R, de Swart B. Towards a standardized assessment procedure for developmental apraxia of speech. European Journal of Disorders of Communication 1997; 32: 37-60.

Thoonen G, Maassen B, Gabreels F, Schreuder R. Validity of maximum performance tasks to diagnose motor speech disorders in children. Clinical Linguistics and Phonetics 1999; 13: 1-23.

Tjaden K, Liss JM. The influence of familiarity on judgements of treated speech. American Journal of Speech-Language Pathology 1995; 4: 39-48.

Tudor C, Selley WG. A palatal training appliance and a visual aid for use in the treatment of hypernasal speech. A preliminary report. British Journal of Communication Disorders 1974 Oct; 9(2): 117-22.

Van Dongen HR, Arts WFM, Yousef-Bak E. Acquired dysarthria in childhood: an analysis of dysarthric features in relation to neurologic deficits. Neurology 1987; 37: 296-9.

Vaughan GR, Clark RM. Speech Facilitation: Extraoral and Intraoral Stimulation Technique for Improvement of Articulation Skills. Springfield, IL: Charles C Thomas, 1979.

Velleman SL. The interaction of phonetics and phonology in developmental verbal dyspraxia: two case studies. Clinics in Communication Disorders 1994; 1: 66-77.

Velleman SL, Shriberg LD. Metrical analysis of the speech of children with suspected developmental apraxia of speech. Journal of Speech, Language and Hearing Research 1999; 42: 1444-60.

Watson B, Gillon G. Responses of children with developmental verbal dypraxia to phonological awareness training. Proceedings of the 1999 Speech Pathology Australia National Conference, 1999; 37-47.

Watson MM, Leahy J. Multimodal therapy for a child with developmental apraxia of speech: a case study. Child Language Teaching and Therapy 1995; 11: 264-72.

Watkins KE, Dronkers NF, Vargha-Khadem F. Behavioral analysis of an inherited speech and language disorder: comparison with acquired aphasia. Brain 2002a; 125: 452-64.

Watkins KE, Vargha-Khadem F, Ashburner J, Passingham RE, Connelly A, Friston KJ. MRI analysis of an inherited speech and language disorder: structural brain abnormalities. Brain 2002b; 125: 465-78.

Wolfe WG. A comprehensive evaluation of fifty cases of cerebral palsy. Journal of Speech and Hearing Disorders 15; 234-51.

Yorkston K, Beukelman D, Bell K. Clinical Management of Dysarthric Speakers. Boston, MA: College Hill Press, 1988.

Yorkston KM, Beukelman DR, Strand EA, Bell KR. Management of Motor Speech Disorders in Children and Adults (second edition). Austin, TX: Pro-Ed., 1999.

Yoss K, Darley FL. Developmental apraxia of speech in children with defective articulation. Journal of Speech and Hearing Research 1974; 17(3): 399-416.

Yoss K, Darley FL. Therapy in developmental apraxia of speech. Language, Speech and Hearing Services in Schools 1994; 5: 23-31.

CHAPTER 11

The evidence base for the treatment of articulation and phonological disorders in children

BEVERLY JOFFE AND TANYA SERRY

Introduction: articulation and phonological problems in context

Articulation and phonological problems are common disorders of speech (or, more generally, communication) in children, which constitute a large proportion of the speech pathologist's caseload (Almost and Rosenbaum, 1998). (In this chapter the term 'speech disorder' is used broadly and interchangeably with 'articulation and phonological disorders'.) There are distinct ramifications to a lack of efficacy in treatment for children exhibiting speech problems. These include the risk of some children developing social interaction problems and/or language learning difficulties.

From clinical experience it is apparent that it is problematic for some children (even those who have relatively few sounds in error) constantly to be asked to repeat words or to be teased for speaking in a 'different' way. Investigators such as Rice et al. (1993) refer to 'social marginalization' of young children with speech differences.

Given potential connections across linguistic levels (Crystal, 1987), ongoing speech disorders would also be expected to affect dimensions such as morphology and syntax, thereby compounding risk factors. Furthermore, there is an urgency to intervene at an early age with children who have speech problems, so that later literacy development is not compromised (Hodsen, 1998). There are longstanding views and cumulative evidence that speech disorders can affect pre-literacy skills and, in turn, scholastic achievement. Stackhouse (1982) identified difficulty with grapheme-phoneme conversions in children with speech disorders, and Dodd et al. (1995) found that children with speech disorders tended to exhibit delayed phonological awareness skills. This highlights the need for timely and effective intervention for children exhibiting speech disorders. How do clinicians ensure they meet such challenges?

One way of striving for efficacy in clinical practice is to access evidence from systematic research (Bannigan, 1997; Sackett et al., 1998). The number of studies published over the years and particularly the changing foci of underlying philosophies represented in these studies contribute to difficulty in accessing information in the area of child speech disorders. Ongoing questions concerning the perceived divide or otherwise, between articulation and phonology, as well as between motor and linguistic approaches, have contributed to a lack of clarity and consistency in the literature. Further, it is not at all straightforward for clinicians to identify which therapeutic management approaches are the most optimal in the literature. The present chapter attempts to shed some light on issues involved in clinical practice and informed decision-making for managing paediatric speech disorders.

Changes have occurred in the area of child speech disorders since the 1960s. Whereas articulation approaches dominated in the 1960s, phonological approaches came strongly to the fore by the end of the 1970s and continued to dominate throughout the 1980s. The linguistic focus or phonological process approach appeared to be afforded greater credibility, in some instances with the unfortunate consequence of 'throwing the baby out with the bathwater'; that is, articulation frameworks were seemingly discarded.

Confusion in terminology and clinical populations became evident in the literature. This confusion in turn affected comparative research as well as clinical practice. In the late 1980s, however, broader views were expressed more frequently in the literature. Thus, it was not considered sufficient to align only with one approach (usually the topical one of a particular decade) nor to use it with all children. Given the heterogeneity of paediatric speech disorders, it is not surprising that any exclusive approach would ultimately be limiting.

The emergence of more speech analysis methods (for example, Ball and Kent, 1997) and the application of psycholinguistic models to child speech (Stackhouse and Wells, 1993; Hewlett et al., 1998; Baker et al., 2001) further supports the need for multiple perspectives instead of one particular approach to clinical reasoning. However, the extent to which new insights has filtered through into practice and in some instances also, across research, is questionable. Oversights with regard to new developments can have a significant effect on the quality of the evidence available in the literature.

Another valuable component of evidence-based practice is clinical expertise (Sackett et al., 1998). Here, the interplay between parameters such as clinicians' previous training, belief systems and time constraints may influence clinical decision-making and, in turn, the efficacy of intervention. Within the clinical expertise 'arm' of evidence-based practice, it is important also to consider novice versus expert practitioners (described by Benner, 1984). The observation that clinicians who work in the area of child speech face the challenge of 'identifying which of these treatments is suited to the individual client' (Baker and McLeod, 2001, p. 101) is an accurate one. This challenge could be particularly pertinent for novice clinicians, whose limited caseload may not have been sufficient to have yet provided them with any sense of salience or tacit knowledge. The ability to integrate foreground factors with tacit knowledge promotes confident clinical decision-making. However, this does not suggest that more experienced clinicians need any less research-based evidence to continue to guide effective decision-making.

Baker and McLeod (2001) point out that a range of articulation and phonology treatment approaches may be suitable for particular children. Here again it would not be unusual to expect that some clinicians with a lot of clinical practice 'know-how' (and prior experience of many different clients and varying outcomes) could alternate, self-assuredly, between a motor-based and a linguistic-based treatment approach, depending on the client's needs. If the nature of such decision-making could be made explicit and documented, this too would contribute to the clinical expertise arm of evidence-based practice. However, in the context of much or little experience, evidence-based practice requires speech pathologists to be up to date with new research, frameworks and strategies as well as to be cognisant of previous literature and practices. Moreover, the evidence-based practitioner would be expected to be able to access, analyse and interpret this information critically in order to be able to select, evaluate and apply optimal treatment approaches for a particular child with speech disorders.

The present chapter briefly outlines the nature of articulation and phonology, and speech problems incorporating these dimensions, as well as clinical practices relating to this field. It then provides an overview of the main treatment approaches and reviews the evidence base for each.

Classification of articulation and phonology and their disorders

Articulation may be construed as the motoric production of speech sounds. 'Articulations' are described as 'gestures of the vocal organs ... to produce speech sounds' (Ladefoged, 2001, p. 5). Generally described at the phonetic level, articulation of speech sounds has been delineated according to 'place of articulation' and 'manner of articulation'. Hence, in the former, for example, a 'tip alveolar' speech sound denotes that the alveolar ridge within the oral cavity is the point of contact for the tongue tip, whereas for the latter, a construct such as 'plosive' or 'stop' may denote an aspect of the manner in which the sound is produced, for instance, involvement of a quick release of the breath stream at the point of articulation.

At the descriptive level, disorders of articulation encompass terminology such as:

- 'Substitutions', for example 'fum' for *thumb* or /wos/ for *wash*.
- 'Omissions', for example /bu/ for *blue*.
- 'Distortions', for example, as in the /s/ in the word *sun* produced with pharyngeal constriction.

Distortions typify, or are relatively straightforward examples of, inaccuracy in pronouncing or articulating speech sounds.

Phonology is associated with the sound system and with rules for combining sounds to form words so as to create different meanings. Clark and Yallop (1991, p. 2) describe phonology as the 'systems and patterns of sounds that occur in particular languages'. The 'phoneme' is considered the most basic unit, where each phoneme has linguistic significance in a word. For example, the use of the final consonant /t/ in the following one-syllable word creates a difference in meaning from exactly the same word, that does not have the final consonant, as in *boat* versus *bow*.

Phonological disorders are conceptualized as involving a lack of contrast (Hewlett, 1985). Take the example once again of the words *boat* versus *bow*. A child might have the /t/ speech sound within his or her phonetic inventory, but be unable to use it in word-final position in order to contrast one word from another, as in the example provided. Phonological disorders may be viewed as problems with 'organization and use of phonological information to signal meaning' (Baker et al., 1999, p. 29). When the speech disorder is conceptualized according to a phonological framework, consistent error patterns across phoneme classes are typically displayed. Commonly, these are referred to as 'phonological processes' and may constitute error types, such as:

- 'Stopping', where all fricatives and affricates are replaced with a stop consonant, produced approximately at the same place as the fricative would have been, for example *soap* becomes /dop/, *shoe* becomes /du/.
- 'Final consonant deletion', for example *coat* becomes /ko/, *rice* becomes /rai/.
- 'Syllable reduction', for example *banana* becomes /nana/, *butterfly* becomes /buflai/.

Over the years, different terminology has been used to identify similar speech production errors, depending on the framework used. For example, at a superficial level, according to the articulatory framework, a child who says /win/ for *ring* may be described as using a 'substitution error', whereas within a phonological framework, the same error may be described as the phonological process of 'gliding'. Hewlett's (1985) proposal to consider articulatory, phonetic and phonological distinctions is an interesting one, as is his suggestion that 'speech characteristics of some disorders might best be explained as resulting from avoidance strategies undertaken at the phonological level in order to circumvent lower level constraints' (Hewlett, 1985, p. 155). The example he provides, of a glottal stop substitution for a coronal voiceless consonant (a sound produced anteriorly in the oral cavity and involving elevation of the tip or blade of the tongue) in conditions involving structural deficits such as cleft palate (instead of it necessarily being a manifestation of a phonological process) makes sense. This example illustrates the complexity of speech disorders and highlights that there is not necessarily a clear-cut dichotomy between articulation and phonological disorders. Accordingly, a superficial approach to construal, clinical management or research would not be optimal and would affect the quality of the evidence base.

Speech sound disorders have more recently been described within the literature increasingly in line with the extended framework of 'non-linear phonology' (for example, Bernhardt and Gilbert, 1992; Bernhardt, 1994; Edwards, 1997; Ingram, 1997). According to such a view, a phonological process of 'stopping' (potentially described as a 'substitution' within an articulation framework) might be construed as a child presenting with the constraint of an inability to produce the feature of continuity when producing consonants. A child exhibiting the phonological process of 'syllable reduction', would be described as potentially having problems with 'syllabification' and hence deleting a syllable boundary or as demonstrating difficulty at the 'onset' (the element that occurs before the peak of a syllable; Bernhardt and Stemberger, 2000) and/or 'rime' (part of the syllable that contains the nuclear vowel and the consonant after the peak of a syllable; Bernhardt and Stemberger, 2000) level of the syllable. Dimensions such as timing units are also considered within this framework, for example a child who produces a singleton consonant because of an inability to produce a consonant cluster may nevertheless be able to retain and produce the word with two timing units.

All the frameworks outlined allow for a range of severity descriptors ranging from mild to severe. Changing frameworks and diverse descriptors contribute to the possibility of terminological confusion and related risks with respect to research and interpretation for clinical application. It is pertinent at this point to consider if there is a level of confidence in relation to how aetiological issues are regarded for speech disorders in children.

Suggested underlying mechanisms in articulation and phonological disorders

Multiple causative factors have been suggested for speech disorders (Weiss et al., 1987). In the presence of obvious anatomical and or physiological involvement of speech structures, the cause of an articulatory problem appears clear. Structural anomalies such as a fistula in the hard palate or abnormally short soft palate obviously affect the processes necessary for optimal speech production in relation to intra-oral breath pressure or requisite closure between velum and pharynx during speech (Spriestersbach and Sherman, 1968).

Similarly, a sensory deficit, like a hearing loss, or a deficit such as a 'tongue thrust' co-existing with a malocclusion are also feasible underlying reasons for an articulatory disorder such as a distorted /s/. Perceiving a sound differently would be expected to affect how it is produced. Menn and Stoel-Gammon (1995) posit an additional reason for children with hearing loss presenting with an impoverished variety of sounds – namely the reduced feedback from hearing oneself talk.

Features of 'cleft palate-type speech' characterized by, for example, pharyngeal constriction during fricative production or nasal release on stops, are relatively clear indicators of a particular underlying mechanism. In this case articulatory distortions may be traced back to behaviours implemented in the attempt to compensate for processes resulting from oral structural and associated functional deficiencies. Other instances of speech-sound disorders are less clear-cut, and for some there is no obvious reason why a child has used an incorrect production of the sound. It is this latter population that forms the largest group of children with speech-sound disorders, and our discussion focuses primarily on this group.

Caution regarding categorical statements on underlying mechanisms is supported by views and findings within the literature. Lancaster and Pope (1989, p. 109) suggest that 'speech disorders are seldom purely motoric or phonological in nature'. Abbs and Kennedy (1982) propose that although there are patterns to articulatory errors suggestive of the influence of linguistic rules in speech-sound production difficulties, it is important not to disregard the influence of sensorimotor control and the motor learning process. These authors cite the phenomenon of speech errors being retained despite the repair of a structural underlying deficit that had been a primary cause, for example cleft palate. Gibbon (1999) posits some form of speech motor control difficulty, even with children with ostensibly mild speech disorders, in that she has noted undifferentiated lingual gestures on electropalatographic recordings of these children. Yet, Fey's (1992, p. 227) premise that something more is required of the child in learning speech than 'just the control over the gestures required for rapid precise articulation', also bears consideration. In addition, potential models of speech breakdown (for example, Hewlett's (1990) two-lexicon framework) have not been sufficiently applied to articulation and phonological disorders. Clearly, the evidence base concerning underlying mechanisms of speech problems still requires extensive research. The findings of such research, in turn, would influence how speech pathologists assess and treat children exhibiting these problems.

Issues in assessing articulation and phonological disorders

Current accepted practice in evaluating speech-sound disorders encompasses administration of a standardized test, with naturalistic sampling and further analyses. Texts (for example, Stoel-Gammon and Dunn, 1985; Elbert and Gierut, 1986) describe protocols including, for instance, required number of utterances and probe words or elicitation of both single words and connected speech, etc. They also provide a step-by-step guide to a series of scans and analyses. Although there is much information to guide clinical practice, there is as yet insufficient systematic exploration of many of these standard practices.

A test such as the *Goldman–Fristoe Test of Articulation* (Goldman and Fristoe, 1986), routinely used in clinical practice and regularly used in research studies (for example, Ruder and Bunce, 1981; Gierut, 1989), has the facility to measure speech-sound errors, not only at the individual sound and word levels but also in connected speech, albeit at a structured sentence level. Although this context is somewhat constrained, it has the advantage of enhancing accuracy of judgements of speech beyond a word level for children who have high unintelligibility. Grunwell (1980), however, drew attention to some of the limitations of this standardized test, including the lack of opportunity to elicit some clusters and to sample clusters in positions other than word-initial position; she questioned the relevance of data obtained from such a measure in terms of clinical utilization.

Clinicians often use screening tests of articulation. However, they too have limitations. Ritterman et al. (1982) suggested there is only modest comparability among such tools. These workers found, for instance, that there was little agreement across different tests (for example, the *Templin–Darley Screening Test of Articulation* (Templin and Darley, 1969);

the *Predictive Screening Test of Articulation* (Van Riper, 1970)) as to identification of the primary speech problem.

Naturalistic sampling also appears in the literature (for example, Bountress et al., 1985; Grunwell's (1985) system, *Phonological Assessment of Child Speech* (PACS)). An advantage of such methods is that the speech sample obtained is likely to be more representative of a child's abilities. Although sampling allows for multiple opportunities for errors to occur, prudence is necessary as well, given that not all combinations of speech sounds will necessarily occur during any one sampling period. Nevertheless, valuable information extracted from the samples may include lists of correct sounds, percentages of sounds in error and notions on the particular pattern of speech errors.

A crucial aspect of the evaluation protocol that can affect the validity of data obtained from speech samples is accuracy of transcription. There is poor agreement between transcribers, highlighting the need for prudence in the consideration of phonetically transcribed samples (Amorosa et al., 1985). A recent article by Powell (2001) highlights important considerations that practitioners need to take into account.

The strong influence of the linguistic approach is noticeable within assessment as well as treatment practices. Although a phonological process analysis is an important and efficient means of establishing patterns of sound errors, it may not always provide requisite sensitivity. More than 20 years ago caution was expressed concerning levels of abstraction within analyses possibly obscuring phonetic facts (Carney, 1979). More recently, the potential for increased sensitivity has been extended via the possibility of complementing standard analysis practices through, for example, a non-linear phonology analysis (considers multiple levels or tiers of information). The potential of the latter to provide additional information pertinent for both research and clinical practice bears consideration.

Non-linear analysis is a method that allows for a fine-grained analysis and has the potential to illustrate, for example, the nature of deficiencies in syllable structures or of restrictions within the onset or rime. It can provide insight into why a child may, for example, delete certain syllables in some multisyllabic words and not others. For instance, syllables may be maintained in strong–weak (within a non-linear phonology framework, segments group into syllables, syllables into feet and feet into words) but in weak–strong contexts. Non-linear analysis also enables determination of strengths and weaknesses and a transparency of treatment targets. For example, if a child presented with restrictions where only vowels were produced within the rime, intervention might focus on increasing the complexity of the rime by adding consonants or shifting features (primary phonological elements that combine to form segments or sounds) (Bernhardt, 1994; Bernhardt and Stemberger, 2000).

Bernhardt and Stemberger (2000), suggest non-linear analysis offers increased sensitivity to identify the nature and levels of breakdown and more sensitive categories to capture these. Features incorporated (which they suggest provide input to the motor component on articulation of a speech sound) are purportedly more sensitive than broader categories of 'fricative' and thus able to capture similarities between sounds.

To date, there is insufficient information regarding the nature of the most evidence-based assessment protocol. Not enough studies have investigated the superiority of one measurement versus another in relation to yielding a true representation of the particular speech disorder. Indeed, no single tool is likely to have the capacity to do so. Instead, a combination of measures (as proposed by Bernhardt and Holdgrafer, 2001) that complement each other would probably constitute best practice. What criteria would be applied in determining the optimal measure for a particular purpose?

McCauley and Swisher (1984) cite ten psychometric criteria that may be used to evaluate standardized tests, including items such as concurrent and predictive validity. Of the five articulation tests that these authors reviewed, only one satisfied three of the ten suggested criteria. According to these researchers, these criteria 'consist of a set of characteristics that should be considered every time a clinician chooses or makes use of a norm-referenced test to evaluate a child's speech and language status' (McCauley and Swisher, 1984, p. 37).

In practice it is possible that the validity of data collected may be compromised by factors inherent within facilities, for example, time constraints. Samples may not be long enough and tests selected may not allow for all permutations of speech sounds to be considered. Non-representative speech samples invalidate diagnoses and also, according to Bernhardt and Holdgrafer (2001), the selection of treatment goals.

Within speech pathology there may have been instances where insufficient consideration has been given to which assessment tools and procedures are optimal. In practice, real circumstances may present constraints that affect the type of equipment that is selected for assessment. Large caseloads may also dictate that only one or two widely available tests are used. Again, there is no clear evidence that any of these tools provide all the necessary data in order to assess the particular speech problem effectively. Other than constraints such as time, sometimes the problem is inaccessibility. For instance, some sites might not have access to instrumentation such as electroplatography or spectography. Electropalatography instrumentation incorporates sensors for use within the oral cavity and a visual feedback mechanism so as to supply information on patterns of tongue and palate contacts during speech. Dent et al. (1995)

found that electropalatography analyses contributed to outcome measurement modes in that they were able to demonstrate visually, different tongue palate contact patterns for individuals following a period of intervention to remediate speech disorders. Clinicians need to ensure that, despite constraints in the workplace, the assessment battery they use is representative, comprehensive and sensitive. Another important consideration is that each assessment procedure is not necessarily all-encompassing and that the important issue is knowing how to obtain all the data and then being able to analyse, interpret and plan a management strategy.

Issues in treating articulation and phonological disorders

Practitioners approach the treatment of articulation and phonological disorders in numerous ways. Conceptualizations relating to disorders of speech have influenced treatment research and practice. In line with the major theoretical perspectives, some adopt more motor-based approaches that incorporate auditory, visual and tactile modalities, motor learning principles and behaviouristic approaches in order to facilitate production of the target sound. Others, who align with a linguistic framework, facilitate correct production by attempting to expand a child's linguistic knowledge. Yet others adopt a combination of these approaches. This eclectic approach has recently been mirrored in the literature (Bowen, 1998). Table 11.1 shows some of the evidence for the common treatment approaches for speech disorders. The review is not exhaustive. Information is presented according to source, study design, participants, measurement, treatment approach, results and evidence level.

It is apparent from Table 11.1 that a variety of treatment approaches have been explored in the literature with varying levels of evidence to support their use. Before contemplating the nature of the evidence base, brief descriptions of some of these strategies are provided. Broadly, strategies are discussed in relation to motor- and linguistic-based approaches. Examples of motor-based approaches include chaining, phonetic placement and cued articulation, whereas examples of linguistic or phonological approaches include minimal pairs therapy and metaphon.

Phonetic placement, which demonstrates the requisite position of the articulators for the production of a particular sound, is commonly incorporated within the traditional approach described in depth by Van Riper (1963). The approach was widely used in the 1960s and early 1970s and to some extent continues to be used to treat speech disorders.

Table 11.1 Evidence for common treatment approaches for speech disorders

Source	Study design	Participants (number and age)	Measurement	Treatment approach	Results	Evidence level
Bankson and Byrne (1972)	Parallel case-studies	n=5, 8–11 years	Speech samples, probes pre- and post-battery	A form of articulation therapy involving reading word lists.	4/5 children improved on one measure of conversation, however error-free speech not maintained.	III.3
Hodsen (1978)	Opinion and observation of application of a preliminary model	n=36, 3–7 years	Qualitative	Auditory stimulation Auditory bombardment Phonological approach to sound remediation.	Increased intelligibility observed. Some overgeneralization apparent.	IV
Schissel and Doty (1979)	Case-study	n=1, 6;6	Pre- and post-battery using McDonald Test of Articulation (1964) and McReynolds and Engmann (1975)	Traditional approach targeting multiple targets.	Improvement scores according to McDonald Test of Articulation (1964) on all sounds except /r/. No data taken in conversation so carry-over not assessed.	IV
Ruder and Bunce (1981)	Parallel case-studies	n=2, 4 years	S1: pre- and post-testing using University of Kansas articulation test S2: repeated administration of Goldman–Fristoe Test of Articulation	Articulation approach using imitative training.	Improvement in sounds targeted and across-sound generalization to production of untrained phonemes.	IV
Weiner (1981)	Parallel single-case designs using a multi-response baseline	n=2, 4;10 and 4;4 years	*Phonological Process Analysis* (Weiner, 1979) Visual inspection of graphs	Minimal pairs contrast procedure.	S1: suppression of all processes in target words S2: partial suppression of processes in target words. Rate of improve-	III.2

					ment was not as rapid as for S1. Measures of generalization to non-target words was less apparent.	III.3
Bountress et al. (1985)	Group design (no partial or random selection)	n=12, two groups	Pre- and post-test battery using Arizona Articulation Proficiency Scale (AAPS) (Fudula, 1970) and conversational speech sampling	Distinctive feature approach versus Costello and Onstine (1976) approach	Statistically similar results for both treatment modalities. 11/12 showed improvement on AAPS (1970) 8/12 showed improvement on conversational speech sampling.	III.3
Monahan (1986)	Parallel case-studies	n=4, 5;5 – 5;8	Pre- and post-test battery using the *Assessment of Phonological Processes* (Hodsen, 1980)	*Remediation of Common Phonological Processes* (Monahan, 1986: 187–98) involving auditory bombardment, conceptualization training and minimal pairs training	All subjects exhibited a decrease in phonological process occurrence post-treatment; generalization to untrained words was observed.	III.3
Schilp (1986)	Case-study	n=1, 8;0	Qualitative description	Cued speech targeting /s/ and /z/	Improved ability to articulate /s/ and /z/.	IV
Tyler et al. (1987)	Parallel case-studies	n=4, 3;1 – 5;1	Generalization probes after approximately six sessions	S1 and S2: minimal pairs approach S3 and S4: modified cycles approach	S1/S2 suppression of target processes with generalization to untrained sounds S3/S4 more processes targeted and marked changes in seven processes with generalization to untrained sounds.	III.3

(contd)

Table 11.1 (contd)

Source	Study design	Participants (number and age)	Measurement	Treatment approach	Results	Evidence level
					Control processes unchanged until targeted with both approaches.	
Young (1987)	Parallel single-case design. Multiple baseline across behaviours.	n=2, 4;4 and 4;5	Measured during baseline period and during treatment phase; percentage sound production correct	Modelling Backward chaining plus rebus (visual picture cues)	Untreated targets did not improve. Both subjects improved on speech sounds that were targeted, that is, they suppressed phonological processes.	III.2
Grunwell and Dive (1988)	Parallel case-studies	n=2, 6;0 and 8;0	Spontaneous speech sample Card naming Phonological Assessment of Child Speech (PACS) (Grunwell, 1985)	Combined articulatory motor and phonological linguistic-based approaches Discrimination Metalinguistics awareness Minimal pairs production	Reorganization of phonological system as evidenced in S1 particularly showing evidence of using more contrasts post-treatment. Also increased realizations of fricatives and affricates.	III.3
Jarvis (1989)	Case-study	n=1, 4;9	Speech and language sample Phonological Assessment of Child Speech (PACS) (Grunwell, 1985)	Minimal pairs Metaphon Teaching contrasts	Increased intelligibility Generalized correct production of target speech sounds into connected speech.	III.3
Gierut (1989)	Single-case study incorporating a multiple baseline design	n=1, 4;7, presenting mainly with initial consonant deletion	Before intervention: • Goldman–Fristoe Test of Articulation (Goldman and Fristoe, 1969) • spontaneous speech	Phonological: maximal opposition approach	Significant improvement in production of initial sounds The number of word-initial omissions decreased and there was evidence of	III.2

Study	Design	Subjects	Assessment	Approach	Results	
					generalization in the subject's phonological system.	
Gierut (1990)	Parallel-case studies incorporating alternating treatments combined with a staggered multiple-baseline design	n=3, all 4;0 Exclusion of at least six sounds from inventory Each subject exposed to both minimal and maximal contrasts for two sound pairs	Before intervention: • Goldman–Fristoe Test of Articulation (Goldman and Fristoe, 1986) • detailed phonological descriptions (Gierut et al., 1987) • Phonological protocol knowledge (Gierut, 1986) sampling Probes administered during intervention	Phonological: comparison between minimal and maximal opposition approaches	Maximal oppositions led to greater improvement in the production of treated sounds as well as a greater number of untreated sounds added to the inventory in 2/3 subjects. Remaining subject displayed comparable learning under both treatment conditions.	III.2
Hoffman, Norris and Monjure (1990)	Parallel-case studies	n=2, 4;1	Assessment of phonological processes	Whole language versus a minimal pairs approach S1: whole-language approach, S2: minimal pairs approach	S1: improved language more than S2. S2: improved phonological performance slightly more than S1.	III.3
Saben and Ingham (1991)	Parallel-case studies: pre- and post-battery	n=2, 4;4 and 3;9, both reduced phonetic inventory and S1 reduced expressive language	Phonological Process Analysis (Weiner, 1979) used to determine which processes were apparent. Word – picture probes were used throughout the treatment process	Phonological: minimal pairs approach with added motoric cues as required	Both subjects successfully passed through the treatment phase of phonological process suppression; however, generalization to untreated words or untreated phonemes did not occur. Minimal pairs treatment was reported not to be successful for these two subjects.	III.3
Bryan and Howard (1992)	Case-study	n=1, 5;0	Pre- and post-test battery Real and non-word repetition sub-test of the test for Receptive Grammar (as control) (Bishop, 1982)	Metalinguistic and discrimination identification segmentation	Increase in accurate realization of consonants and in generating syllable structures.	III.3

(contd)

Table 11.1 (contd)

Source	Study design	Participants (number and age)	Measurement	Treatment approach	Results	Evidence level
			Auditory Discrimination and Attention Test (Morgan Barry, 1988)		Significant improvement in accuracy of sounds in real-word repetitions and picture naming. Increased auditory discrimination skills.	
Abraham (1993)	Parallel-case studies Alternating treatment design	n=4, 5:0–10:5 years with pre-linguistic moderate to severe hearing impairment	Articulation measures: • *Goldman–Fristoe test of Articulation* (Goldman and Fristoe, 1969) • *Test of Minimal Articulatory Competency* (Secord, 1981) • PCC Phonological process measures: • *Phonological Process Analysis* (Weiner, 1979) • *Kahn–Lewis Phonological Analysis* (Kahn and Lewis, 1986)	Phonetic placement approach compared with minimal pairs approach	Tendency toward improvement with phonemic approach. All children improved with minimal pairs training and they were able to generalize the rule to untrained words. Results were more variable for phonetic placement training and generalization showed a similar trend.	III.2
Bernhardt (1994)	Conceptual	–	–	Non-linear phonology	–	IV
Dagenais et al. (1994)	Parallel-case studies	n=2, 8;8 and 8;6	*Goldman–Fristoe Test of Articulation* (Goldman and Fristoe, 1986) *McDonald Test of Articulation* (1969)	Electropalatography Use of visual representation to enhance oral sensory feedback associated with	S1 achieved accurate production of /s/ and generalized S2 did not evidence any changes according to the	III.3

			Audio-taped recordings judged by raters Pre- and post-treatment palatography results	linguapalatal contact patterns	*Goldman–Fristoe Test of Articulation* and showed a decrease in production accuracy according to the McDonald Test of Articulation.	IV
Penney et al. (1994)	Case study	n=1, 4;11	Adaptation of Pollock and Keiser (1990) stimulus word list	Traditional: motor plus discrimination targeting vowel accuracy Oral placement Bubble blowing Lip rounding Traditional type sequence	Improvement according to overall percentage of correct vowels.	
Rvachew (1994)	Randomized controlled trial	n=27, 42–66 months	Pre–post-test battery initially tested using: • computer analysis of phonological processes (Hodson, 1985) • sheet-X-sheet word identification test (p. 350) Post-test: • sheet-X-sheet word identification test (p. 350)	Traditional articulation training to remediate /S/ 'sh' along with computer-driven speech perception training	Results from this study indicate that computer-driven speech perception training provided concurrently with articulation training is beneficial for some phonologically impaired children. Further research is required to ensure optimal stimuli content and presentation.	II
Stringfellow and McLeod (1994)	Case-study	n=1, 5;0	Probes	Approximation Co-articulatory transitions Splitting syllables Carrier phrases and key words Facilitatory phonetic contexts Phonetic placement with key word approach	Achieved target production Subject realized /l/ and /j/ as two distinct phonemes. Generalized to conversational speech.	III.3

(contd)

Table 11.1 (contd)

Source	Study design	Participants (number and age)	Measurement	Treatment approach	Results	Evidence level
Dent et al. (1995)	Group	n=23	Perceptual evaluation by examiners. Analyses of tongue palate contact patterns according to electropalatograph	Computer-based biofeedback and electro-palatography as a visual tool to assist subject detect changes	Different tongue plate contacts post-treatment with some characteristics of a model pattern.	III.3
McLeod and Isaac (1995)	Single-case study	n=1	Spectrographic analysis prior to current treatment phase in this study; spectrographic analysis was also conducted during and at the end of the intervention	Phonological process approach to remediate gliding of / l / (see Stringfellow and McLeod, 1994)	Subject was able to produce and maintain a correct / l / Spectrographic analysis assisted in determining formant frequency changes that could not easily be detected using perceptual analysis.	III.3
Gierut et al. (1996)	Parallel-case studies and group study - conducted consecutively Studies 1 and 2 - both staggered multiple base-line across subjects designs	n=9 Study 1 (three cases) Study 2 (three cases participating in one condition (e.g. with particular phonemes targeted) versus three cases participating in another condition)	*Goldman–Fristoe Test of Articulation* (Goldman and Fristoe, 1986) Visual inspection of graphs	Imitation and spontaneous production	For Study 1: greater accuracy in production for subjects where later acquired phonemes were targeted. Study 2: no differences with moderate improvement for two subjects in each of groups.	III.2
Klein (1996)	Group design Retrospective	n=36,	*Pre-articulation Proficiency Scale* (Fundula, 1970) *Goldman–Fristoe Test of Articulation* (Goldman and Fristoe, 1986)	Comparison of phonemic versus phonetic approach Imagery plus minimal pairs versus phonetic placement, speech discrimination and imitation	Subjects who had undergone phonology treatment had a lower mean severity score post-treatment and participated in fewer sessions in treatment.	III.3

Study	Design	Sample	Assessment	Approach	Outcome	Level
Almost and Rosenbaum, (1998)	Randomized controlled trial of groups of children randomly assigned to two treatment groups.	n=26, Mean age = 42 months Group 1: four months' intervention cycle followed by four months of no intervention cycle Group 2: reverse procedures	• *Assessment of Phonological Processes - Revised* (Hodsen, (1986) • *Goldman–Fristoe Test of Articulation* (Goldman and Fristoe, 1986) • PCC • MLU	Modified cycles approach based on a minimal pairs approach	Group 1 showed greater improvement than no Group 2 during first cycle. During second cycle Group 1 continued to improve and were significantly better on conversational PCC.	II
Bowen and Cupples (1998)	Case study	n=1, 4;4	Metaphon screening system (Dean et al., 1990) Severity Rating Scale (Bowen, 1996)	Eclectic comprising linguistic and traditional approaches	All phonological processes suppressed.	IV
Bowen and Cupples (1999)	Group design – treatment and control (no treatment)	n=22, 2;11–4;9 14 (treatment); 8 (control – no treatment)	*Severity Rating Scale* (Bowen, 1996) Metaphon resource pack screening assessment (Dean et al., 1990) PACS (Grunwell, 1985) Independent relational analysis (Stoel-Gammon, 1985)	Eclectic approach comprising metalinguistic tasks, phonetic production procedures, multiple exemplars, minimal pairs, bombardment, structured programme for parents to follow	Accelerated improvement in phonological patterns compared with untreated children.	III.2
Dodd and Bradford (2000)	Parallel-case studies	n=3, 3;0, 3;4 and 4;3	Pre and post treatment assessment battery Speech sample (phonetic inventory, percentage consonants correct, phonological processes) *Goldman–Fristoe Test of Articulation* (Goldman and Fristoe, 1986)	Comparison of three approaches: phonological contrast; core vocabulary; prompt	Phonology rules help children who have consistent errors; core vocabulary helps children who are inconsistent.	III.3

(contd)

Table 11.1 (contd)

Source	Study design	Participants (number and age)	Measurement	Treatment approach	Results	Evidence level
Hesketh et al. (2000)	Semi-randomized comparative group design	n=61, 3;6–5;0	Modified Metaphon Screening Assessment (Dean et al., 1990) Articulation test (Edinburgh Articulation test) Spontaneous speech measures Individual probes Phonological awareness measure developed by authors (MAB)	Comparison of metaphonological therapy versus phonetic placement and its significance to phonological awareness skills	Children in both intervention groups made significant gains in both phonological output and metaphonological skills and no significant group differences were apparent on virtually all measures.	II.2

Essentially, it focuses on targeting production of individual speech sounds, on a sound-by-sound basis and encompasses work on perception and production. Therapy incorporates the use of a range of modalities, for example, both tactile and proprioceptive modalities are involved, with the visual modality. The traditional treatment approach typically involves a hierarchical and sequential approach commencing with a focus on the isolated sound and advancing to the next level of complexity only when a high level of accuracy has been attained. The approach is didactic and incorporates a large amount of imitation and practice in order that the sound becomes automatic. The approach is effective when there are a limited number of errors and particularly at the establishment and stabilization phases of treatment. Van Riper's (1963) classic text on principles and methods of speech correction was used in a prescriptive manner, with clinicians reporting good outcomes, particularly where only one or two sounds were in error. The text also addressed the issue of generalization, a phenomenon that continues in the present century to be a challenge. It is apparent from anecdotal information and observations that clinical practice has outpaced clinical research but with insufficient empirical data to support the positive findings observed in clinics.

Consistent with the cognitive linguistic approach, the framework for conceptualizing speech impairments became a linguistic construct where speech errors were analysed according to the rule-based sound system of phonology. In line with phonology principles, intervention was 'designed to effect change in one or more major areas of the phonological system, i.e., over several segments and word positions' (Bernhardt and Gilbert, 1992, p. 123).

The 'minimal pairs' approach is a commonly cited linguistic intervention technique. According to Baker (1997, p. 17) it remains 'the most frequently researched intervention approach'. Baker (1997) summarized this approach as part of her review of phonological therapy techniques. Essentially, this approach involves providing a child with word pairs that are homophones in the dysfunctional phonological system and teaching the child to make the distinction between the two words. For example, a child may be presented with a pair of words, such as *she* and *sea*, in which /S/ ➜ /s/ and /s/ ➜ /s/. The intervention method draws on linguistic knowledge to facilitate correct articulation rather than motoric placement of articulators. Real words are typically used as the stimuli (*see* Baker (1997) for further details).

The 'maximal pairs' approach (Elbert and Gierut, 1986), another linguistic-based approach, is similarly focused in its use of phonological contrasts in the absence of perceptual and motoric instruction. In this approach, however, word pairs contain maximal oppositions in an attempt to expand the child's phonological knowledge. In this instance, nonsense words may be used but they are given lexical significance (Baker, 1997).

Some authors, who have aligned with the linguistic 'phonological process' approach, have taken strong views against the traditional approach (for example, Klein, 1996). Others, such as Camaratta (1995), have decried the fact that treatment for speech has persisted with drill-type activities characteristic of motor approaches. Notwithstanding such views, others have documented how despite a clinician's ostensible support for the linguistic approach they tend to still use some motor cues (Fey, 1992). This reflects the eclectic approach that is manifest in clinical research and practice.

Irrespective of the decades in which they practise, clinicians clearly aim to provide the most optimal and efficient treatment. Yet it is likely that they are also strongly influenced by their training and access to ongoing research. Some longstanding management decisions in relation to speech disorders have involved practices such as targeting earlier developing sounds first or working in one-to-one settings within clinics, for example. Whereas some of these practices have been questioned and altered, others have continued.

Gierut (2001) clearly extracts factors identified in previous research that are likely to influence progress, for example selection of targets that have greater markedness properties, that occur more frequently and that have greater articulatory phonetic complexity. Many of these factors are counter to what has been suggested in texts over the years. Gierut (2001) particularly highlights the need for clinicians to keep abreast of current rigorous research and to bring established opinions and practices into question, especially if they have not been tested empirically.

Table 11.1 demonstrates that the majority of treatment studies in the areas of articulation and phonology were empirical case studies that incorporated experimentation. Many case studies incorporated A–B, pre- and post-treatment designs. It is also apparent from Table 11.1 that there are other case studies that incorporate more qualitative description. However, there are few which appear to have used particularly rigorous forms of qualitative inquiry. There are a number of single-case designs that are carefully controlled, for example multiple-baseline across behaviours. In a number of instances where case studies or single-case designs were used, more than one subject was involved; hence the descriptor, 'parallel' in Table 11.1.

Few studies employing group designs are reflected in this table. Some of these had small sample sizes (Bankson and Byrne, 1972; Bountress et al., 1985; Abraham, 1993). Some had samples sizes of at least 25 (Rvachew, 1994; Almost and Rosenbaum, 1998) and there were isolated treatment studies involving substantial subject sizes (Hesketh et al., 2000). Some larger group studies also were reported as incorporating randomized controls or semi-randomized controls.

Although randomized control designs are held as the gold standard (Sackett et al., 1998), few such designs are noted in the speech pathology area for articulation and phonology treatment studies. Closer inspection of the available group studies, reveal inherent difficulties in conducting these studies because of an intrinsically heterogeneous population that is characteristic of children with speech disorders. Other factors that may have detracted in relation to the dearth of group studies could be lack of feasibility strategically in setting up rigorous experimental design and treatment features across multiple subjects. A further factor that would contribute to lack of homogeneity for group comparisons involves the anticipated variation in children's responses to treatment and differing rates of progress over time. The same issues are likely to exist even if an attempt were made to involve subjects in a series of small treatment groups; the feasibility of the latter presenting problems given extraneous variables that are inherent in any attempt to replicate treatment contexts. It is interesting to note that no studies involving group therapy treatment were found.

It is understandable that single-case studies predominate, given some merit in single-case studies because of the heterogeneity of speech disorders in children. The overwhelming majority of intervention studies fell at the 'lower' end of evidence according to Briggs (2001). No study was categorized as a Level I, which uses 'systematic review of all relevant randomised controlled trials'. Fitz-Gibbon (1986) argues for both randomized controlled trials as well as case studies, albeit with a different clinic population type. Nevertheless, there is probably a need to question the reasons for trends toward the lower levels of evidence and to consider if and what additional types of evidence are possible.

Sommers et al. (1992) conducted a critical review of treatment research related to articulation and phonological disorders spanning the decades of the 1970s and 1980s. These workers reported more simple group designs from the 1970s, whereas case studies tended to predominate in the 1980s. Single-subject designs using either withdrawal or multiple-baseline also appeared in the literature in equal amounts over both these decades. They reported further that there was a notable paucity of other designs, such as matched-group designs. Our review revealed a similar trend in the 1990s following on from the previous decade with some emerging larger group studies.

The question at this point is whether the current literature provides sufficient evidence for intervention with childhood speech sound disorders? The answer to this is complex. If we adopt both the view of Sackett et al. (1998) of what constitutes a gold standard and Briggs' (2001) notion of what constitutes the 'highest level of evidence', the current body of literature, on the whole, does not meet the criteria. According to the Briggs (2001) framework, the majority of the literature in this field is at the lower end of the levels of evidence. This implies that the evidence for much of the intervention for speech disorders in children is relatively weak. Nevertheless, there is a solid body of literature that has 'unfolded' as theories and practices have evolved. Much of this has come about because of sound information gained via rigorous single-case study design. It is worthy to consider single-case study design for its own merits rather than as a reactive substitute because of constraints, such as an heterogeneous population. Furthermore, studies complying with a large sample size and randomized controlled design may have inherent problems when reporting on a fundamentally heterogeneous group. An added challenge within a single-case study design however, is the issue of the extent that change could be attributed to treatment variables, given potential for generalization (albeit a desired outcome from a therapeutic perspective).

The papers reviewed here typically reported positive outcomes following treatment. A case has been presented in this chapter (as well as by other authors) to support the use of single-case reporting as a means of investigating treatments for speech disorders in children. However, the worth of this design must also be balanced against some potential limitations. First, the lack of control in some studies that do not use a multiple-baseline approach or perhaps a matched control from a waiting list; second, the incomplete reporting of therapy techniques in some studies and also including what instruction may have occurred to parents (that is, were some children receiving support at home and not others); and third, the lack of longer-term follow-up in some studies, an extremely important consideration. Omission of information on generalization and use of diverse methodologies have contributed to the difficulty in comparing and interpreting studies. Certainly, there is a need for a more consistent attempt to provide longitudinal results for subjects investigated in the research.

Perhaps what is lacking in the literature is a greater number of replication studies on various treatments. Pring (1986), aligning with the single-case methodology, supports our premise by stressing the value of replication to strengthen the case for various intervention approaches.

Conclusion: future directions

There is a need for a more consistent way of measuring speech and speech changes across the literature to foster a more consistent approach to measurement procedures and analysis of data across studies. In fact, as a precursor, it would be invaluable to investigate the internal validity and rigour of various assessment approaches. This, in turn, would allow for a more consistent methodology in measurement of speech production. Larger-scale investigations across clinic sites, irrespective of study design type, that is, single-case or group, could increase consistency in measurement approaches and assist rigorous comparative research.

It is important to foster a culture whereby clinicians are encouraged to report on cases to build to the body of literature with a strong clinical focus. Again, this is not a new point and is captured well in the following quotation, 'to encourage the use of some relatively simple single-case designs in clinical practice, thus returning to the individual therapist the means to evaluate and refine treatment interventions' (Pring, 1986, p. 104).

Documentation of each clinic case as a research exercise, the failures as well as the successes, would contribute to the evidence base, provide clinically feasible applications and alert clinicians to potential pitfalls. Also, the anecdotal evidence provided by many clinicians who refer to 'tried and true' strategies ought to be measured dispassionately and shared via the literature. Clinical impressions of improvement are important, but alone are not enough to attribute efficacy; the need for rigour and sensitivity in measurement remains indisputable.

This chapter has provided an overview of the status quo with respect to the management of articulation and phonological disorders as well as the challenges in meeting the needs of children exhibiting such problems. A call is made for clinicians to access research in this area continually as well as to evaluate, interpret and integrate it with experience from clinical practice and also translate findings from rigorous research studies that do exist into their clinical practice. Moreover, clinicians are encouraged to document their own practices, thereby contributing themselves to the evidence base for managing speech disorders.

Some of the reasons that may have mitigated against routine adoption of evidence-based practice for child speech disorders to date were identified. Issues such as the increasing volume of research, yet ongoing need for intervention studies, were highlighted. The terminological confusion and seeming superficial integration of constructs and the uncertainty regarding underlying mechanisms were also considered.

Lags in adopting increasingly sensitive assessment and analysis systems are touched upon to illustrate the observation that so-called straightforward communication problems involving speech sounds are, in fact, only so at face value and that the actual complexity probably necessitates more considered approaches. Certainly, there is a need now to conduct and access research that looks at the area of articulation and phonology in an integrated manner and against potential theoretical perspectives. Theory needs to inform practice and vice versa. An over-arching perception shared by the authors is that articulation and phonological disorders need to be addressed in an integrated manner.

References

Abbs JA, Kennedy JG. Neurophysiological processes of speech movement control. In: Lass NJ, McReynolds LV, Northern JL, Yoder DE. Speech, Language and Hearing. Philadelphia, PA: WB Saunders, 1982; 84-108.

Abraham S. Differential treatment of phonological disability in children with impaired hearing who are trained orally. American Journal of Speech-Language Pathology 1993; 2: 23-30.

Ainoda N, Okazaki K. Results of systematic speech sound monitoring in children with cleft palate. Folia Phoniatrica et Logopaedica 1996; 48: 86-91.

Almost D, Rosenbaum P. Effectiveness of speech intervention for phonological disorders: a randomized controlled trial. Developmental Medicine and Child Neurology 1998; 40: 319-25.

Amorosa H, von Benda U, Wagner E, Keck A. Transcribing phonetic detail in the speech of unintelligible children: a comparison of procedures. British Journal of Disorders of Communication 1985; 20: 281-7.

Anthony A. The Edinburgh Articulation Test. Edinburgh: ES Livingstone, 1971.

Baker E. Phonological intervention: An overview of five current approaches. Australian Communication Quarterly 1997; Autumn: 17-20.

Baker E, McLeod S. Aligning practice with research: making informed clinical decisions when managing phonological impairments in children. In L Wilson and S Hewat Proceedings of the Speech Pathology Australian National Conference, 2001; 101-9.

Baker E, Croot K, McLeod S, Paul R. Psycholinguistic models of speech development and their application to clinical practice. Journal of Speech and Hearing Research 2001; 44: 685-702.

Baker E, Croot K, van Doorn J, Reed V. In search of a sound theory: Investigating articulation and phonology. In: McLeod S, McAllister L (eds). Proceedings of the Speech Pathology Australian National Conference, 'Towards 2000: Embracing Change, Challenge and Choice'. Melbourne: Speech Pathology Australia, 1999; 29-36.

Ball MJ, Kent RD. The New Phonologies: Developments in Clinical Linguistics. San Diego, CA: Singular Publishing Group Inc., 1997.

Bankson NW, Byrne MC. The effect of a timed correct sound production task on carryover. Journal of Speech and Hearing Research 1972; 15: 160-168.

Bannigan K. Clinical effectiveness: systematic reviews and evidence-based practice in occupational therapy. British Journal of Occupational Therapy 1997; 60: 479-83.

Benner P. From Novice to Expert: Excellence and Power in Clinical Nursing Practice. Menlo Park: Addison Wesley, 1984.

Bernhardt B. Phonological intervention techniques for syllable and word structure development. Clinical Communication Disorders 1994; 4: 54-65.

Bernhardt B, Gilbert J. Applying linguistic theory to speech language pathology: the case for nonlinear phonology. Clinical Linguistics and Phonetics 1992; 6: 123-145.

Bernhardt BH, Stemberger JP. Workbook in Nonlinear Phonology for Clinical Application. Austin, TX: Pro-Ed., 2000.

Bernhardt BH, Holdgrafer G. Beyond the basics I: the need for strategic sampling for in-depth phonological analysis. Language, Speech and Hearing in the Schools 2001; 32: 18-27.

Bishop DVM. Test for Reception of Grammar. Cambridge: MRC Applied Psychology Unit 1982.

Bountress NG, Bountress MG, Nussbaum JL. Modification of articulation error using a multiple-context, distinctive-feature treatment program. Perceptual and Motor Skills 1985; 61: 792-4.

Bowen C. Developmental Phonological Disorders: A practical guide for families and teachers. Melbourne: Australian Council for Education Research Ltd, 1998.

Bowen C. Evaluation of a Phonological Therapy with Treated and Untreated Groups of Children. Sydney: Macquarie University 1996.

Bowen C, Cupples L. A tested phonological therapy in practice. Child, Language Teaching and Therapy 1998; 10: 29-50.

Bowen C, Cupples L. Parents and children together (PACT): a collaborative approach to phonological therapy. International Journal of Language and Communication Disorders 1999; 34: 35-83.

Briggs J. Evidence based practice information sheets for health professionals: appraising systematic reviews. Changing Practice 2001; 2: 1-6.

Bryan A, Howard D. Frozen phonology thawed: the analysis and remediation of a developmental disorder of real word phonology. European Journal of Disorders of Communication 1992; 27: 343-65.

Camaratta S. A rationale for naturalistic speech intelligibility intervention. In: Fey ME, Windsor J, Warren SF (eds). Language Intervention: Preschool through Elementary Years. Baltimore, MD: Paul Brooks, 1995.

Carney E. Inappropriate abstraction in speech-assessment procedures. British Journal of Disorders of Communication 1979; 14: 123-35.

Clark J, Yallop C. An Introduction to Phonetics and Phonology. Oxford: Basil Blackwell, 1991.

Costello J, Onstine JM. The modification of multiple articulation errors based on distinctive feature theory. Journal of Speech and Hearing Disorders 1976; 41(2): 199-215.

Crystal D. Towards a 'bucket' theory of language disability: taking account of interactions between levels. Clinical Linguistics and Phonetics 1987; 1: 7-22.

Dagenais PA, Critz-Crosby P, Adams JB. Defining and remediating persistent lateral lisps in children using electropalatography: preliminary findings. American Journal of Speech–Language Pathology 1994; 3: 67-76.

Dean EC, Howell J, Hill A, Waters D. Metaphon Resource Pack. Windsor: NFER-Nelson, 1990.

Dent H, Gibbon F, Hardcastle B. The application of electropalatography (EPG) to the remediation of speech disorders in school-aged children and young adults. European Journal of Disorders of Communication 1995; 30: 264-77.

Dodd B, Bradford A. A comparison of three therapy methods for children with different types of developmental phonological disorder. International Journal of Language and Communication Disorders 2000; 35: 189-209.

Dodd B, Gillon G, Oerlemans M, Russell T, Syrmis M, Wilson H. Phonological disorder and the acquisition of literacy. In: Dodd B (Ed.). Differential Diagnosis and Treatment of Children with Speech Disorder. London: Whurr Publishers, 1995.

Edwards ML. Historical overview of clinical phonology. In: Hodsen BW, Edwards ML. Perspectives in Applied Phonology. Maryland: Aspen, 1997; 1-17.

Elbert M, Gierut J. Handbook of Clinical Phonology: Approaches to Assessment and Treatment. London: Taylor & Francis, 1986.

Fey ME. Articulation and phonology: inextricable constructs in speech pathology. Language, Speech and Hearing Services in Schools 1992; 23: 225-32.

Fitz-Gibbon CT. In defence of randomised controlled trials, with suggestions about the possible use of meta-analysis. British Journal of Disorders of Communication 1986; 21: 117-24.

Gibbon F. Towards a better understanding of abnormal lingual articulation in children with speech disorders. In: McLeod S, McAllister L (eds). Proceedings of the Speech Pathology Australian National Conference, 'Towards 2000: Embracing Change, Challenge and Choice'. Melbourne: Speech Pathology Australia, 1999; 13-23.

Gierut ME. Handbook of Clinical Phonology: Approaches to assessment and treatment. London: Taylor and Francis, 1986.

Gierut J. Maximal opposition approach to phonological treatment. Journal of Speech and Hearing Disorders 1989; 54: 9-19.

Gierut J. Differential learning of phonological oppositions. Journal of Speech and Hearing Research 1990; 33: 540-9.

Gierut JA. Complexity in phonological treatment: clinical factors. Language, Speech and Hearing Services in Schools 2001; 32: 229-41.

Gierut JA, Morrisette ML, Hughes MT, Rowland S. Phonological treatment efficacy and developmental norms. Language, Speech and Hearing Services in Schools 1996; 27: 215-30.

Goldman R, Fristoe M. Goldman–Fristoe Test of Articulation. Minneapolis, MN: American Guidance Services, 1969.

Grunwell P. Procedures for child speech assessment: a review. British Journal of Disorders of Communication 1980; 15: 189-203.

Grunwell P. Phonological Assessment of Child Speech PACS. Windsor: NFER-Nelson, 1985.

Grunwell P, Dive D. Treating 'cleft palate speech': Combining phonological techniques and functional articulation therapy. Child Language Teaching and Therapy 1988; 4: 193-210.

Harbers HM, Paden EP, Halle JW. Phonological awareness and production: changes during intervention. Language, Speech and Hearing Services in Schools 1999; 30: 50-60.

Hesketh A, Adams C, Nightingale C, Hall R. Comparison of metaphonological therapy and articulatory training in phonologically disordered children. International Journal of Communication Disorders 2000; 35: 337-354.

Hewlett N. Phonological versus phonetic disorders: some suggested modifications to the current use of the distinction. British Journal of Disorders of Communication 1985; 20: 155-164.

Hewlett N. Processes of development and production. In: Grunwell P (Ed.). Developmental Speech Disorders. Edinburgh: Churchill Livingstone, 1990.

Hewlett N, Gibbon F, Cohen-McKenzie W. When is a velar an alveolar? Evidence supporting a revised psycholinguistic model of speech production in children. International Journal of Language and Communication Disorders 1998; 33: 161-176.

Hodsen BW. A preliminary hierarchical model for phonological remediation. Language, Speech and Hearing Services in Schools 1978; 9: 236-240.

Hodsen BW. Computer analysis of phonological processes. Stonington, IL: Phonocomp, 1985.

Hodsen BW. Research and practice: applied phonology. Topics in Language Disorders 1998; 18: 58–70.

Hoffman PR, Norris JA, Monjure J. Comparison of process targeting and whole language treatments for phonologically delayed preschool children. Language, Speech and Hearing Services in Schools 1990; 21: 102–9.

Ingram D. The categorization of phonological impairment. In: Hodsen BW, Edwards ML. Perspectives in Applied Phonology. Maryland: Aspen, 1997; 19–41.

Jarvis J. Taking a metaphon approach to phonological development: a case study. Child Language Teaching and Therapy 1989; 5: 16–32.

Kahn L, Lewis N. Kahn-Lewis Phonological Analysis. Circle Pines, MN: American Guidance Service, 1986.

Klein ES. Phonological/traditional approaches to articulation therapy: a retrospective group comparison. Language, Speech and Hearing Services in Schools 1996; 27: 314–23.

Ladefoged P. Vowels and Consonants: An Introduction to the Sounds of Languages. Oxford: Blackwell Publishers, 2001.

Lancaster G, Pope L. Working with Children's Phonology. Bicester: Winslow Press, 1989.

Menn L, Stoel-Gammon C. Phonological development. In: Fletcher P, MacWhinney B. The Handbook of Child Languge. Boston, MA: Blackwell Publishers Ltd., 1995.

McCauley RJ, Swisher L. Psychometric review of language and articulation tests for preschool children. Journal of Speech and Hearing Disorders 1984; 49: 34–42.

McDonald ET. Articulation Testing and Treatment: A sensory motor approach. Pittsburgh, PA: Stanwix House, 1964.

McLeod S, Isaac K. Use of spectrographic analyses to evaluate the efficacy of phonological intervention. Clinical Linguistics and Phonetics 1995; 9: 229–234.

McReynolds LV, Engmann DC. Distinctive Feature Analysis of Misarticulation. Baltimore, MD: University Park Press, 1975.

Monahan D. Remediation of common phonological processes: Four case studies. Language, Speech and Hearing Services in Schools 1986; 17: 199–206.

Morgan Barry R. The Auditory Discrimination and Attention Test. Windsor: NFER-Nelson, 1988.

Penney G, Fee J, Dowdle C. Vowel assessment and remediation: A case study. Child Language Teaching and Therapy 1994; 10: 47–66.

Pollack KE, Keiser NJ. An examination of vowel errors in phonologically disordered children. Clinical Linguistics and Phonetics 1990; 4: 161–78.

Powell TW. Phonetic transcription of disordered speech. Topics in Language Disorders 2001; 21: 52–72.

Pring TR. Evaluating the effects of speech therapy for aphasics: developing the single case methodology. British Journal of Disorders of Communication 1986; 21: 103–15.

Rice ML, Hadley PA, Alexander AL. Social biases towards children with specific language impairment: a correlative, causal model of language limitations. Applied Psycholinguistics 1993; 14: 443–72.

Ritterman SI, Zook-Herman SL, Carlson RL, Kinde S. The pass/fail disparity among three commonly employed articulatory screening tests. Journal of Speech and Hearing Disorders 1982; 47: 429–33.

Ruder KF, Bunce BH. Articulation therapy using distinctive feature analysis to structure the training program: two case studies. Journal of Speech and Hearing Disorders 1981; 46: 52-8.

Rvachew S. Speech perception training can facilitate sound production learning. Journal of Speech and Hearing Research 1994; 37: 347-57.

Saben CB, Ingham JC. The effect of minimal pairs treatment on the speech-sound production of two children with phonologic disorders. Journal of Speech and Hearing Research 1991; 34: 1023-40.

Sackett DL, Richardson WS, Rosenberg W, Haynes RB. Evidence Based Medicine: How to Practise and Teach EBM. London: Churchill Livingstone, 1998.

Schilp CE. The use of cued speech to correct misarticulation of /s/ and /z/ sounds in an 8-year-old boy with normal hearing. Language, Speech and Hearing Services in Schools 1986; 17: 270-5.

Schissel RJ, Doty MH. Application of the systematic multiple phonemic approach to articulation therapy: A case study. Language, Speech and Hearing Services in Schools 1979; 10: 178-84.

Secord WA. Test of Minimal Articulatory Competency. Columbus, OH: Charles E. Merrill, 1981.

Sommers RK, Logsdon BS, Wright JM. A review and critical analysis of treatment research related to articulation and phonological disorders. Journal of Communication Disorders 1992; 25: 3-22.

Spriestersbach DC, Sherman D. Cleft Palate and Communication. New York, NY: Academic Press, 1968.

Stackhouse J. An investigation of reading and spelling performance in speech disordered children. British Journal of Disorders of Communication 1982; 17: 53-60.

Stackhouse J, Wells B. Psycholinguistic assessment of developmental speech disorders. European Journal of Disorders of Communication 1993; 28: 331-48.

Stoel-Gammon C, Dunn C. Normal and Disordered Phonology in Children. Baltimore, MD: University Park Press, 1985.

Stringfellow K, McLeod S. Using a facilitating phonetic context to reduce an unusual form of gliding. Language, Speech and Hearing Services in Schools 1994; 25: 191-3.

Templin MC, Darley FL. The Templin-Darley Test of Articulation. Second ed., IA: University of Iowa, 1969.

Tyler AA, Edwards ML, Saxman JH. Clinical application of two phonological based treatment approaches. Journal of Speech and Hearing Disorders 1987; 52: 393-409.

Van Riper C. Speech Correction: Principles and Methods (fourth edition). Englewood Cliffs, NJ: Prentice-Hall, 1963.

Van Riper C. Predictive Screening Test of Articulation.

Weiner F. Effects of listener uncertainty on articulatory inconsistency. Journal of Speech and Hearing Disorders 1979; 4: 487-93.

Weiner F. Treatment of phonological disability using the method of meaningful minimal contrast: Two case studies. Journal of Speech and Hearing Disorders 1981; 46: 97-103.

Weiner F. Phonological Process Analysis. Baltimore, MD: University Park Press, 1989.

Weiss CE, Gordon ME, Lillywhite HS. Clinical Management of Articulatory and Phonologic Disorders (second edition). Baltimore, MD: Williams & Wilkins, 1987.

Wells B. Junction in developmental speech disorder: a case study. Clinical Linguistics and Phonetics 1994; 8: 1-25.

Young EC. The effects of treatment on consonant cluster and weak syllable reduction processes in misarticulating children. Language, Speech and Hearing Services in Schools 1987; 18: 23-33.

CHAPTER 12

The evidence base for augmentative and alternative communication

TERESA IACONO

Introduction

Augmentative and alternative communication (AAC) presents a unique challenge to the task of gathering an evidence base as a result of its comprehensive nature, early developmental stage and multidisciplinary influences. AAC can take many forms, such as the use of gestures by a child with severe and multiple developmental disability, a basic eye-gaze chart by an adult with a spinal cord injury in an intensive care unit, or an electronic voice output communication aid with word prediction by an adult with cerebral palsy in an office setting. Similarly, the goals of AAC may vary from providing a tool within an early language-based intervention to a means of addressing both communication and literacy activities across home, school or work and social environments.

As a result of the particular nature of AAC, and the early stage of development of the field, questions arise about the appropriateness of applying standards of evidence used with other clinical fields. Concerns about strategies to ensure control (such as randomization), in particular, become evident when research in AAC is considered within the contexts of its forms and components, models of assessment and intervention and history.

Defining AAC

The definition of AAC as proposed by the American Speech–Language–Hearing Association (ASHA) is:

> An area of clinical practice that attempts to compensate (either temporarily or permanently) for the impairment and disability patterns of individuals with severe expressive communication disorders (i.e., the severely speech–language and writing impaired). (ASHA, 1989, p. 107)

This early and widely accepted definition focused on levels of impairment and disability. According to a previous World Health Organization (WHO) classification of impairments, disabilities and handicaps (WHO, 2000), an 'impairment' is the level of abnormality – psychological, physiological or anatomical structure or function and a 'disability' is the level of ability to perform daily tasks. The WHO also referred to 'handicap', which is the level of societal disadvantage resulting from the individual's impairment or disability. As AAC has evolved, the field has included the third level of handicap as an outcome target (Blackstone, 1995; Beukelman and Mirenda, 1998). Recently, the WHO revised its classification, with the resulting *International Classification of Functioning, Disability and Health* (referred to as 'ICF') in which the terms 'activity limitations' replaced 'disability' and 'participation restrictions' replaced 'handicap' (WHO, 2000).

AAC as a multi-component system

When attempting to address the three ICF levels of impairment, activity and participation, AAC for an individual has come to be seen as a comprehensive system of the following components:

- The individual's extant communication skills (for example, gestures, vocalizations, facial expressions).
- Symbols (for example, signs, graphic line drawings, traditional orthography).
- Aids (for example, low-technology communication boards, high-technology voice output communication devices).
- Strategies (for example, incidental teaching, physical guidance, writing composition tasks).
- Techniques (for example, gesturing, signing, direct selection, scanning) (Beukelman and Mirenda, 1998).

Clinical decisions in developing an AAC system rely on knowledge of the evidence of how each component, individually and in combination, may affect a person. This effect may occur at any of the three levels of impairment, activity limitation and/or participation restriction.

Models of assessment and their implications for intervention

The focus of AAC on the three ICF levels has resulted from an evolutionary process, beginning with traditional models of assessment and intervention. Early popular assessment frameworks were borrowed from the general area of communication disorders, with a focus on prerequisite skills that were thought to be necessary for a person to be able to use an AAC system. These communication process models required the assessment of speech and language skills, with outcomes guiding movement through a matrix of steps to a final decision regarding the adoption and type of AAC system (Chapman and Miller, 1980; Shane and Bashir, 1980; Owens and House, 1984), with AAC often viewed as a last resort (Shane and Bashir, 1980). These assessment models, based on the notion of candidacy for AAC, were argued to be inappropriate, given the lack of research to substantiate the relationship between particular cognitive skills (for example, those seen at Piaget's Sensorimotor Stage 5) and use of a non-speech symbol system (Kangas and Lloyd, 1988; Reichle and Karlan, 1988). Furthermore, these developmental models were often inappropriately applied to adults, often functioning to exclude individuals who were most in need of AAC. Instead, these individuals were relegated to lengthy periods of unsuccessful and non-functional 'speech' or cognitive skills training (Reichle and Karlan, 1988).

For adults with acquired communication impairment, AAC assessment usually occurs within a rehabilitation setting or an intensive care unit in a hospital. In both situations, the goal of intervention is rarely to 'normalize communication' (Beukelman et al., 1985, p. 6), but rather, to identify the communication needs of the user across various daily environments or, in an intensive care unit, to facilitate medical management (Mitsuda et al., 1992). With consideration of these issues, needs assessments were developed in the context of AAC interventions for adults with acquired disability (Beukelman et al., 1985); they have also been applied to children with acquired disability (Light et al., 1988). Similarly, as interventionists realized the failure of traditional approaches for both adults and children with developmental disability (in particular, autism and intellectual disability), there was a call to 'rescue' them from skill-based interventions to those that aimed at increasing functional outcomes in everyday contexts (Calculator, 1988; Romski and Sevcik, 1988). Such functional outcomes are the intervention goals that emerge from a needs assessment that addresses the level of activity limitation by focusing on identification of the communication tasks that individuals must perform each day.

The move of people with disability from institutions to the community, which began in the 1970s and continues today (Malony and Taplin, 1988; Young et al., 1998), has required the factoring of community participation into intervention goals. Barriers to such participation must be assessed. Beukelman and Mirenda (1998, p. 147) refer to a participation model that 'provides a systematic process for conducting AAC assessments and designing interventions based on the functional participation requirements of peers without disabilities of the same chronological age as the potential

AAC user'. This model incorporates both a skill-based assessment (referred to as a 'capability assessment') and extends the needs assessment by including the observation of peers in the settings in which the AAC user wishes to participate and carry out communication tasks.

These assessment models provide the basis on which to determine the efficacy of intervention, wherein the benefits are derived under ideal conditions (as in an experimental study) (Blackstone, 1995). Such efficacy studies shed light on the effect of an AAC intervention on an individual's impairment (for example, increasing expressive language skills) and activity requirements (for example, providing access to the internet). Recently in the AAC literature, there has also been a call for studies into the effectiveness of interventions, wherein the benefits are derived under typical or everyday conditions (Blackstone, 1995). According to this definition, effectiveness studies address the generalization of skills, in addition to determining the direct effect of intervention on outcomes (Schlosser and Braun, 1994). They also provide information on the social validity of interventions, but only if measurement of outcomes extends to identifying the effect on participation in the community.

Development of the evidence base

Zangari et al. (1994) provided an historical perspective of the development of the field of AAC. These authors noted that, although use of AAC systems was documented as early as the 1950s, it was not until the 1960s and 1970s that anecdotal reports appeared in the literature on the successful use of signs and picture systems with children with autism (Creedon, 1973; Miller and Miller, 1973) and intellectual disability (Kopchick et al., 1975; Murphy et al., 1977). These brief reports appeared at a time when research was demonstrating that signs and abstract symbols could be taught to primates (Gardner and Gardner, 1969; Premack, 1971). These findings were applied to teaching early requesting (Romski et al., 1988) and language skills (Carrier, 1974) to people with intellectual disability; in fact, this research base continues to influence current AAC interventions for this group (see Romski et al., 1994; Romski and Sevcik, 1996).

According to Zangari et al. (1994), it was towards the end of the 1970s that AAC emerged as an area of specialization. Developments in the 1980s, such as the introduction of Blissymbols to children with cerebral palsy at the Ontario Crippled Children's Center in Canada and the appearance of other symbol sets (for example, COMPIC in Australia, PicSyms in the USA) and technological advances that culminated in the first electronic communication systems to be commercially available, created a need for greater specialization and sharing of expertise. This need resulted in the formalization of the field into cohesive entities and a proliferation of publications devoted to AAC.

In Australia, the Australian Group on Severe Communication Impairment (AGOSCI) was formed in 1981 (http://members.iinet.net.au/~sharono/AGOSCI/), soon followed by the International Society of Augmentative and Alternative Communication (ISAAC) in 1983 (Zangari et al., 1994). Both organizations produced newsletters as a means of sharing information among professionals, and later, consumers. In addition, a number of books dedicated to AAC were published in this decade (Schiefelbush, 1980; Silverman, 1980; Beukelman et al., 1985; Goossens' and Crain, 1985a, 1985b; McNaughton, 1985; Blackstone, 1986; Musselwhite and St Louis, 1988). Other developments in the 1980s included the proliferation of research into various aspects of AAC in multidisciplinary journals. It was in 1985, however, that the first edition of a journal dedicated to this specialized area was published: *Augmentative and Alternative Communication*. With this dedicated AAC journal came the realization that the field needed to examine the efficacy of the growing clinical and educational applications of AAC, and thereby to create an evidence base (McNaughton, 1985; Calculator, 1988; Light, 1988; Musselwhite and St Louis, 1988; Zangari et al., 1988).

Locating the evidence base

With the first issue of *Augmentative and Alternative Communication* came a call for empirically based studies addressing all aspects of AAC, along with clinically based case studies and conceptual papers that furthered the theoretical basis for clinical practice (Yoder, 1985). As the journal evolved, so did the evidence base, with researchers and practitioners submitting papers in response to the first and subsequent editors' requests. *Augmentative and Alternative Communication* has become the key source of scholarly work in the field, supplemented by research in other peer-reviewed journals, further texts and publications devoted to AAC. A review of articles appearing from 1985 to 2000 documents the development of the evidence base: a preponderance of early descriptions of clinical practice was gradually replaced by rich case studies, controlled single-case and group studies, and reviews of the literature. This journal thereby provides the key source for the current review of the evidence in AAC. Papers appearing over these 15 years were reviewed and included if they were descriptive or experimental studies dealing with efficacy or effectiveness of symbol or technology aspects of AAC systems, and included the impact on each of the three ICF levels of impairment, activity or participation. These studies were supplemented by key studies appearing in other peer-reviewed journals.

The evidence

System design

Technological developments have allowed increasingly sophisticated features to be incorporated into aided high-technology systems. These features were mostly the result of decisions by manufacturers with little guidance from research, at least in the early days, regarding the choice of symbol types, layout and aspects of voice output. Instead, researchers have attempted to evaluate features frequently provided in such devices according to learner performance. As a result, a large body of research has been devoted to issues of symbol learning (for example, signs and various graphic symbols), intelligibility and comprehensibility of commercial speech synthesizers, selection techniques (for example, direct selection and various types of scanning options) and rate enhancement strategies (for example, options for encoding messages). (The issues addressed in this body of research are summarized in Table 12.1.)

Table 12.1 Issues explored in research addressing selection of AAC components

Component	Issues	Source
Symbol Learnability •signs	Factors of motoric requirements, symmetry, iconicity and translucency on sign learnability and recall	Coelho and Duffy (1986) Doherty (1985) Granlund et al. (1989)
•Bliss symbols	Comparisons with other graphic systems and methods of teaching (eg., paired associated learning, teaching meaning of elements, teaching within story narratives)	Fuller (1997) Luftig and Bersani (1985) Mizuko (1987) Schlosser and Lloyd (1997) Shepherd and Haaf (1995)
Speech synthesis	Comparison of commercially available speech synthesizers for word and sentence level intelligibility and user preferences	Crabtree et al. (1990) Fucci et al., (1995) Mirenda and Beukelman (1987, 1990)
	Recent studies focused on impact on message comprehension using sentence verification tasks	Koul and Hanners (1997) Raghavendra and Allen (1993)

(contd)

Table 12.1 (contd)

Component	Issues	Source
Selection techniques	Comparison amongst options (direct selection, various scanning types, and input methods) for physical and cognitive demands	Mizuko and Esser (1991) Mizuko et al. (1994) Peterson et al. (2000) Szeto et al. (1993)
Rate enhancement	Comparison of strategies for effectiveness and ease of learning, and trade-offs with cognitive and perceptual demands and motor requirements	Horstmann Koester and Levine (1996) Light and Lindsay (1992) Light et al. (1990)

The proliferation of high- and low-technology AAC systems on the market, and the types of systems that may be custom designed by practitioners for individual AAC users creates a challenge for research to guide design or to assess the efficacy of existing systems. The complexity of the task is seen in the tendency for studies into system design to predominantly include people without disability (for example, Crabtree et al., 1990; Mizuko et al., 1994; Schlosser and Lloyd, 1997; Reynolds and Jefferson, 1999). As a result, the adoption of control procedures (such as random allocation to treatment and no-treatment groups) has been possible. Mizuko et al. (1994) for example, randomly assigned 22 children to one of two experimental conditions to determine the short-term memory requirements of direct selection versus row–column scanning. As with this study, other researchers attempting to apply control procedures have tended to include relatively few subjects (Crabtree et al., 1990; Schlosser and Lloyd, 1997). For studies involving people with disability, subject numbers have been even smaller (Light et al., 1990; Light and Lindsay, 1992; Horstmann Koester and Levine, 1996; Koul and Hanners, 1997); for example, Light et al. (1990) used a repeated-measures group design to compare rates of accessing messages for three message encoding strategies for six AAC users.

The inclusion of participants with, versus those without, disabilities has resulted in some controversy in the field. Higginbotham (1995) argued that non-disabled participants are more accessible and less expensive, and their inclusion over people with disability results in fewer potential confounds. Bedrosian (1995), on the other hand, argued that there is insufficient evidence to indicate the generalizability of findings from non-disabled participants to AAC users. Certainly, most studies into aspects of system design await replication with AAC users.

Effect on the AAC user

AAC interventions have been used with individuals across the lifespan with varied developmental and acquired disorders. These interventions have been documented in published case studies, whereas attempts to establish their efficacy have been the focus of empirical studies. The breakdown of the research according to the effect of AAC on the ICF levels of impairment, activity and participation is presented in Table 12.2. In addition, the nature of the research is indicated in the table according to case studies, experimental single-case studies and group studies.

Impairment

Interventions that target changes in speech, cognition and language skills address the level of impairment. Inspection of Table 12.2 indicates that a total of 13 case studies relating to impairment were located. These case studies documented the use of AAC, both unaided (for example, signs and gestures) and aided (for example, communication boards with graphic symbols and electronic devices), in teaching vocabulary and basic sign or symbol combinations to children with intellectual disability (Kouri, 1989) and cerebral palsy (Bruno, 1989). In addition, pre-symbolic children with disability, including dual visual–hearing impairment, have learned cause–effect skills within AAC interventions (Schweigert and Rowland, 1992). Case studies at the level of impairment involving people with acquired disorders were more limited in number. The three case studies represented in Table 12.2 demonstrated the teaching of high-technology AAC to adults with aphasia (King and Hux, 1995; Rostron et al., 1996; Waller et al., 1998).

Similar target structures to those taught in case studies involving people with congenital disorders have been the focus of most of the 11 experimental

Table 12.2 Summary of the AAC research base

	ICF levels					
Study design	Impairment		Activity limitation		Participation restriction	
	Disorder					
	Developmental	Acquired	Developmental	Acquired	Developmental	Acquired
Case study	10	3	24	15	6	0
ESCD	9	2	16	2	5	1
Group	3	0	2	1	7	0

ESCD = Experimental single-case design.

single-case studies represented in Table 12.2. Experimental single-case studies, such as the use of ABA (Schweigert, 1989) and multiple-baseline designs (Harris et al. 1996) have been used to demonstrate whether AAC intervention *per se* results in increases in language skills. Comparison of AAC systems and strategies are best conducted with alternating-treatments designs, given the suitability and specificity of this design to comparing two or more treatments (Barlow et al., 1984). Iacono et al. (1993), for example, compared sign+speech to a VOCA+speech condition in teaching two-word combinations to two children with intellectual disability. By use of a mutliple-baseline study design, treatment efficacy for both approaches was demonstrated, whereas use of an alternating-treatment design within the multiple-baseline study design demonstrated an advantage for the VOCA+speech intervention for one child.

Only two experimental single-case design studies were located at the impairment level for acquired disorders. Steele et al. (1989) evaluated the effect of a computer-based visual communication system in teaching vocabulary and syntax to five adults with aphasia. Unfortunately, data were presented for only one participant within a multiple-baseline design, with the target limited to the teaching of prepositions. Few details of the procedures and no data on reliability were provided, preventing any attempt to replicate the study. Because performance of the other participants was presented descriptively, the true efficacy of the AAC intervention cannot be evaluated. Conducting a more controlled study, Koul and Harding (1998) also used a multiple-baseline study design to evaluate the effects on communication skills of adults with aphasia of a computer-based symbol system. All participants improved their ability to produce symbols and symbol combinations as a result of treatment.

Group studies at the impairment level have been limited, with only three studies located (see Table 12.2) (Osguthorpe and Li-Chang, 1988; Watkins et al., 1993; Wilkinson and Romski, 1994). All three studies included participants with developmental disorders, with two demonstrating the effectiveness of AAC intervention for increasing symbol or sign acquisition (Osguthorpe et al., 1988; Watkins et al., 1993). The study by Wilkinson and Romski (1994) was a group comparison of 13 youths involved in a longitudinal project into the effects of the programme known as 'system for augmenting language'. Participants were divided into those who combined graphic symbols (lexigrams*) and those who used single symbols only. The findings of the study indicated that the symbol-combiners reflected semantic combinations characteristic of normal language development. In addition, no

---

*Lexigrams are opaque graphic symbols constituted by combining a set of geometric elements.

differences in input provided by conversational partners were found to account for differences in the language skills between the two groups. Such group studies provide information on potential outcomes for participants grouped according to inherent or learnt traits (for example, users of single versus combined symbols). They fail, however, to demonstrate treatment efficacy because of the absence of experimental manipulation.

Activity restriction

Early in the evolution of *Augmentative and Alternative Communication*, concern was expressed about the lack of functional outcomes resulting from AAC interventions (*see* Schlosser and Braun, 1994). Calculator (1988), for example, argued the need for assessing the efficacy of AAC by examining the effect of interventions on a person's functioning in naturalistic situations, rather than skills that could be demonstrated only in clinics or experimental settings. This call for functional outcomes reflected a move in the general field of communication disorders, wherein the value of didactic procedures in clinical settings was questioned in the face of a failure of skills to generalize to everyday environments (Fey, 1986).

In AAC, researchers and practitioners responded to the concern for functional outcomes, as indicated by the number of case studies, and experimental single-case and group studies represented in Table 12.2. Case studies (39 in total) demonstrated the focus on signs and symbols with functional value (for example, to request leisure or make choices) (Mirenda and Dattilo, 1987) and to provide a means to engage in conversational interactions (Buzolich and Lunger, 1995). The case studies at the ICF activity level represent a wide range of AAC systems used with individuals across the age span and with varied disorders. They demonstrate the clinical application of AAC not only for people with developmental disability (Stephenson and Linfoot, 1995) or adults with aphasia (Garrett et al., 1989) but also to provide basic and more advanced systems to children with developmental verbal apraxia (Cumley and Swanson, 1999) or traumatic brain injury (DeRuyter and Donoghue, 1989) and adults with degenerative diseases, such as amyotrophic lateral sclerosis (Yorkston, 1989) and multiple sclerosis (Honsinger, 1989).

Experimental, single-case designs are far fewer than case or descriptive studies at the level of activity limitation (total of 18) (Table 12.2). Multiple-baseline study designs and their variant, multiple-probe designs, have been favoured to demonstrate the effect of teaching AAC in facilitating the use of signs or symbols for basic pragmatic functions (for example, Soto et al., 1993; Sigafoos et al., 1996) or to teach conversational participation by high-tech users (Buzolich et al., 1991; Datillo and Camarata, 1991). In these latter studies, researchers attempted to overcome problems identified in earlier case studies that indicated the passive roles of AAC users in conversational interactions (Calculator and Dolloghan, 1982; Calculator and Luchko, 1983). (*See also* Light et al., 1985 for a detailed study of the interaction patterns between young aided system users and their caregivers.)

Not represented in Table 12.2 are the number of studies that perhaps best exemplify successful functional use of AAC; that is, aided and unaided AAC in functional communication training to reduce or eliminate challenging behaviours in individuals with severe disability. A large body of research has established the efficacy of functional communication training in providing individuals with alternatives to challenging behaviour. The studies have been predominantly experimental single-case designs in which behaviour analysis has preceded AAC intervention. Most of these studies have appeared in journals focusing on behavioural analysis or intellectual disability, with few appearing in *Augmentative and Alternative Communication* (*see* Durand (1993) for an exception). Mirenda (1997) reviewed 21 studies in which functional communication training or AAC intervention efficacy was demonstrated in individuals aged from 1;3 to 36 years, with severe to profound intellectual disability or autism. These studies have enabled the identification of key principles to successful functional communication training, including matching AAC messages to the response function of the challenging behaviour, and choosing AAC responses that are easy to produce, are readily recognizable and to which people will respond promptly.

For people with acquired disorders, only two case studies addressing the ICF level of activity limitation were located from peer-reviewed journals. Purdy et al. (1994) used a multiple-baseline study design to determine the effects of communication board use by two adults with Broca's aphasia. The communication board was used for requesting and providing personal information, but the participants demonstrated a preference for vocalisations and gestures for social messages. Garrett and Beukelman (1995) demonstrated the usefulness of a strategy for adults with aphasia. The strategy 'written choice communication' is a dynamic low-technology procedure involving the communication partner in providing written choices during conversations.

Only three group studies addressing the level of activity were located. For people with developmental disability, group studies are limited to two based on the system for augmenting language longitudinal study referred to above. Adamson et al. (1992) and Romski et al. (1994) investigated aspects of vocabulary and contexts in terms of outcomes for their participants with intellectual disability. A similar dearth of group studies is evident for acquired disability, with the one study by Purdy et al. (1994) suggesting that their adults with non-fluent aphasia preferred use of their own vocalizations to AAC modalities. Fox and Fried-Oken (1996) queried the usefulness of this study because of methodological problems (including a failure to randomly select participants, and differences in training tasks across communication modalities) and the researchers' failure to explore reasons for modality preferences.

Participation

Interventions at the level of participation address issues relating to the individual accessing and interacting in life situations. From Table 12.2, it is evident that there are few case studies addressing this level, with none that focus specifically on acquired disorders. Three of the case studies provided descriptions of interventions involving conversational interactants (McNaughton and Light, 1989), thereby demonstrating a shift in focus from the AAC user to both communication partners. The other three case studies provided programme outcome information, in which AAC partners or parents have responded to surveys about their perceptions of the effect of AAC on an individual or family (McCall et al., 1997).

Experimental single-case studies addressing participation restrictions (a total of six) have, as with the few case studies, focused on communication partner training in enhancing interactions with AAC users. Partners, both adults and children, have been taught to provide more communication opportunities (Stiebel, 1999) or to use strategies to facilitate AAC users to become more active participants in conversations (Hunt et al., 1991; Light et al., 1992; Carter and Maxwell, 1998). Of note from these studies is that very brief instruction of peers appears to result in increases in conversational turns by AAC users (Hunt et al., 1991; Carter and Maxwell, 1998). Training conversational partners was also found to be effective in the only experimental single-case study addressing participation of people with acquired disorders. Bourgeois (1992) trained carers of patients with Alzheimer's disease to facilitate their use of memory wallets. Treatment efficacy was demonstrated by use of a multiple-baseline study design, with most of the six participants increasing their on-topic conversations and accurate responses following the implementation of treatment.

A factor argued to affect individuals' participation in life situations is attitudes of peers or others (Beukelman and Mirenda, 1998). The seven group studies represented in Table 12.2 address the issue of attitudes towards people who use different types of AAC. Factors such as the use of high- versus low-technology or unaided systems (Gorenflo and Gorenflo, 1991), the quality of speech output (Gorenflo et al., 1994) and the length of messages produced (Bedrosian et al., 1992; Hoag and Bedrosian, 1992) have been manipulated in these studies. Findings indicate that these factors affect the attitudes of people observing interactions between AAC users and natural speakers.

A controversial issue: facilitated communication

The need for evidence to support practice in AAC has been most strongly felt in an area that has caused much controversy – that of facilitated communication. Facilitated communication is the provision of physical support to allow an individual to directly access a communication system (for example, picture, word or alphabet board, computer keyboard or electronic device). According to Crossley (1992, p. 47), facilitated communication 'is a teaching strategy used with people with SCI requiring aided communication who are not yet able to access a communication aid independently but for whom direct access with their hands is a realistic and desirable goal'. The strategy has been reported to be useful for people with autism and others with severe communication impairment (Crossley, 1992; Crossley and Remington-Gurney, 1992).

The controversy surrounding facilitated communication comes from concerns about whether communication produced through it originates with the individual or the facilitator, in addition to claims of unexplained literacy and communication skills (Biklen et al., 1992; Crossley and Remington-Gurney, 1992; Eberlin et al., 1993) and Biklen's hypothesis that the communication difficulty of many individuals presenting with low-functioning autism is the result of apraxia, or a movement disorder, which may underlie disorders of hand function (see Crossley and Remington, 1992).

The issue of the author of communication produced through facilitated communication is perhaps the most serious one, causing concern not only among researchers and practitioners but also legal bodies. Facilitated communication achieved international notoriety following court cases in which individuals with severe communication impairment, through facilitated communication, alleged crimes, such as sexual abuse by carers (see Archer, 1992; Crossley, 1992; Bligh and Kupperman, 1993; Calculator and Hatch, 1995). Attempts have been made to validate the communication of the individual with severe communication impairment. Strategies have included having the facilitator look away from the communication aid when the response was formulated (Crossley, 1992). In addition, the facilitator's responses were compared according to whether or not they were informed of the questions (for example, Calculator and Hatch, 1995). However, these attempts have been unsuccessful, resulting in court hearings being terminated.

Support for the successful use of facilitated communication has come largely from qualitative studies, characterized by rich data from varied sources (for example, Biklen et al., 1992; Sabin and Donnellan, 1993). From these studies, evidence that messages through facilitated communiation are authored by the individual with severe communication impairment are based on observations, such as the production of typographical and phonetic spelling errors unique to the individual, the production of unusual sentences unlikely to be produced by a facilitator and the production of content that is not known to the facilitator. Except for an investigation by the Intellectual Disability Review Panel (1989), in which one of three individuals passed an experimentally controlled task of message passing with and without the facilitator being informed of the message, quantitative studies with objective measures have not provided support for the validity of the strategy. In fact, the evidence points to facilitators influencing message content (Datlow Smith and Belcher, 1993; Hudson et al., 1993; Moore et al., 1993; Moore, Donovan and Hudson, 1993).

In one of few experimental studies in this area, Bebko et al. (1996) used multiple methods to determine if facilitated communication enhanced communication in people with autism or pervasive developmental disorder (aged 6–21 years) in comparison to independent communication, and if facilitators influenced communication. Their results and those of other studies (Bomba et al., 1996; Simon et al., 1996) have failed to find an advantage of facilitated communication over independent communication.

Proponents of facilitated communication have argued that quantitative research strategies are inappropriate, given the unique characteristics of facilitated communication as a collaborative process, requiring rapport and trust between the individual and facilitator (Duchan, 1993), features that cannot be captured using experimental procedures in non-naturalistic settings. In addition, the potential for facilitators to influence communication has been acknowledged (Crossley, 1992). Factors that might affect facilitator influence would appear better documented through qualitative than quantitative means. Although anecdotal reports suggest that, at least for some individuals, the true test of validation has been achieved through independent communication after training in facilitated communication (Crossley and Remington-Gurney, 1992), longitudinal qualitative studies that document progress from early stages have been lacking in the published literature base.

Summarizing the state of the art

Recent reviews in AAC have indicated a continued call for empirical evidence to support practice (Calculator, 1999; Granlund and Olsson, 1999; Light, 1999). It seems that despite the burgeoning of research in the area, much AAC practice is grounded in clinical experience, rather than validation through research. Of particular concern is a lack of research into the effectiveness of interventions, or the impact of AAC in typical or daily environments, with few studies addressing generalization and maintenance of effects. In the current review, studies that included assessment of the generalization and/or maintenance of effects were few (examples include Bellaire et al., 1991; Buzolich et al., 1991; Iacono et al., 1993; Soto et al., 1993; Turnell and Carter, 1994; Reichle, 1997; Stiebel, 1999). More comprehensive data on generalization and maintenance effects may be found in the recent meta-analysis by Schlosser and Lee (2000). From an exhaustive review of the AAC literature from 1976 to 1995, these authors located 50 studies that included data on the effects of intervention, generalization and maintenance. Schlosser and Lee (2000) found that most researchers did not include specific generalization or maintenance strategies, adopting a 'train and hope' approach rather than a strategy of training multiple exemplars. Fortunately, the 'non-strategy' approach appeared effective, with 85% of interventions found to result in generalization across stimuli, people, settings or a combination. Data for maintenance were less positive, with only 46% of the interventions found to result in maintenance of learning outcomes.

Limitations and strengths of the evidence base

If the gold standard of clinical evidence is the use of group experimental studies with randomized allocation of participants to treatment and no-treatment groups, experimenter manipulation of independent variables and control over the conduct of the experiment as a means of establishing cause–effect (Fox and Fried-Oken, 1996) then the evidence base in AAC is grossly deficient. In few of the studies reviewed was this design adopted, with the exceptions addressing issues of attitudes towards AAC users (for Hoag and Bedrosian, 1992; Gorenflo and Gorenflo, 1997), technology design (Light et al., 1990; Mizuko et al., 1994) or symbol learnability (Fuller, 1997; Schlosser and Lloyd, 1997). The lack of experimental group studies to assess treatment efficacy and effectiveness reflects the apparent overall inappropriateness of this design in AAC, given the low incidence and heterogeneity within the AAC population (Light, 1999).

More appropriate to questions of efficacy of AAC interventions are experimental single-case designs, which are well suited to analysing individual performance while controlling for confounding variables. In fact, multiple-baseline designs feature prominently in the research reviewed (Buzolich et al., 1991; Hunt et al., 1991; Iacono et al., 1993; Koul and Harding, 1998). Alternating-treatments designs also feature in this literature base (Goodman and Remington, 1993; Iacono and Duncum, 1995), allowing for the comparison of treatments (Schlosser, 1999). Similarly, multiple-baseline and alternating-treatment designs dominated the 50 studies reviewed by Schlosser and Lee (2000).

The flexibility of experimental single-case designs is demonstrated in those studies in which basic designs have been modified in order to address specific research questions (Iacono et al., 1993). When learning is the target outcome, multiple-baseline and alternating-treatment study designs, and their variations, appear more suitable than basic withdrawal designs, such as ABA and ABAB designs, which rely on return to baseline levels in order for treatment effects to be demonstrated (Barlow et al., 1984). This problem was evident in the study by Kouri (1988) in which participants were taught signs within an ABAB design. Although treatment performance tended to be stronger in the B phases than in baseline, performance in the second baseline was higher than the first across the five participants, thereby weakening the demonstration of treatment effects.

The heterogeneity of the populations served by AAC, the multiple components of AAC intervention (for example, customization of systems, instructional strategies for AAC users and facilitators) and the levels at which AAC may have an effect (impairment, activity and participation) result in dependent and independent variables that are difficult to define (Light, 1999). In fact, AAC intervention was described by Light (1999, p. 16) as 'complex, "messy" processes', whereas Calculator (1999) cautioned researchers about the need to ensure that, by unravelling variables that are intertwined in their natural state, research does not become socially invalid. As an example, Calculator, in commenting on his own difficulty in conducting research in one typical context, the classroom, noted:

> it has proven difficult, if not impossible, to isolate the precise role AAC plays with respect to functional outcomes in the chaotic milieus of public school education and elsewhere. The introduction of AAC occurs in a changing context of attitudes, perceptions, resources, experiences, consultants, and so forth. (Calculator, 1999, p. 8)

Some researchers have attempted to identify factors that affect the successful use of AAC in everyday contexts, such as attitudes of peers (Blockberger et al., 1993), or to gather social validation data on outcomes; for example, Garrett and Beukelman (1995) asked the adult AAC user in their study about the effect of the written choice AAC strategy and found that he did not perceive any changes in his communication effectiveness. The paucity of research into social validation of outcomes, in addition to the overall lack of research addressing the participation level, are indicative of the field's early stage in effectiveness research.

Despite its limitations, the AAC literature is strong in its documentation of clinical applications of AAC to individuals whose severe communication impairment arises from a large variety of causes. In addition to case studies appearing in journals are texts devoted to case presentations and exploration of AAC with individuals with developmental (for example, von Tetzchner and Hygum Jensen, 1996) and acquired disorders (for example, Beukelman et al.,

1985). Although case studies do not provide empirical evidence for treatment effects, they have been argued to play a valuable role in the development of clinical fields by developing hypotheses for research, informing theory and providing a vehicle for sharing expertise amongst practitioners and consumers (McEwan and Karlan, 1990). Given the complexity of AAC interventions, case studies, such as the longitudinal documentation of an evolving AAC intervention by Light and colleagues (1988) of a young girl with a traumatic brain injury, provide guidance to clinical decision-making and the changing role of AAC for an individual over time.

The results of surveys conducted in Australia (Russell and McAllister, 1995; Balandin and Iacono, 1998), the UK (Udwin and Yule, 1991; McCall et al., 1997) and the USA (Matas et al., 1985; Ratcliff and Beukelman, 1995) have indicated a lack of awareness or knowledge of AAC. These studies speak to a need for ongoing education of families and professionals about the range of AAC options, its value at various stages of intervention or rehabilitation, and appropriate intervention goals and strategies. Case studies provide documentation that is perhaps most accessible to practitioners and families. These descriptive accounts require parallel investigations into the efficacy of each aspect of AAC intervention. As noted, the AAC field has achieved some level of success in demonstrating treatment efficacy, at least for people with developmental disability, and at the ICF levels of impairment and activity. This evidence has been provided largely at the evidence level of experimental single-case studies, thereby allowing determination of both research and clinical effects of treatment. Still needed, however, is evidence to support the efficacy of AAC for people with acquired disorders (Fox and Fried-Oken, 1996) and also evidence of its effectiveness, through a focus on issues of generalization and maintenance of changes occurring in controlled treatment settings to typical and natural settings (Calculator, 1999; Schlosser and Lee, 2000).

A pragmatic motivation for expanding the evidence base

In an era of cost rationalization, governments and other agencies that control spending on special education, rehabilitation and other clinical services require documentation to support the cost of devices and intervention, thereby providing a powerful force to drive the expansion of the AAC evidence base. In a field in which device abandonment has been problematic (Allaire et al., 1991; Fisher et al., 1993; Culp et al., 1996; Bebb and Raghavendra, 2000), practitioners must provide strong justification for the purchase of devices and therapy time. This need was recently demonstrated in the USA. Strategies were implemented by a group of AAC professionals to expedite a review conducted by the Healthcare Financing and Administration (HCFA) of the coverage offered through Medicare, the largest health care programme in the country (Blackstone, 2000). Following pressure from the AAC community, the HCFA agreed to review its policy of not offering coverage for AAC. According to Blackstone (2000), a working party gathered written documentation of the efficacy and outcomes of AAC and submitted it to HCFA. The documentation, comprising published research articles (case studies and controlled studies) contributed to HCFA lifting its prohibition on AAC coverage (Moore, 2000).

In Australia, funding for AAC varies across states, with few offering a formal system. An exception is Victoria, in which the state government considers funding of AAC devices for individuals who meet certain eligibility requirements through its Aid and Equipment Program for Aids (http://hnb.dhs.vic.gov.au/ds/disabilitysite.nsf/pages/pub_aids). Extending this funding to low-technology systems, and the establishment of similar schemes in other states or through private health insurance is likely to be facilitated by a strong evidence base.

Conclusion

The evidence for AAC intervention is comprehensive, given the range in the needs, skills and life situations of people with permanent or temporary severe communication impairment. Case studies have demonstrated the range of potential applications in a process that evolves with each individual. As a result, no longer is AAC seen as the last-resort intervention for people who have 'failed' in traditional speech pathology. Rather, AAC serves to enhance communication along an intervention continuum from functioning as a short-term intervention strategy to providing varied means of meeting all communication requirements across life situations.

The case studies have been supplemented by an increase in experimental studies, mostly single-case, that have demonstrated the efficacy of AAC intervention, in particular for addressing activity limitations in people with developmental disability. The gaps in evidence are most notably studies demonstrating the efficacy of AAC for people with acquired disorders (for example, aphasia, TBI, degenerative diseases) and the effectiveness of AAC in naturalistic settings, thereby addressing the level of participation restrictions. Convincing the community beyond those who have chosen to specialize in AAC, either through professional options or life circumstances, is dependent on continued investigation into factors affecting AAC intervention success in enhancing full communication participation. Research addressing these issues will, by virtue of the nature of AAC and the populations who benefit from it, rely on small-scale studies, with a focus on the individual. For AAC, then, convincing evidence lies in small controlled studies, with attention to replication and generalization strategies.

References

Adamson L, Romski MA, Deffebach K, Sevcik R. Symbol vocabulary and the focus of conversations: augmenting language development for youth with mental retardation. Journal of Speech and Hearing Research 1992; 35: 1333-43.

Allaire J, Gressard R, Blackman J, Hostler S. Children with severe speech impairments: caregiver survey of AAC use. Augmentative and Alternative Communication 1991; 7: 248-55.

American Speech-Language-Hearing Association (ASHA). Competencies for speech-language pathologists providing services in augmentative communication. ASHA 1989; 31: 107-10.

Archer A. Where is the 'facile' in 'facilitated communication'? Communicating Together 1992; 10: 5-7.

Balandin S, Iacono T. AAC and Australian speech pathologists: results of a national survey. Augmentative and Alternative Communication 1998; 14: 239-49.

Barlow D, Hayes S, Nelson, R. The Scientist Practitioner: Research and Accountability in Clinical and Educational Settings. New York, NY: Pergamon Press, 1984.

Bebb M, Raghavendra, P. Predictors of Device Abandonment in Students who Transition from School to the Community. Paper presented at the Australian Cerebral Palsy Association, Melbourne, November 2000.

Bebko J, Perry A, Bryson S. Multiple method validation study of facilitated communication: II. Individual differences and subgroup results. Journal of Autism and Developmental Disorders 1996; 26: 19-42.

Bedrosian J. Limitations in the use of nondisabled subjects in AAC research. Augmentative and Alternative Communication 1995; 11: 6-10.

Bedrosian J, Hoag L, Calculator S, Molineux B. Variables influencing perceptions of the communicative competence of an adult augmentative and alternative communication system user. Journal of Speech and Hearing Research 1992; 35: 1105-13.

Bellaire K, Georges J, Thompson, C. Establishing functional communication board use for nonverbal aphasic subjects. Clinical Aphasiology 1991; 19: 219-27.

Beukelman D, Mirenda P. Augmentative and Alternative Communication: Management of Severe Communication Disorders in Children and Adults (second edition). Baltimore, MD: Paul H Brooks, 1998.

Beukelman D, Yorkston K, Dowden P. Communication Augmentation: A Casebook of Clinical Management. San-Diego, CA: College-Hill Press, 1985.

Biklen .D, Winston Morton M, Gold D, Gerrigan C, Swaminathan S.Facilitated communication: implications for individuals with autism. Topics in Language Disorders 1992; 12: 1-28.

Blackstone S. Augmentative Communication: An Introduction. Rockville, MD: American Speech-Language-Hearing Association, 1986.

Blackstone S. AAC outcomes: definitions and the WHO. Augmentative Communication News 1995; 8: 1-3.

Blackstone S. Making a difference for people who rely on AAC: the Medicare story. Augmentative Communication News 2000; 12: 1-2.

Bligh S, Kupperman P. Brief report: facilitated communication evaluation procedure accepted in a court case. Journal of Autism and Developmental Disorders 1993; 23: 553-7.

Blockberger S, Armstrong R, O'Connor A, Freeman R. Children's attitudes toward a nonspeaking child using various augmentative and alternative communication techniques. Augmentative and Alternative Communication 1993; 9: 243-50.

Bomba C, O'Donnell L, Markowitz C, Holmes D. Evaluating the impact of the communicative competence of fourteen students with autism. Journal of Autism and Developmental Disorders 1996; 26: 43-58.

Bourgeois M. Evaluating memory wallets in conversations with persons with dementia. Journal of Speech and Hearing Research 1992; 35: 1344-57.

Bruno J. Customizing a MinspeakTM system for a preliterate child: a case example. Augmentative and Alternative Communication 1989; 5: 89-100.

Buzolich M, King J, Baroody S. Acquisition of the commenting function among system users. Augmentative and Alternative Communication 1991; 7: 88-99.

Buzolich M, Lunger J. Empowering system users in peer training. Augmentative and Alternative Communication 1995; 11: 37-48.

Calculator S. Evaluating the effectiveness of AAC programs for persons with severe handicaps. Augmentative and Alternative Communication 1988; 4: 177-9.

Calculator S. AAC outcomes for children and youths with severe disabilities: when seeing is believing. Augmentative and Alternative Communication 1999; 15: 4-12.

Calculator S, Dolloghan C. The use of communication boards in a residential setting: an evaluation. Journal of Speech and Hearing Disorders 1982; 47: 281-7.

Calculator S, Hatch E. Validation of facilitated communication: a case study and beyond. American Journal of Speech-Language Pathology 1995; 4: 49-58.

Calculator S, Luchko, C. Evaluating the effectiveness of a communication board training program. Journal of Speech and Hearing Disorders 1983; 185-91.

Carter M, Maxwell K. Promoting interaction with children using augmentative and alternative communication through peer-mediated intervention. International Journal of Disability, Development and Education 1998; 45: 75-96.

Carrier J. Nonspeech noun usage training with severely and profoundly retarded children. Journal of Speech and Hearing Research 1974; 17: 510-17.

Chapman R, Miller J. Analyzing language and communication in a child. In: Schiefelbusch R (Ed.). Nonspeech Language and Communication: Acquisition and Intervention. Baltimore: University Park Press, 1980; 159-96.

Coelho C, Duffy R. Effects of iconicity, motoric complexity, and linguistic function on sign acquisition in severe aphasia. Perceptual and Motor Skills 1986; 63: 519-30.

Crabtree M, Mirenda P, Beukelman D. Age and gender preferences for synthetic and natural speech. Augmentative and Alternative Communication 1990; 6: 256-61.

Creedon M. (1973). Language Development in Non-verbal Autistic Children Using a Simultaneous Communication System. Paper presented at the Society for Research in Child Development. Philadelphia, PA, 1973.

Crossley R. Getting the words out: case studies in facilitated communication training. Topics in Language Disorders 1992; 12: 46-59.

Crossley R, Remington-Gurney J. Getting the words out: facilitated communication training. Topics in Language Disorders 1992; 12: 29-45.

Culp D, Ambrosi D, Berninger T, Mitchell K. Augmentative communication aid use - a follow-up study. Augmentative and Alternative Communication 1996; 2: 19-24.

Cumley G, Swanson S. Augmentative and alternative communication options for children with developmental apraxia of speech: three case studies. Augmentative and Alternative Communication 1999; 15: 110-25.

Datlow Smith M, Belcher R. Brief report: facilitated communication with adults with autism. Journal of Autism and Developmental Disorders 1993; 23: 175-83.

Datillo J, Camarata S. Facilitating conversation through self-initiated augmentative communication treatment. Journal of Applied Behavior Analysis 1991; 24: 369-78.

DeRuyter D, Donoghue K. Communication and traumatic brain injury: a case study. Augmentative and Alternative Communication 1989; 5: 49-54.

Doherty J. The effects of sign characteristics on sign acquisition and retention: an integrative review of the literature. Augmentative and Alternative Communication 1985; 1: 108-21.

Duchan J. Issues raised by facilitated communication for theorizing and research on autism. Journal of Speech and Hearing Research 1993; 36: 1108-19.

Durand M. Functional communication training using assistive devices: effects on challenging behavior and affect. Augmentative and Alternative Communication 1993; 9: 168-76.

Eberlin M, McConnachie G, Ibel S, Volpe L. Facilitated communication: a failure to replicate the phenomenon. Journal of Autism and Developmental Disorders 1993; 23: 507-30.

Fey M. Language Intervention with Young Children. London: Taylor & Francis, 1986.

Fisher P, Toczek M, Seeger B. Technology for people with disabilities: a survey of needs. Assistive Technology 1993; 5: 106-18.

Fox L, Fried-Oken M. AAC Aphasiology: partnership for future research. Augmentative and Alternative Communication 1996; 12: 257-71.

Fucci D, Reynolds M, Bettagere R, Gonzales, M. Synthetic speech intelligibility under several experimental conditions. Augmentative and Alternative Communication 1995; 11: 113-17.

Fuller D. Initial study into the effects of translucency and complexity on the learning of Blissymbols by children and adults with normal cognitive abilities. Augmentative and Alternative Communication 1997; 13: 30-39.

Gardner R, Gardner B. Teaching sign language to a chimpanzee. Science 1969; 165: 664-72.

Garrett D, Beukelman D, Low-Morrow D. A comprehensive augmentative communication system for an adult with Broca's aphasia. Augmentative and Alternative Communication 1989; 5: 55-61.

Garrett K, Beukelman D. Changes in the interaction patterns of an individual with severe aphasia given three types of partner support. Clinical Aphasiology 1995; 23: 237-51.

Goodman J, Remington B. Acquisition of expressive signing: comparison of reinforcement strategies. Augmentative and Alternative Communication 1993; 9: 26-35.

Goossens C, Crain S. Augmentative Communication: Assessment Resource. Wauconda, IL: Don Johnston Developmental Equipment, Inc., 1985a.

Goossens C, Crain S. Augmentative Communication: Intervention Resource. Wauconda, IL: Don Johnston Developmental Equipment, Inc., 1995b.

Gorenflo C, Gorenflo D. The effects of information and augmentative communication technique on attitudes towards nonspeaking individuals. Journal of Speech and Hearing Research 1991; 34: 19-26.

Gorenflo D, Gorenflo C. Variations on the written choice strategy for individuals with severe aphasia. Augmentative and Alternative Communication 1997; 13: 87-91.

Gorenflo C, Gorenflo D, Santer S. Effects of synthetic voice output on attitudes toward the augmented communicator. Journal of Speech and Hearing Research 1994; 37: 64–8.

Granlund M, Olsson C. Efficacy of communication intervention for presymbolic communicators. Augmentative and Alternative Communication 1989; 15: 25-37.

Granlund M, Strom E, Olsson C. Iconicity and productive recall of a selected sample of signs from Signed Swedish. Augmentative and Alternative Communication 1999; 5: 173-82.

Harris L, Skarakis-Doyle E, Haaf R. Language treatment approach for users of AAC: experimental single-subject investigation. Augmentative and Alternative Communication 1996; 12: 230-43.

Higginbotham DJ. Use of nondisabled subjects in AAC research: confessions of a research infidel. Augmentative and Alternative Communication 1995; 11: 2-5.

Hoag L, Bedrosian J. Effects of speech output type, message length, and reauditorization on perceptions of the communicative competence of an adult AAC user. Journal of Speech and Hearing Research 1992; 35: 1363-66.

Honsinger M. Midcourse intervention in multiple sclerosis: an inpatient model. Augmentative and Alternative Communication 1989; 5: 71-3.

Horstmann Koester H, Levine S. Effect of a word prediction feature on user performance. Augmentative and Alternative Communication 1996; 12: 155-68.

Hudson A, Melita B, Arnold N. Brief report: a case study assessing the validity of facilitated communication. Journal of Autism and Developmental Disorders 1993; 23: 165-73.

Hunt P, Alwell M, Goetz L. Interacting with peers through conversation turntaking with a communication book adaption. Augmentative and Alternative Communication 1991; 7: 117-26.

Iacono T, Duncum J. Use of an electronic device in a multi-modal language intervention for a child with developmental disability: a case study. Augmentative and Alternative Communication 1995; 11: 249-59.

Iacono T, Mirenda P, Beukelman D. Comparison of unimodal and multimodal AAC techniques for children with intellectual disabilities. Augmentative and Alternative Communication 1993; 9: 83-94.

Intellectual Disability Review Panel. Report to the Director-general on the Reliability and Validity of Assisted Communication. Melbourne: Department of Community Services.

Kangas K, Lloyd L. Early cognitive skills as prerequisites to augmentative and alternative communiation use: what are we waiting for? Augmentative and Alternative Communication 1988; 4: 211-21.

King J, Hux K. Intervention using talking word processing software: an aphasia case study. Augmentative and Alternative Communication 1995; 11: 187-92.

Kopchick G, Rombach D, Smilovitz R. A total communication environment in an institution. Mental Retardation 1975; 13: 22-3.

Koul R, Hanners J. Word identification and sentence verification of two synthetic speech systems by individuals with intellectual disabilities. Augmentative and Alternative Communication 1997; 13: 99-107.

Koul R, Harding R. Identification and production of graphic symbols by individuals with aphasia: efficacy of a software application. Augmentative and Alternative Communication 1998; 14: 11-23.

Kouri T. Effects of simultaneous communication in a child-directed treatment approach with preschoolers with severe disabilities. Augmentative and Alternative Communication 1988; 4: 222-32.

Kouri T. How manual sign acquisition relates to the development of spoken language: a case study. Language, Speech, and Hearing Services in Schools 1989; 20: 50-62.

Light J. Interaction involving individuals using augmentative and alternative communication systems: state of the art. Augmentative and Alternative Communication 1988; 4: 66-82.

Light J. Do augmentative and alternative communication interventions really make a difference? Augmentative and Alternative Communication 1999; 15: 13-24.

Light J, Beesley M, Collier B. Transition through multiple augmentative and alternative communication systems: a three-year case study of a head injured adolescent. Augmentative and Alternative Communication 1988; 4: 2-14.

Light J, Collier B, Parnes P. Communicative interactions between young nonspeaking physically disabled children and their primary caregives: Part 1 - Discourse patterns. Augmentative and Alternative Communication 1985; 1: 74-83.

Light J, Lindsay P, Siegel L, Parnes P. The effects of message encoding techniques on recall by literate adults using AAC. Augmentative and Alternative Communication 1990; 6: 184-201.

Light J, Dattilo J, English J, Gutierrez L, Hartz J. Instructing facilitators to support the communication of people who use augmentative communication systems. Journal of Speech and Hearing Research 1992; 35: 865-75.

Luftig R, Bersani H. An investigation of two variables influencing blissymbol learnability with nonhandicapped adults. Augmentative and Alternative Communication 1985;1: 32-37.

Malony H, Taplin J. Deinstitutionalisation of people with developmental disability. Australia and New Zealand Journal of Developmental Disabilities 1988; 14: 109-22.

McCall F, Markova I, Murphy J, Moodie E, Collins S. Perspectives on AAC systems by the users and their communication partners. European Journal of Disorders of Communication 1997; 32: 235-56.

McEwan I, Karlan G. Case studies: why and how. Augmentative and Alternative Communication 1990; 6: 69-75.

McNaughton D, Light J. Teaching facilitators to support the communication skills of an adult with severe cognitive disabilities: a case study. Augmentative and Alternative Communication 1989; 5: 35-41.

McNaughton S (Ed.). Communicating with Blissymbolics. Toronto: Blissymbolics Communication Institute, 1985.

Miller A, Miller E. Cognitive development training with elevated boards and sign language. Journal of Autism and Childhood Schizophrenia 1973; 3: 65-85.

Mirenda P. Supporting individuals with challenging behavior through functional communication training and AAC: research review. Augmentative and Alternative Communication 1997; 13: 207-25.

Mirenda P, Beukelman D. A comparison of speech synthesis intelligibility with listeners from three age groups. Augmentative and Alternative Communication 1987; 3: 120-7.

Mirenda P, Beukelman D. A comparison of intelligibility among natural speech and seven speech synthesizers with listeners from three age groups. Augmentative and Alternative Communication 1990; 6: 61-8.

Mirenda P, Dattilo J. Instructional techniques in alternative communication for students with severe intellectual handicaps. Augmentative and Alternative Communication 1987; 3: 143-52.

Mitsuda P, Baarslag-Benson R, Hazel K, Therriault T. Augmentative communication in intensive and acute care settings. In: Yorkston K (Ed.). Augmentative Communication in the Medical Setting. Tuscon, AZ: Communication Skill Builders, 1992; 5-57.

Mizuko M. Transparency and ease of learning of symbols represented by Blissymbolics, PCS, and Picsyms. Augmentative and Alternative Communication 1987; 3: 129-36.

Mizuko M, Esser J. The effect of direct selection and circular scanning on visual and sequential recall. Journal of Speech and Hearing Research 1991; 34: 43-8.

Mizuko M, Reichle J, Ratcliff A, Esser J. Effects of selection techniques and array sizes on short-term visual memory. Augmentative and Alternative Communication 1994; 10: 237-244.

Moore M. Medicare moves closer to coverage for AAC devices. ASHA 2000; 5: 15 (Leader).

Moore S, Donovan B, Hudson A. Brief report: facilitator-suggested conversational evaluation of facilitated communication. Journal of Autism and Developmental Disorders 1993; 23: 541-52.

Murphy G, Steele K, Gilligan T, Yeow J, Spare D. Teaching a picture language to a non-speaking retarded boy. Behavior Research and Therapy 1977; 15: 198-201.

Musselwhite C, St Louis KS. Communication Programming for Persons with Severe Handicaps. Boston, MA: College-Hill, 1988.

Osguthorpe R, Li-Chang L. The effects of computerized symbol processor instruction on the communication skills of nonspeaking students. Augmentative and Alternative Communication 1988; 4: 23-34.

Osguthorpe RT, Eiserman WD, Shisler L, Top BL, Scruggs TE. Students with handicaps as tutors: Learning by teaching. Counterpoint 1988; 8(3): 5-7.

Owens R, House L. Decision-making processes in augmentative communication. Journal of Speech and Hearing Disorders 1984; 49: 18-25.

Peterson K, Reichle J, Johnston S. Examining preschoolers' performance in linear and row-column scanning techniques. Augmentative and Alternative Communication 2000; 16: 27-36.

Premack D. Language in chimpanzees? Science 1971; 172: 808-22.

Purdy M, Duffy R, Coelho C. An investigation of the communicative use of trained symbols following multimodality training. Clinical Aphasiology 1994; 22: 345-56.

Raghavendra P, Allen G. Comprehension of synthetic speech with three text-to-speech systems using a sentence verification paradigm. Augmentative and Alternative Communication 1993; 9: 126-33.

Reichle J. Communication intervention with persons who have severe disabilities. Journal of Special Education 1997; 31: 110-34.

Reichle J, Karlan G. Selecting augmentative communication interventions: a critique of candidacy criteria and a proposed alternative. In: Scheifelbush R, Lloyd L (eds). Language Perspectives: Acquisition, Retardation, and Intervention (second edition). Baltimore, MD: University Park Press, 1988; 321-9.

Reynolds M, Jefferson L. Natural and synthetic speech comprehension: comparison of children from two age groups. Augmentative and Alternative Communication 1999; 15: 174-82.

Romski M, Sevcik R. Breaking the Speech Barrier: Language Development through Augmented Means. Baltimore. MD: Paul H. Brookes, 1996.

Romski M, Sevcik R, Robinson B, Bakeman R. Adult-directed communications of youth with mental retardation using the system for augmenting language. Journal of Speech and Hearing Research 1994; 37: 617-28.

Romski MA, Sevcik R. Augmentative and alternative communication systems: considerations for individuals with severe intellectual disabilities. Augmentative and Alternative Communication 1988; 4: 83-93.

Romski MA, Sevcik R, Wilkinson K. Peer-directed communicative interactions of augmented language learners with mental retardation. American Journal of Mental Retardation 1994; 98: 527-38.

Rostron A, Ward S, Plant R. Computerised augmentative communication devices for people with dysphasia: design and evaluation. European Journal of Disorders of Communication 1996; 31: 11-30.

Russell A, McAllister S. Use of AAC by individuals with acquired neurologic communication disabilities: results of an Australian survey. Augmentative and Alternative Communication 1995; 11: 138-46.

Sabin L, Donnellan A. A qualitative study of the process of facilitated communication. Journal of the Association for Persons with Severe Handicaps 1993; 18: 200-11.

Schiefelbush R (Ed.). Nonspeech Language and Communication. Baltimore, MD: University Park Press, 1980.

Schlosser R. Comparative efficacy of interventions in augmentative and alternative communication. Augmentative and Alternative Communication, 1999;15: 56-68.

Schlosser R, Braun U. Efficacy of AAC interventions: methodological issues in evaluating behavior change, generalization, and effects. Augmentative and Alternative Communication 1994; 10: 207-23.

Schlosser R, Lee D. Promoting generalization and maintenance in augmentative and alternative communication. Augmentative and Alternative Communication 2000; 16: 208-26.

Schlosser R, Lloyd L. Effects of paired-associate learning versus symbol explanations on Blissymbol comprehension and production. Augmentative and Alternative Communication 1997; 13: 226-38.

Schweigert P. Use of microswitch technology to facilitate social contingency awareness as a basis for early communication skills. Augmentative and Alternative Communication 1989; 5: 192-8.

Schweigert P, Rowland C. Early communication and mocrotechnology: instructional sequence and case studies of children with severe multiple disabilities. Augmentative and Alternative Communication 1992; 8: 273-86.

Shane H, Bashir A. Election criteria for the adoption of an augmentative communication system: preliminary considerations. Journal of Speech and Hearing Disorders 1980; 45: 408-14.

Shepherd T, Haaf R. Comparison of two training methods in the learning and generalization of Blissymbolics. Augmentative and Alternative Communication 1995; 11: 154-64.

Sigafoos J, Laurie S, Pennell D. Teaching children with Rett syndrome to request preferred objects using aided communicaiton: two preliminary studies. Augmentative and Alternative Communication 1996; 12: 88-96.

Silverman F. Communication for the Speechless. Englewood Cliffs, NJ: Prentice-Hall, 1980.

Simon E, Whitehair P, Toll D. A case study: follow-up assessment of facilitated communication. Journal of Autism and Developmental Disorders 1996; 26: 9-18.

Soto G, Belfiore P, Schlosser R, Haynes C. Teaching specific requests: a comparative analysis of skill acquisition and preference using two augmentative and alternative communication aids. Education and Training in Mental Retardation 1993; 26: 169–78.

Steele R, Weinrich M, Wertz R, Kleczewska R, Carlson G. Computer-based visual communication in aphasia. Neuropsychologia, 1989; 27: 409–26.

Stephenson J, Linfoot K. Choice-making as a natural context for teaching early communication board use to a ten year old boy with no spoken language and severe intellectual disability. Australia and New Zealand Journal of Developmental Disabilities 1995; 20: 263–86.

Stiebel D. Promoting augmentative communication during daily routines: a parent problem-solving intervention. Journal of Positive Behavior Interventions 1999; 1: 159–69.

Szeto A, Allen E, Littrell M. Comparison of speed and accuracy for selected electronic communication devices and input methods. Augmentative and Alternative Communication 1993; 9: 229–42.

Turnell R, Carter M. Establishing a repertoire of requesting for a student with severe and multiple disabilities using tangible symbols and naturalistic time delay. Australia and New Zealand Journal of Developmental Disabilities 1994; 19: 193–207.

Udwin O, Yule W. Augmentative communication systems taught to cerebral palsied children – a longitudinal study. II. Pragmatic features of sign and symbol use. European Journal of Disorders of Communication 1991; 26: 149–62.

von Tetzchner S, Hygum Jensen M (eds). Augmentative and Alternative Communication: European Perspectives. London: Whurr Publishers, 1996.

Waller A, Dennis F, Brodie J, Cairns A. Evaluating the use of TalksBac, a predictive communication device for nonfluent adults with aphasia. International Journal of Language and Communication Disorders 1998; 33: 45–70.

Watkins T, Sprafkin J, Krolikowski D. Using videotaped lessons to facilitate the development of manual sign skills in students with mental retardation. Augmentative and Alternative Communication 1993; 9: 177–83.

Wilkinson K, Romski MA. Responsiveness of male adolescents with mental retardation to input from nondisabled peers: the summoning power of comments, questions, and directive prompts. Journal of Speech and Hearing Research 1994; 38: 1045–53.

World Health Organization. International Classification of Functioning, Disability and Health – ICF. Albany, NY: World Health Organization, 2000.

Yoder D. Editorial. Augmentative and Alternative Communication 1985; 1: 1.

Yorkston K. Early intervention in amyotrophic lateral sclerosis: a case presentation. Augmentative and Alternative Communication 1989; 5: 67–70.

Young L, Sigafoos J, Suttie J, Ashman A, Grevell P. Deinstitutionalisation of persons with intellectual disability: a review of Australian studies. Journal of Intellectual and Developmental Disability 1998; 23: 155–70.

Zangari C, Kangas K, Lloyd L. Augmentative and alternative communication: a field in transition. Augmentative and Alternative Communication 1988; 4: 60–5.

Zangari C, Lloyd L, Vicker B. Augmentative and Alternative Communication: an historical perspective. Augmentative and Alternative Communication 1994; 10: 27–59.

Part Three
Examining Practice and
Future Directions

CHAPTER 13

Translating evidence into practice

MIRANDA ROSE AND STACEY BALDAC

Introduction

This chapter describes essential characteristics necessary for speech pathologists to become evidence-based practitioners, and suggests ways in which professional preparation and continuing education programmes can prepare their participants for such practice. The challenges of, and barriers to, the successful implementation of evidence-based practice are discussed and suggestions made to overcome them.

What are the necessary skills and essential steps for evidence-based practice?

Little has been written about the skills and steps necessary for speech pathologists to implement evidence-based practice. Sackett et al. (1997), writing from a medical perspective, suggested four essential requirements for evidence-based practitioners:

1 Mastery of the clinical skills of patient interviewing, history-taking and physical examination in order to generate diagnostic hypotheses (the beginning) and integrate valid, important evidence with patients' values and expectations (the end).
2 The practice of continuous, life-long, self-directed learning.
3 Humility, without which we become immune both to self-improvement and to advances.
4 Enthusiasm and irreverence.

Practitioners then must form a clinical question so that it may be answered, must search for the best external evidence, must critically

317

appraise the evidence for its validity and importance, must apply it in practice and must evaluate their performance as evidence-based practitioners.

Why is evidence-based practice not implemented routinely by speech pathologists?

Most speech pathology university programmes would assert that they equip their graduates with the necessary skills and experience to enable them to be evidence-based practitioners. It is our contention, albeit gleaned from extensive interaction with practitioners rather than from detailed investigative study that, once practising, speech pathologists fluctuate in their commitment to and implementation of evidence-based practice. Several factors that potentially contribute to this situation in speech pathology have been identified:

- Knowledge–practice gap.
- Tradition of trial-and-error problem-solving.
- Characteristics of the discipline.
- Nature of speech pathology 'problems'.
- Types of evidence.
- Threats to professional autonomy and the need for marketing.

We have also looked to other allied health professions for data from which we may infer.

Knowledge–practice gap

There is a growing gap between research-based (propositional) knowledge, taught in professional schools, and the practical knowledge and skill-based competencies required of practitioners in the field. Schon (1987) suggested that this gap is a result of the knowledge explosion, the rapid change in the nature and demands of the contexts in which professionals are acting, and the uncertainty of the professional workplace. Professional training courses frequently respond to the pressure of including large amounts of new theory and factual information into already over-full curricula by reducing practical and skill-based activities. In contrast, new graduates are confronted by a rapidly changing workplace where high levels of skill are required on entry, and the time and opportunity for reflection, supervision and client contact-free activity is minimal. Such a dichotomy may induce practitioners to act from habit and past knowledge rather than to research, reflect and update practice.

Tradition of trial-and-error problem-solving

The strong tradition of trial-and-error practice in speech pathology contributes to poor implementation of evidence-based practice behaviours after graduation. Early practitioners needed to innovate and experiment with what worked best for the individual client at hand, as there was little research evidence on which to base practice. Consequently, a culture of self-reliance was established, whereby clinicians had to reason from fundamental principles and apply logic to clinical problem-solving. Such 'experimentation' leads to the development and valuing of professional craft knowledge (Higgs and Titchen, 2000). This knowledge was handed down to practitioners through workplace practice with an associated respect for intuition and artistry. Speech pathologists valued skilled practitioners in the 'apprenticeship' model and looked to such experts as a source of knowledge, perhaps as much as to textbooks or research journals.

Characteristics of the discipline

The concept of learning style may have application in this situation. Learning styles are conceptualized as the preference or habitual strategy used by individuals to process information for problem-solving (Katz and Heimann, 1991). It has been suggested that particular professions have a tendency towards particular styles of learning. The learning styles of speech pathologists focus on people and doing (accommodation, divergence) rather than on theory and abstraction (assimilation, convergence) (McLeod et al., 1995). Perhaps these preferences predispose speech pathologists to revert to comfortable behaviours on graduation, relying on expert peers and trial-and-error approaches to problem solving, rather than on more abstract sources of knowledge, such as journals, texts and information technology.

Nature of speech pathology 'problems'

A potential barrier to evidence-based practice in speech pathology includes the nature of the clinical problems the profession works with and the research strategies required to investigate them adequately. Communication skills are cognitively, physically and socially complex, and highly individual, and hence their breakdown and remediation are equally variable. The gold standard for speech pathology research may not be the randomly assigned control trial, so useful in medicine and promoted as the ideal evidence in evidence-based practice (Robey and Schultz, 1998) (see Chapter 2). Research in speech pathology does not only focus on large group design studies but also on multiple single-case experimental designs and qualitative research methodologies, which attempt to take into account the huge variance existing in communication systems. Therefore, speech pathologists are unlikely to be able to consult a single source, such as a meta-analysis study, in order to gain accurate and recent empirical evidence about a problem. Further, evidence is likely to be published across wide fields of inquiry; for example, linguistics, psychology, education, medicine, rehabilitation, sociology and semiotics. Such a wide distribution of information may discourage practitioners from initiating a search.

Types of evidence

Speech pathologists need to acknowledge that differing professions value differing types of evidence (Wilby and Elwyn, 1999). The scientific approach, sometimes equated with epidemiology and biostatistics, is just one approach to patient care. Speech pathologists must take into account patient perspectives, and the emotional realities in diagnosis and treatment decision-making. This suggests the need for a more eclectic and less reductionist approach to evidence-based practice (Smith and Taylor, 1996; Colyer and Kamath 1999). Speech pathologists may reject the perceived narrow, black and white constructs associated with current models of evidence-based practice.

Threats to professional autonomy and the need for marketing

Evidence-based practice has been criticized for medicalizing health care (Clarke, 1999; French, 1999), for focusing on quantitative measures (French, 1999) and for threatening professional autonomy (Dubouloz et al., 1999). Like Monaghan (1999), writing in dentistry, speech pathologists may perceive that adopting evidence-based practice guidelines will lead to a loss of professional autonomy and to greater control by service administrators, thereby dictating the nature and frequency of service delivery. This is not necessarily the case. The proponents of evidence-based practice emphasize the need for individual practitioners to use the best available evidence in the context of individual clients' needs. Speech pathologists, like the allied health practitioners in the study by Wilby and Elwyn (1999), may require convincing of this. Furthermore, in the face of no available, high-quality evidence, practice must still continue and the practitioners in the study by Wilby and Elwyn (1999) reported heightened anxiety in such circumstances. As Wilby and Elywn (1999) stated, it would be a shame if good practice, based on sound clinical reasoning, problem-solving and repeated experience, is lost owing to lowered morale, fear and a reluctance to intervene without good evidence. Clearly, there is a need for open and frank discussion of the perceived threats and limitations of evidence-based practice in speech pathology.

Equally, there is a need to market evidence-based practice. Monaghan (1999) suggested evidence-based practice should be renamed 'patient-centred practice' and French (1999) recommended that it should be seen as consistent with the philosophy of continuous quality improvement.

The following discussion of factors that potentially limit speech pathologists' uptake of evidence-based practice is speculative and based on inference from the limited evidence in allied fields.

What is required for successful implementation of evidence-based practice?

Kitson et al. (1998) suggested that for the successful implementation of evidence-based practice, practitioners not only require excellent evidence but also a context ready for such practice and a method to facilitate the changed practice. Table 13.1 presents a framework developed by the Royal College of Nursing Institute in London, which illustrates the complex factors in play.

Table 13.1 Conditions for evidence, context and facilitation*

Evidence		
Research	Low High	
	Anecdotal evidence	Randomized controlled trials
	Descriptive information	Systematic reviews
		Evidence-based guidelines
Clinical experience	Low High	
	Expert opinion divided	High levels of consensus
	Several 'camps'	Consistency of view
Patient preferences	Low High	
	Patients not involved	Partnerships
Context		
Culture	Low High	
	Task-driven	Learning organization
	Low regard for individuals	Patient-centred
	Low morale	Valuing people
	Little or no continuing education	Continuing education

(contd)

Table 13.1 (contd)

Leadership	Low — High	
	Diffuse role	Clear roles
Lack of team roles		Effective team work
	Poor organization or management of services	Effective organizational structure
	Poor leadership	Clear leadership
Measurement	Low — High	
	Absence of: audit and feedback; peer review; external audit; performance review of junior staff	Internal measures used routinely
		Audit or feedback used routinely
		Peer review
		External measures
Facilitation		
Characteristics	Low — High	
	Respect	Respect
	Empathy	Empathy
	Authenticity	Authenticity
	Credibility	Credibility
Role	Low — High	
	Lack of clarity around: access; authority; position in organization successfully negotiated; change agenda	Access
		Authority
		Change agenda
Style	Low — High	
	Inflexible	Range and flexibility of style
	Sporadic	
	Infrequent	Consistent and appropriate
	Inappropriate	presence and support

(*Kitson et al., 1998, p. 151.)

Successful implementation is conceptualized as a function of the relation between the nature of the evidence, the context in which a proposed change is to be implemented and the mechanism by which a change is facilitated. According to this framework, rather than perceiving these dimensions in a hierarchy or linearity of cause and effect, each of the dimensions must be considered simultaneously. Kitson et al. (1998) asserted that if implementation is to be successful, as much attention to detail as was given to preparation of the evidence must be paid to preparing the context and selecting the implementation method. The model suggests that the more that evidence, context and facilitation dimensions are located towards the 'high' end of each continuum, the more likely that evidence will be implemented successfully.

The effectiveness of the framework in predicting successful implementation of evidence-based practice was trialled by Kitson et al. (1998) in four situations where the evidence was rated at the high end of each continuum, but the context and facilitation dimensions varied. When evidence was high but the context was rated low, successful implementation was predicted by high facilitation parameters. The utility of the model is yet to be fully researched but it offers a window into the complexity of implementation.

Other current authors have identified factors that contribute to the successful implementation of evidence-based practice. Three parameters identified are:

- Nature of the evidence.
- Context in which it is to be implemented.
- Facilitation method used.

These recommendations are summarized under the framework of Kitson et al. (1998) as follows.

Nature of the evidence

Evidence needs to be:

- Presented in an accessible and friendly medium (Law and Baum, 1998).
- Presented by trusted information sources (Law and Baum, 1998).
- Easy to read (Law and Baum, 1998).
- Supported with professional position papers (Dobson, 1998).
- Presented in the context of current practice issues (Law and Baum, 1998).

In addition, valued sources of evidence need to be acknowledged (Dubouloz et al., 1999).

Context of implementation

The context in which evidence-based practice is to be implemented needs to include:

- Commitment of the organization to provide ongoing support (Law and Baum, 1998; Wilby and Elwyn, 1999).
- The involvement of all stakeholders (French, 1999).
- A process of promoting research to implementation (French, 1999).

Facilitation method

The facilitation method used needs to:

- Use opinion leaders and peer feedback (Law and Baum, 1998).
- Develop relationships between researchers, service-providers, funding bodies and consumers (Law and Baum, 1998).

Helping graduate speech pathologists to become evidence-based practitioners

Law and Baum (1998) highlighted that, in order to transfer the concepts of evidence-based practice into practice, an analysis of potential barriers needs to be undertaken so that implementation procedures may be customized for individuals and organizations. These authors suggested evaluating barriers at an individual and system level. Here, by use of Law and Baum's (1998) framework, barriers have been reframed into statements and suggestions provided to encourage successful implementation.

Barriers at an individual level

Barrier

Limited time to search for evidence.

Suggestions

- Develop a speech pathology-specific research database.
- Make search results available to the profession electronically and in written format through national level speech pathology professional bodies to reduce duplication.
- Use search assistants, for example librarians or allied health assistants.

Barrier

Limited skills in searching for and interpreting research information.

Suggestions

- Incorporate skill development activities into continuing education

programmes, special interest groups and departmental activities.
- Use self-learning or distance education packages, for example *Evidence-based Health Care: An Open Learning Resource for Health Care Practitioners* (CASP/HCLU, 1999).
- Use skilled individuals within the organization.

Barrier

Lack of ability and comfort in implementing research findings.

Suggestions

- Use colleagues as professional mentors or supervisors.
- Discuss successes and failures of implementation with colleagues.

Barriers at a system level

Barrier

Lack of support from administration.

Suggestions

- Develop human resource policies to support evidence-based practice, for example in job descriptions highlight the expectation that evidence-based practice principles are to be used in client management.
- Fund and plan for resources to access evidence, for example information technology.
- Fund staff development programmes.
- Focus on quality of care not just quantity of clients.

Barrier

Limited access to research studies.

Suggestions

- Provide membership to libraries.
- Provide computer access to facilitate searches.
- Provide subscriptions to journals.
- Attend speech pathology and other professions' journal club meetings.
- Support attendance at conferences.

Barrier

No time allocated to search for and implement evidence.

Suggestions

- For the purposes of statistics-based funding, the time taken to search and implement evidence should be able to be credited as direct client care time.
- Job descriptions should specify that time is to be allocated to performing searches to improve the quality of care to clients.
- Departmental heads or supervisors need to monitor and encourage employees to allocate time to search for information.

Other barriers

In addition, individual bias and skills in interpretation and implementation of research information has been reported as a potential threat to evidence-based practice (DiFabio, 1999; Monaghan, 1999). The way in which the research evidence is presented or framed has been reported to influence readers' interpretation of the information (Clarke, 1999; Monaghan, 1999). To deal with these potential shortcomings DiFabio (1999) suggested that information from research studies needs to be balanced with other forms of evidence, such as clinical experience and expertise. In addition, DiFabio (1999) highlighted the need to recognize that different interpretations exist and differences should be embraced to facilitate the development of less biased interpretations.

Preparing undergraduates to become evidence-based practitioners

There is a need to prepare future professionals to be good consumers of research (Olson, 1996). This requires the ability to question accepted practices (Rambur, 1999) and to have the required skills to evaluate research information (Olson, 1996). Fostering such skills at undergraduate level requires re-evaluating the student–teacher dyad (Rambur, 1999), developing assessment techniques to evaluate the application of evidence-based practice (Bradley and Humphris, 1999), supporting evidence-based practice in clinical practice and addressing the barriers to teaching evidence-based practice (Olson, 1996).

Rambur (1999) highlighted that traditional teaching modalities do not foster the critical evaluation skills required to promote evidence-based practice. Rambur (1999) indicated that learning pre-arranged informational facts undermines the ability to discard outdated information. In addition, with the increasing quantity of research information, conflicting viewpoints may result in ambiguity. Rambur (1999) suggested the need for a curriculum revolution to support evidence-based practice. The student–teacher dyad needs to be reconceptualized from recipient and provider to 'student–teacher partnerships'. Rambur (1999) described a course for nursing students aimed at teaching them to be seekers of information. In so doing, they learn, in a supported environment, that contradictory information and lack of empirical research is a problem. This exposes students to real-life issues that face practitioners and highlights that accepted practices can be challenged. Olson (1996) described a course to facilitate evidence-based practice by focusing on teaching students skills in locating and evaluating different forms of research evidence. In a structured environment students are required to investigate a specific problem about which they have been exposed to divergent opinions. Students learn how to evaluate information critically and to develop an appreciation of how presentation of information may affect opinions. Therefore, the challenge for educators is to develop a curriculum that promotes a questioning culture and to teach the required skills to be able to discriminate between the types of evidence presented.

The curricula developed between need to be consistent with evidence-based practice processes and to have appropriate assessment techniques. Law and Baum (1998) suggested use of a problem-based format to facilitate evidence-based practice. Problem-based curricula have been reported to facilitate a deep approach to learning and to prepare students to become life-long learners (David and Harden, 1999). Norman and Schmidt (1992), in their review of the evidence on problem-based learning from a psychological perspective, concluded that a problem-based format may increase retention of knowledge, enhance transfer and integration of concepts into clinical practice and enhance self-directed learning skills.

Olson (1996) identified potential barriers to teaching evidence-based practice. These included non-compliance of staff owing to scepticism and personal preferences, perceived threats associated with the use of a different teaching modality, frustration that can result from a lack of evidence to support and answer questions, and additional time and energy that may be required in preparation activities. In order to overcome such barriers, staff leaders and managers may need to pay particular attention to the context parameters discussed by Kitson et al. (1998).

Conclusions: the way forward

In this chapter it has been argued that, although speech pathologists may agree with the rationale behind the use of evidence-based practice and have many of the skills and attributes required of the evidence-based practitioner, many fail to implement such practice consistently. Such low implementation may reflect the knowledge–practice gap, a tradition of trial-and-error problem-solving behaviour, specific discipline characteristics, the complexity of speech pathology problems, the types of evidence speech pathologists value and perceived threats to professional autonomy. Successful implementation of evidence-based practice in speech pathology requires attention to education principles and methods in undergraduate programmes, as well as to the context and facilitation processes for clinicians in the workplace. Furthermore, the complex nature of speech pathology problems requires a broad frame of reference when defining what constitutes gold standard evidence. Lastly, a lack of empirical evidence about speech pathologists' understanding of, reactions to and implementation of evidence-based practice was identified. Future empirical study into the perceptions, attitudes and practices of speech pathologists was encouraged with respect to the understanding and implementation of evidence-based practice. Such study is a necessary starting point to enable better uptake of evidence-based principles and practices in speech pathology.

References

Bradley P, Humphris G. Assessing the ability of medical students to apply evidence in practice: the potential of the OSCE. Medical Education 1999; 33: 815-17.

Critical Appraisal Skills Programme and the Health Care Libraries Unit (CASP/HCLU). Evidence-Based Health Care: An Open Learning Resource for Health Care Practitioners. Oxford: Update Software, 1999.

Clarke JB. Evidence-based practice: a retrograde step? The importance of pluralism in evidence generation for the practice of health care. Journal of Clinical Nursing 1999; 8: 89-94.

Colyer H, Kamath P. Evidence-based practice. Journal of Advanced Nursing 1999; 29: 188-93.

David M, Harden R. AMEE medical education guide 15: Problem-based learning. A practical guide. Medical Teacher 1999; 21: 130-40.

DiFabio RP. Myths of evidence-based practice. Journal of Orthopedic and Sports Physical Therapy 1999; 29: 632-4.

Dobson AM. Moving towards evidence-based practice. Journal of Human Nutrition and Dietitics 1998; 11: 189.

Dubouloz C, Egan M, Vallerand J, Zweck C. Occupational therapists' perceptions of evidence-based practice. American Journal of Occupational Therapy 1999; 53: 445-53.

French P. The development of evidence-based nursing. Journal of Advanced Nursing 1999; 29: 72-8.

Higgs J, Titchen A. Knowledge and reasoning. In: Higgs J, Jones M (eds). Clinical Reasoning in the Health Professions (second edition). Oxford: Butterworth-Heinemann, 2000.

Katz N, Heimann N. Learning styles of students and practitioners in five health professions. Occupational Therapy Journal of Research 1991; 11: 238-45.

Kitson A, Harvey G, McCormack B. Enabling the implementation of evidence-based practice: a conceptual framework. Quality in Health Care 1998; 7: 149-58.

Law M, Baum C. Evidence-based occupational therapy. Canadian Journal of Occupational Therapy 1998; 65: 131–5.

McLeod S, Lincoln M, McAllister L, Maloney D, Purcell A, Eadie P. A longitudinal investigation of the learning styles of speech pathology students. Australian Journal of Human Communication Disorders 1995; 23: 13–25.

Monaghan N. Human nature and clinical freedom, barriers to evidence-based practice? British Dental Journal 1999; 186: 208–9.

Norman GR, Schmidt H.G. The psychological basis of problem-based learning: a review of the evidence. Academic Medicine 1992 Sept; 67(9): 557–65.

Olson E. Evidence-based practice: a new approach to teaching integration of esearch and practice in gerontology. Educational Gerontology 1996; 22: 523–37.

Rambur B. Fostering evidence-based practice in nursing education. Journal of Professional Nursing 1999; 15: 270–4.

Robey R, Schultz M. A model for conducting clinical outcome research: an adaptation of the standard protocol for use in aphasiology. Aphasiology 1998; 12: 787–810.

Sackett D, Scott Richardson W, Rosenberg W, Hynes R. Evidence-based Medicine. How to Practise and Teach EBM. New York, NY: Churchill Livingstone, 1997.

Schon D. Educating the Reflective Practitioner. San Francisco, CA: Jossey-Bass, 1987.

Smith B, Taylor R. Medicine – a healing or a dying art? British Journal of General Practice 1996; 46: 249–51.

Wilby P, Elwyn G. The evidence-based workshop experience: a 10 month follow-up study. Journal of Interprofessional Care 1999; 1: 190–1.

CHAPTER 14

Evidence-based practice in speech pathology – future directions

SHEENA REILLY, JENNI OATES AND JACINTA DOUGLAS

> Education is not completed at the medical school: it is only begun.
> William Welch

Evidence-based practice and speech pathology: the way forward

Historically, many aspects of health care (including speech pathology) have been founded on tradition, assumption and precedence. However, in the last two decades, health care has moved towards a culture whereby it is expected that every level of clinical service will be informed by scientifically derived findings (*see* www.rch.unimelb.edu.au/outcomes/EBPnurse.htm). In this chapter we pose and attempt to answer four important questions:

- What evidence exists in speech pathology?
- Where does the speech pathology profession stand in relation to evidence-based practice?
- What are the aims of the speech pathology profession in relation to evidence-based practice?
- How is the speech pathology profession going to achieve these aims?

What evidence exists in speech pathology?

Part 2 of this book (Chapters 3–12) highlighted that speech pathology is a diverse profession made up of numerous subspecialities, only some of which are addressed here. When reviewing the evidence for each subspeciality, methodological shortcomings that threaten the validity of the available evidence were identified. For example, in Chapter 3, we learned that of all the group clinical outcome studies of aphasia treatment, 46% provided inadequate quantitative information and only 19% of published single-subject design studies presented quantifiable outcomes. These findings indicate that such methodological shortcomings need to be addressed if the quality, level and types of evidence in speech pathology are to improve.

After reviewing Chapters 3–12, and following discussion with colleagues in the profession, we have generated a list of methodological priorities (see Box 14.1 below) as well as two priority areas requiring further research in subspeciality areas (see Table 14.1). The methodological priorities outlined below demand careful consideration in the design of future studies in speech pathology, whether they address questions about intervention, prognosis, diagnosis or whether they form an economic evaluation.

Box 14.1 Methodological priorities

- Ensure research designs are grounded in the principles of epidemiology
- Include adequate controls and/or comparisons in intervention trials
- Ensure unbiased allocation of clients to the conditions compared in controlled intervention
- Ensure adequate baseline evaluation in single-case intervention trials
- Ensure adequate (replicable) specification of the assessment and treatment procedures under investigation
- Identify and evaluate outcomes that are relevant to people with communication disorders, and their families, and that extend beyond changes in impairment levels
- Systematically evaluate outcomes over short and long periods of time after discharge
- Employ complementary quantitative and qualitative methodologies
- Ensure adequate subject numbers are included to detect treatment effects
- Report exact statistics in results to enable application of meta-analytic statistical procedures
- Systematically replicate positive results
- Develop systematic research programmes to identify how much of which interventions, in what delivery format, optimize outcomes in a given type of patient with a communication disorder

---

Methodological shortcomings in speech pathology

For some time now researchers and clinicians have been undertaking intervention studies in some subspecialities (for example, verbal dyspraxia) with limited understanding of the natural history and progression of the disorder. In some conditions there is a distinct lack of agreement about what

Table 14.1 EBP priorities in speech pathology

Subspecialty	Identified research priorities	
Aphasia after stroke	Establish systematic research programmes evaluating: (i) type, duration and intensity of intervention, and (ii) short- and long-term effects of intervention	Identify and evaluate outcomes that are relevant to people with aphasia and their families
Cognitive communicative disorders	Develop reliable outcome measures that reflect meaningful changes in performance of everyday activities in the community	Evaluate different interventions by use of well-designed and controlled group trials and single-case studies
Stuttering	Intervention trials with adequate control/comparisons	Elucidation of the aetiological pathways leading to stuttering
Voice disorders	Conduct well-designed intervention studies comparing different treatment methods with adequate controls/comparisons	Increase the range of conditions/disorders studied
Dysphagia	Establish the validity and reliability of tools used for screening and diagnosis	Conduct well-designed outcome studies where longer term, clearly defined and measurable outcomes are included
Child language disorder	Epidemiological study of the natural history of developmental language disorders	Elucidation of the exact nature of processing deficits of children with developmental language disorders
'Late talkers'	Epidemiological study of the natural history of developmental language disorders	Conduct well-designed intervention trials with adequate control/comparisons
Motor speech disorders in children	Define the clinical phenotype(s)	Epidemiological study of the natural history of speech disorders in children

Table 14.1 (contd)

Subspecialty	Identified research priorities	
Phonological and articulation disorders	Establish the validity and reliability of measurement tools	Conduct well-designed intervention trials with adequate control/comparisons
Augmentative and alternative communication (AAC)	Effectiveness of AAC in naturalistic settings	Efficacy of AAC for people with acquired disorders

constitutes the condition (for example, the clinical or behavioural phenotype) and therefore no agreed clinical diagnostic entity (for example, paediatric motor speech disorders). As a result, poorly developed causal models have hampered the development of research hypotheses. Some populations commonly seen in speech pathology (for example, Rett syndrome, amyloidosis of the larynx, sulcus vocalis) are low prevalence, rare conditions where it will never be possible to conduct studies such as randomized controlled trials. However, it is possible to conduct good intervention studies (by use of non-randomized trials, single-case or multiple-baseline study designs) that include adequate controls or control periods, thereby addressing what, to date, have been methodological shortcomings in speech pathology research.

It is not necessary to convince speech pathologists that communication and/or swallowing disorders affect both individuals and their families and result in a significant burden. The measurement of outcomes has moved significantly in the last 5-10 years and tools have been, or are being, developed that have established validity and reliability, and measure outcomes across multiple domains. However, the tools still require further development and remain focused on the individual. In many speech pathology subspecialities, the burden on the carers is enormous and intervention often involves not just the patient with a communication and/or swallowing disorder, but the family as well. Few attempts have been made to measure these aspects of intervention.

It is the experience of many speech pathologists that tension between quantitative and qualitative methodologies arises most often because of misunderstanding and ignorance. To argue about the relative values of one or the other is to miss the point and detracts from a more important issue: that of choosing the correct design to answer the question posed. Those researchers who understand both quantitative and qualitative methodologies, and utilize them effectively, recognize that they are complementary (Giacomini and Cook, 2000). The choice of methodology is predicted entirely by the research question posed.

Readers should keep in mind that as well as focused questions about evidence in subspecialities there are other broader issues, about which very little is known, that may well affect the validity of the evidence. For example, in much of the research appraised here, only short-term outcomes have been studied. Few studies have included long-term outcomes following treatment. Little is known about how we should best deliver treatment. Are groups effective and if so, for whom? What dose is most effective or how many treatment sessions are required in order to reach the desired outcome? Is intensive treatment always better? Other important questions about the delivery of treatment include: For individuals with multiple problems, what is the best intervention approach? Should all techniques be applied at once (referred to as the 'shotgun' approach) or should a stepped or hierarchical approach be adopted in therapy?

Many of the methodological shortcomings identified above are not limited to speech pathology; they are problems common to many other areas of medical, allied health and nursing research. The shortcomings help to explain, in part, why variable levels of evidence exist across some of the subspecialities in speech pathology. However, there has been a pitiful amount of research undertaken in some subspecialities, where it is an issue of quantity rather than quality.

Some good advice was given to an audience at an evidence-based practice workshop recently: 'Only read research that has used the right design to answer the question.' If a focused hypothesis has been developed, the research design has been carefully chosen (regardless of whether it is a qualitative or quantitative methodology, a randomized controlled trial or a multiple-baseline single-subject design) and the outcomes clearly defined, speech pathology can benefit from the good quality evidence. Much current speech pathology practice is underpinned by evidence, although the quality and strength of the evidence varies amongst subspecialities.

Where does the speech pathology profession stand in relation to evidence-based practice?

Throughout this book (see in particular Chapters 1, 2 and 13) the barriers that speech pathologists face in becoming evidence-based practitioners have been proposed and discussed. Although some barriers were common to medical, allied health and nursing professions, others were discipline specific (for example, 'Tradition of trial and error problem-solving' and 'Characteristics of the discipline', Chapter 13).

Chapter 1 argued strongly for practice to be evidence-based; however, is there any evidence to date that evidence-based practice has had any impact on clinical practice, the education of speech pathologists and/or research direction in speech pathology? Until recently, there was almost no literature on the use of evidence-based practice in speech pathology. It was impossible, therefore, to know what effect, if any, evidence-based practice has had on the clinical practice and education of speech pathologists. Although there was increasing information about the barriers that existed that prevented the professions of medicine and nursing from embracing the principles of evidence-based practice, no such information was available in speech pathology.

Speech pathologists' awareness of, attitudes to and barriers regarding evidence-based practice

Two recent surveys conducted in the UK and Australia (Metcalfe et al., 2001; Brener et al., 2003) report some interesting findings. Brener et al. (2003) conducted a pilot study of 53 speech pathologists attending a masterclass in paediatric dysphagia, with regard to their knowledge of evidence-based practice. (In an ongoing study the same team in partnership with Speech Pathology Association Australia (SPAA), has surveyed Victorian Branch members about their views on evidence-based practice.) Brener et al. (2002) reported some good news: the majority of speech pathologists surveyed had heard of evidence-based practice (81%) and just under half (46%) said they used or tried to apply evidence-based practice to their practice but reported that there were barriers to its implementation (such as those as highlighted in Chapter 13).

Metcalfe et al. (2001) explored potential barriers to implementing the evidence base in the professions of dietetics, occupational therapy, physiotherapy and speech pathology. Both studies confirmed that many of the barriers highlighted in Chapter 13 exist in speech pathology. There were a number of similarities between the UK (Metcalfe et al., 2001) and Australian (Brener et al., 2003) samples. Both studies cited the lack of time available as a main barrier. Guyatt and Rennie (2002) highlighted that after more than a decade with evidence-based practice, one of the biggest challenges, the limited time available, has not changed. However, Guyatt and Rennie (2002) discussed the fact that innovative changes are rapidly taking place and many new resources are emerging that will hopefully assist clinicians to overcome this barrier.

In addition to the time barrier, 57% of UK clinicians and 52% of Australian clinicians stated that inadequate facilities (for example, access to desktop computers) were a barrier. Many of the Australian speech pathology clinicians who had access to a computerized database for literature searching (for example, MEDLINE, CINAHL) stated that they did not access it regularly (50% reported accessing this technology on a monthly basis).

The two surveys (Metcalfe et al., 2001; Brener et al., 2002) also examined attitudes to research. The majority of respondents (97% of the UK sample; 75% of the Australian sample) believed that research findings were of importance in the development of professional practice. Interestingly, 98% of the speech pathologists surveyed rated the importance of research highly, and speech pathologists as a group rated the importance of research significantly higher than did their colleagues in occupational therapy and physiotherapy (Metcalfe et al., 2001). These findings indicated that speech pathologists know about evidence-based practice and they think it is important. Few reported that they had no interest in research findings (just 5% of the UK sample said they were not interested in reading research findings). However, many clinicians indicated that conducting research was not a high priority (56%) and that treating patients was more important than research (45.5%) or reading about research (33%) (Metcalfe et al., 2001).

A number of barriers to the implementation of evidence-based practice were documented by both Brener et al. (2003) and Metcalfe et al. (2001). Many speech pathologists said that research findings had little impact on their clinical practice (about one-third in the study by Brener et al., 2003). The barriers (explored in Chapter 13) are clearly important factors that might explain the disparity between believing that research was important but stating that it had little effect on clinical practice. Metcalfe et al. (2001) uncovered some interesting findings in relation to speech pathologists' reading of and interpretation of the literature and in the quality of the evidence found, which might offer further explanation. About 78% of respondents said they had difficulty understanding the statistics reported and about 66% said the implications for practice were not made clear. A common comment was that the literature was dispersed over a wide number of journals and could not be found in one or two places. The existing evidence was often conflicting, suffered from methodological problems and could not be generalized (Metcalfe et al., 2001).

The studies discussed and described above provide essential information and give direction for the changes needed to become an evidence-based profession. However, this can only be achieved if the barriers and problems are tackled by use of a co-ordinated strategy involving clinical practice, education and research. Change will be a fundamental part of the process.

What are the aims of the speech pathology profession in relation to evidence-based practice?

The speech pathology profession should aim to become an evidence-based profession in which clinical services are informed by scientifically derived findings. In order to achieve this, a coordinated effort to change is required and this will involve professional associations, universities and employers as well as individual clinicians and practitioners. All have critical responsibilities and roles to play. Although each will be discussed in turn, the divisions are somewhat artificial, as many of the changes require an integrated effort on the part of professional bodies, university staff, clinical managers and clinicians (*see* Table 14.3).

Professional bodies

Professional bodies, such as the Speech Pathology Association of Australia (SPAA) and the Royal College of Speech and Language Therapists (RCSLT), state that the establishment and monitoring of professional standards (competence and high standards of clinical practice and ethics) is a key component of their work. The RCSLT, SPAA and the American Speech, Language and Hearing Association (ASHA) have made statements about the need for speech pathologists to keep abreast of current evidence, and to maintain the provision of high-quality services for patients. In the UK, in 1994, the College of Occupational Therapists (COT), the Chartered Society of Physiotherapy (CSP) and the RCSLT issued a position statement that contained recommendations concerning priorities for the future development of research amongst the three professions. These included:

- greater involvement in research and development committees and groups
- management support to recognize and value the contribution of researchers
- education and training
- career infrastructure
- greater understanding of research methodologies relevant to therapy research
- involvement in dissemination and implementation initiatives.

Although the recommendations were research priorities, they are pertinent to the development of a culture in which evidence-based practice is the norm.

The websites of the RCSLT, SPAA and ASHA were reviewed with regard to evidence-based practice initiatives and it was disappointing to find few resources listed. The RCSLT website had a two-page section entitled 'Clinical Effectiveness: Getting the Evidence into Practice' (www.rcslt.org/ effective.shtml). The ASHA website (www.asha.org) had some excellent resources available relating to clinical trials as well as reference lists concerning efficacy in subspecialities. (These may be found in the special interest section.) The ASHA website also offered the ASHA online literature review, to which individuals may subscribe. Similar services are available from many different sources; for example, subscribers may have the contents pages from favourite journals delivered to them by email on a regular basis so they do not even have to search new issues. If the library subscribes to an online version, readers can download that article and print it: instant evidence delivered to your clinical workstation. On the SPAA website (www.speechpathologyaustralia.org.au) no references to evidence-based practice were found. It was disappointing that the websites did not contain statements about evidence-based practice, nor was there any evidence that the principles of evidence-based practice had been incorporated into the coursework or structure of continuing professional education events (more about this later).

Establishing guidelines

Mead (1998) emphasized that when aiming to support the delivery of effective clinical services, professional bodies must ensure that national standards are met. Mead (1998) discussed the need for nationally developed clinical guidelines that are based on the very best available evidence. In the UK the development of clinical guidelines is the responsibility of the appropriate professional body because they contribute to the role of setting and maintaining clinical standards.

What are clinical guidelines? Clinical guidelines are 'systematically developed statements which assist clinicians and patients in making decisions about appropriate treatment for specific conditions' (NHS Executive, 1996). Guidelines may be developed at the national or local level and may differ according to the country in which they are devised, the region, type of hospital or clinic.

Evidence-based guidelines rely on a critical and systematic appraisal of best evidence following extensive consultation on a variety of levels. The consultation process includes the following stages.

- Consultation occurs with a group of experts and decision-makers who may have been involved in the critical appraisal (although some would argue that this should be conducted independently).
- Front-line clinicians are consulted and asked to review the guidelines for applicability and practicability.
- User groups (patients and self-help groups) are involved in careful appraisal of the guidelines and asked to comment on the guidelines' implications and acceptability.

The first two consultation stages above should also involve representation from multidisciplinary groups, as speech pathology interventions often affect other health professionals. For example, the *Post-Stroke Rehabilitation*

Clinical Practice Guideline (Gresham et al., 1995; produced by the Agency for Health Care Policy and Research in the USA) was developed with input from all the disciplines involved in rehabilitation of people who experience stroke. Patients and families also played a role in the development process. Thus, this guideline includes recommendations specific to speech pathology practice in a multidisciplinary context across the continuum from acute care to community rehabilitation and across the subspecialities of aphasia, dysphagia, dysarthria, apraxia and cognitive impairment. Similarly, clinical guidelines for the management of the late talking child would include liaison with maternal and child health nurses, paediatricians and general practitioners; professional voice care would include liaison with ENT specialists, speech pathologists, singers, voice and singing teachers, gastroenterologists, physiotherapists and surgeons.

When developing guidelines, there should be a statement in the text about the level, quality, relevance and strength of evidence and the recommendations should reflect this statement. Because the evidence in speech pathology subspecialities is variable, turning this into a clinically useful recommendation will depend on the judgement, good sense and the skill of the guideline developers.

In May 1998 the RCSLT published a set of guidelines entitled *Clinical Guidelines by Consensus for Speech and Language Therapists* (RCSLT, 1998). The guidelines were the culmination of three years' work and were based where possible on existing research and the knowledge and experience of clinicians and practitioners. The *Guidelines* state that 'where research evidence does not yet exist consensus advice of the highest standard is available to improve the quality of care offered to users of all speech and language therapy services'. When publishing the *Guidelines* the RCSLT undertook to expand and review them in 2001. The *Guidelines* covered eight areas, including:

- adults with acquired dysphasia
- adult dysphagia
- cleft palate and velopharyngeal anomalies
- clinical voice disorder (dysphonia)
- dysarthria
- fluency disorders
- pre-school children with speech and language disorders
- school-aged children with speech and language disorders.

To our knowledge these are the only guidelines developed by a professional speech pathology body. SPAA has published position papers, but the guidelines contained in the position papers were based mainly on the knowledge and experience of practitioners rather than on evaluations of research evidence. In the introduction to the RCSLT *Guidelines* the methodology used is explained fully and, in general, follows the principles outlined above, although clear statements are not made about the strength and quality of the evidence underpinning the guidelines in each subspeciality.

Clinical guidelines are important, not only because they are one of the keys to effective clinical practice but because they help to bridge some of the barriers outlined in Chapter 13. For example, if developed in accordance with agreed procedures, clinical guidelines bring benefits to all aspects of clinical care. Some of these benefits include the following.

- Reducing the amount of time spent searching for the evidence because best practice guidelines are based on the best available evidence following a systematic review and a critical appraisal.
- Providing a collection of evidence that may have been gathered from diverse sources. (Diversity of sources is often cited as a barrier.)
- Providing advice where evidence is limited or unavailable, of poor quality or conflicting because in such situations the views of experts, patients and other professionals' experience would be taken into account to form a consensus.
- Improving patient care by streamlining referral and discharge processes (adapted from the Healthcare Bulletin; NIH, 1994).
- Encouraging patient participation in the clinical decision-making process (adapted from the Healthcare Bulletin; NIH, 1994).
- Promoting best practice by providing criteria or standards against which care may be monitored (for example, clinical and quality audit) (adapted from the Healthcare Bulletin; NIH, 1994).

Information about the development of clinical guidelines may be obtained from a variety of sources, including documents published by the Health Advisory Committee of the National Health and Medical Research Council (NHMRC); the UK NHS briefing documents and the JAMA guides, in particular, Eddy (1990), Hayward et al. (1995) and Barratt et al. (1999).

A word of warning: guidelines can be dangerous if they are 'set in stone' and not reviewed on a regular basis in line with emerging evidence. As indicated in the RCSLT *Guidelines*, review dates must be set and updates published. (For a full discussion on the advantages and disadvantages of guidelines see Macdonald, 2001.)

Speech pathology professional bodies have a responsibility to become involved in the development of clinical guidelines such as those developed by the RCSLT. They should also look to the examples set by other professional bodies (for example, the Royal College of Paediatrics and Child Health in the UK; the American Academy of Pediatrics and the Canadian Task Force) in developing guidelines, and critically appraised topics for distribution among members. Physiotherapists in Australia have developed PEDro, the Physiotherapy Evidence Database (http://ptwww.cchs.usyd.edu.au/CEBP/), which is an initiative of the Centre for Evidence-Based Physiotherapy (CEBP) in Sydney. The rationale behind the development of the database was to provide 'rapid access to bibliographic details and abstracts of randomised controlled trials and systematic reviews in physiotherapy'. The majority of trials on the database have undergone 'quality control' to allow readers to discriminate quickly 'between trials which are likely to be valid and interpretable and those which are not'.

Professional bodies must also undergo the cultural change needed in order to become an evidence-based profession and be prepared to set standards, not only in the continuing professional education of its members but also in setting the research agenda.

Universities: education and research

For the speech pathology profession to produce evidence-based practitioners, attention will have to be paid to education methods. How many undergraduate courses contain more than a cursory lecture (or two) on evidence-based practice? Are lecture streams underpinned by evidence-based practice or do they continue to be based on 'expert opinion'? In Chapter 13, Rose and Baldac discussed the preparation of undergraduates so that they understand and use the principles of evidence-based practice. The authors pointed out that curricula consistent with evidence-based practice processes need to be developed and indicate that application of problem-based learning principles provides a mechanism to accomplish this outcome.

Problem-based learning

The compatibility between the principles of problem-based learning and those of evidence-based practice is compelling. In Chapter 1 five steps to becoming an evidence-based practitioner were outlined (Sackett et al., 1997):

- convert a clinical need into an answerable question
- search for and find the best evidence
- critically evaluate the evidence
- apply the results to your practice
- evaluate your performance.

The typical sequence of steps associated with problem-based learning is outlined in Table 14.2. Clearly, all five steps described by Sackett et al. (1997)

Table 14.2 Typical sequence of steps in problem-based learning

Steps	Associated questions
Trigger/clinical scenario	What is the trigger for the clinical case? *Note:* the trigger/clinical scenario can relate to any aspect of practice: diagnosis, management, service delivery, research, professional development or education
Identify cues	What have you observed?
Formulate problem(s)	What is the problem (something that needs further clarification, attention, analysis, etc.)? How would you prioritize these problems?
Generate hypotheses	What are the possible causes for the problem? How would you prioritize these hypotheses? *Note:* Use broad categories to begin with. One hypothesis may explain several problems
Explain hypotheses	Why have you chosen these hypotheses? What is your thinking process? How does your hypothesis lead to (or cause) the problem? *Note:* This is a key step. It leads to recall and application of prior knowledge and generation of questions as students reach the limitation of their understanding
Identify learning issues	What information is needed to help make one of your hypotheses more or less likely? Do you need knowledge of mechanisms, functions, processes, treatment, research designs, etc.? Do you need history information, test results, language/speech sample, etc.? How will the information obtained help you assess the likelihood of your hypotheses?
Obtain new information and plan enquiry	How will you get the information? How will you plan the inquiry and identify resources?
Individual study	What learning issues will individual/group study be guided by? What information and evidence can you gather and share?
Generate and evaluate solutions	Based on the information and evidence you have gathered, what solutions can you generate and evaluate?
Solution/decision	What is the best possible solution or decision you can reach?
Summary	What were the learning objectives/issues that were met/not met?
Evaluation	How did the group process work for this problem?

are involved in this process. The use of problem-based learning provides students at all levels of training with an opportunity to develop their professional knowledge base and skills using a process that prepares graduates for life-long learning and self-assessment in their professional practice. Problem-based learning is certainly not new and has been used in medical curricula since the 1960s. However, comprehensive problem-based learning curricula have only recently been introduced into speech pathology training (for example, Bachelor of Speech Pathology programme, Hong Kong, 1998; Master of Speech Pathology programme, La Trobe University, Australia, 2000). Ongoing evaluation and the development of training programmes are essential ingredients for the development of an evidence-based practice culture in speech pathology.

Continuing professional education

Continuing professional education events include conferences, workshops and special interest groups. Education occurs through the dissemination of material in journal articles and publications in professional magazines. Strong evidence has emerged to suggest that even when clinicians do their very best to keep up to date, these traditional education methods do not necessarily result in improved learning outcomes (Davis et al., 1995; Thompson et al., 1998). used the randomized controlled trial to test the efficacy of continuing education programmes for doctors. These authors discovered that traditional methods in common use failed to modify clinical performance, although there was no doubt that traditional methods increased the knowledge level of the participants substantially (Davis et al., 1995). There was minimal carryover into patient care and clinical decision-making. The researchers concluded that traditional methods of clinical education were judged ineffective in improving the health outcomes of the patients concerned and did not address the problem of declining clinical competence.

None of the above findings are surprising when they are considered alongside the findings of the studies discussed earlier (Metcalfe et al., 2001; Brener et al., 2003). Even when research evidence is primarily disseminated through journal articles, many clinicians may have problems interpreting the research findings. In addition, some clinicians do not consider reading about research as important as treating patients. Yet if we are to meet the aim stated at the outset of this chapter, 'every level of clinical service will be informed by scientifically derived findings', then reading, interpreting and applying research findings to clinical practice must be seen as an integral part of clinical practice – not as a separate activity. Closing this gap will be a major challenge.

Some effective strategies have been identified that may be used to close the gap between research and clinical practice. These involve active implementation that includes outreach visits, the development of 'local opinion leaders', prompts and reminders, patient-mediated interventions and multifaceted interventions (Davis et al., 1995; Thomson et al., 1998). Current styles of continuing professional education need to be examined to take account of these findings. The evidence regarding educational approaches should be integrated into continuing professional education events. Clearly, this is not the sole responsibility of universities, rather it is the joint responsibility of all organizations involved.

Research

Research questions are often generated from clinical practice (through client contacts and discussion with others). In order to generate, shape and answer such questions, an interface is required between an academic (usually based in a university) and a clinical department (where patient access will be facilitated). This will help to shape the question and focus the hypotheses, and crucially, choose the appropriate design and methods. Interaction between the clinical and academic departments is crucial at every step. Dissemination of the results will be through both academics and clinicians and channelled into undergraduate teaching, continuing professional education events and publication of findings in journals. For this cycle to be dynamic and successful, it is essential that the triage of teaching, clinical service and research roles of the profession are equally valued.

There has been a move toward the conduct of research that is clinically relevant. To achieve this many countries have established national research policies to ensure research has clinical relevance. One example is the NHS Research and Development (R&D) programme in the UK, which has led to greater involvement of clinicians in setting research priorities and also led to the establishment of a programme to evaluate different methods of promoting the implementation of research findings. The concept of 'payback' on research has been developed, resulting in a framework that may be used to assess the benefits that arise from research programmes.

The speech pathology profession has responsibility at all levels to influence the development of research policies. This may begin with lobbying of the need for systematic reviews in specific areas of speech pathology.

Employers: employing bodies and clinical managers

Two recent studies in nursing (Caine and Kendrick, 1997; Closs et al., 2000) examined the barriers to evidence-based practice in nursing practice. The findings suggested that clinical managers need to be involved in facilitating change because extrinsic organizational barriers exist that may prevent the implementation of evidence-based practice. This is exemplified in a study by

Rousseau et al. (2001) that investigated the use of a well-known intervention programme (the Lidcombe programme) for young stutterers by speech pathologists in Australia. As explained in Chapter 1, the researchers set out to ascertain the extent to which the Lidcombe programme was used, as well as to determine the level of satisfaction among users and uncover potential barriers to its use. Only half of the clinicians questioned reported that they used the programme as recommended, largely because of workplace restrictions. Specifically, service delivery was set up to offer a prescribed number of sessions, not necessarily on a weekly basis as recommended in the programme. Furthermore, the Lidcombe programme also exceeded the time allocated per case and therefore was not delivered as recommended, nor as had been shown to be effective in published studies. Clearly, the evidence was not getting into practice because of what Caine and Kendrick (1997) and Closs et al. (2000) describe as 'extrinsic' organisational or service barriers.

The benefits of evidence-based clinical guidelines: a scenario

Evidence-based clinical guidelines are necessary for the development and planning of clinical services. Imagine that you are the manager of an inner city community centre with mixed social demographics but little cultural diversity. The results of the survey about the use of the Lidcome programme (Rousseau et al., 2001) have been fed back to you. You talk to your line manager, who is not particularly helpful and says, *'There aren't any more resources you will just have to make do'*, and adds, *'Don't think of lengthening the waiting list.'* In a throwaway line your manager mutters something about following your clinical practice guidelines. The message is clear: sort it out. You are newly arrived in your post and there are no clinical guidelines as yet.

Consultation with your professional body reveals the lack of a national guideline in this subspeciality. You talk to your colleagues who give you some literature on guideline development and generously loan you some of their local examples in other subspecialities. How would you go about the development of a guideline regarding best practice for intervention with pre-school children who stutter and require speech pathology services? There are numerous steps involved and readers are directed to numerous documents on guideline development (see pp. 338–41).

The following steps would be required.

- Define the problem. What is stuttering in pre-school children? How many pre-school children begin to stutter? How many recover? How many require treatment?
- Define best practice. This will begin with an appraisal of the literature to identify if any guidelines already exist, if there are any systematic reviews,

randomized controlled trials or other treatment trials to guide practice. If a guideline already exists you might decide to adopt that or adapt it for use in your setting. You will also appraise any other evidence that exists or has been published recently and may not therefore be included in the existing guidelines or review. Each of the questions raised in defining the problem will need to be considered as there will almost certainly be different types of services required (for example, monitoring versus intensive treatment).

- Define the resources that are required to meet best practice in each of these areas. First, the epidemiology of the 'population', preschool stutterers, should be considered; for example, how many preschool children stutter and how many require treatment? The staff required to deliver the treatment (recommended in defining the problem) may be estimated along with the need to involve other multidisciplinary professionals in service delivery. At the same time any external influences and resources required, such as special equipment, will also need to be considered.
- How does current clinical practice compare to best practice as defined in your guideline?
- What changes would need to be made in order to meet best practice?
- What are the implications of such changes? Can they be met within current service provision or will this require negotiation with other services and with your line manager?

The development of best practice clinical guidelines often highlights discrepancies between current practice and best practice. Once guidelines are developed, a criterion-based audit may be implemented. This type of audit uses the guideline as the standard against which practice may be benchmarked or measured. For example, if best practice, as indicated in the guideline, stipulates 11 sessions, then it is relatively easy to measure this against what each pre-school child might receive in your service. The information from the research project (Rousseau et al., 2001) suggested that only four to six sessions were available per child. This results in a number of problems rather than solutions. In auditing clinical service delivery, however, you may uncover inefficiencies or areas where resources might be employed differently and in a more cost-efficient manner. For example, a telephone monitoring service for children who begin to stutter may reduce the need to assess each child individually as some may have recovered by the time they receive an assessment. It may also be possible to fast-track children at higher risk (for example, family history of stuttering) who might be predicted to recover spontaneously. However, in the scenario described above it appears that an increase in resources may be required and, although your line manager may not appreciate it, lengthening waiting lists may be inevitable. Is there any benefit to delivering poor or inadequate treatment (in this case fewer sessions than have been shown to be effective) and what costs are involved?

Clinical managers have considerable responsibilities in ensuring that their services are designed to promote rather than hinder evidence-based practice. As well as tackling service delivery issues they must also ensure that the facilities and support are in place to facilitate evidence-based practice. This includes providing access for staff to the online databases they require, and assessing and monitoring the training staff need to become evidence-based practitioners (such as library training in searching, research and methods training). In addition, value must be attached to finding, appraising and valuing research to overcome the barriers cited in the study by Metcalfe et al. (2001). In particular, it is crucial to ensure that clinicians consider the interpretation and application of research to their practice as being as important as treating patients (as highlighted earlier). Ultimately it is the manager's responsibility to ensure that clinicians are equipped to become participants in, and users of, research even though they may never be active researchers.

Clinicians

The clinician's responsibility, as highlighted in the four steps proposed by Sackett et al. (1997) (see Chapter 13), seems a relatively simple one. However, time, skill and expertise is required to formulate clinical questions and search for evidence. It is critical appraisal that presents the greatest challenge to clinicians in all professions; that is, appraisal of the validity and importance of the evidence found. As highlighted by Metcalfe et al. (2001), the majority of clinicians have problems accessing and understanding the literature and its implications for practice. (Fault may also lie with the authors of the papers who may not make the implications clear.) In order to be evidence-based practitioners clinicians need to be able to:

- find, read and interpret published research
- identify learning needs (for example, literature searching, research methodology, etc.)
- keep up to date
- integrate research findings with practice
- implement research findings
- take every opportunity to influence management about areas of practice that are not evidence-based
- conduct audit and measure outcomes
- develop clinical questions that need to be researched and discuss how these might be answered with academic colleagues

- develop stronger links with the nearest university department – encourage honours and research students to conduct clinical research in your department, hospital or centre.

There is no doubt that many clinicians will require in-service training and continuing education on research design and methodology, and library training to meet these needs.

Conclusion: how is the profession going to achieve these aims?

There is a variety of methods through which the speech pathology profession could respond to the challenges outlined in this chapter. It requires a coordinated and strategic effort from all the branches of the profession and strong professional leadership (see roles and responsibilities in Table 14.3). Collaborations with other international speech pathology professional bodies may facilitate the process.

Professional bodies have a responsibility to influence and reinforce a culture of evidence-based practice both nationally and internationally. It is disappointing that, unlike our colleagues in nursing and physiotherapy for example, no such visible initiatives exist in speech pathology. Clear statements are needed from professional bodies about evidence-based practice. There may be benefits to joining our colleagues in nursing and other allied health professions to lobby government concerning the need to overcome barriers to evidence-based practice within the professions.

The speech pathology profession must set a clear research agenda for the profession and identify research priorities. In Table 14.1 two research priorities from the subspecialities reviewed in Part Two of this book were identified. Such priority areas should be communicated by speech pathologists to all relevant funding bodies and potential collaborators. It is only through such methods that the profession will influence funding bodies and key decision-makers.

Conducting research within discipline-specific 'silos' is no longer feasible or desirable. Strong multidisciplinary collaborations are essential; it is at the intersection of disciplines that the future scientific advances in speech pathology will be made. However, such collaborations should be under the leadership of speech pathologists. Because the cycle of research is dependent on a successful clinical practice–research–teaching interface, it is important that research is clinically relevant and not conducted in 'ivory towers'. Lastly, it is vital that the profession pays attention to the methodological shortcomings that have bedevilled the quality of evidence in the profession.

Table 14.3 Roles and responsibilities in moving towards a culture of evidence-based practice in speech pathology

	Professional bodies	Universities		Clinical managers	Clinicians
		Researchers	Educators		
Adopt and foster a culture of evidence-based practice	✔	✔	✔	✔	✔
Train in research methods and searching skills	✔	✔	✔	✔	✔
Change the format and structure of continuing professional education	✔	✔	✔	✔	✔
Add 'value' to the time needed to become an evidence-based practitioner	✔			✔	
Incorporate reading the literature as part of the 'treatment' of each patient	✔		✔	✔	✔
Ensure facilities and resources available in workplace	✔			✔	✔
Develop evidence-based clinical guidelines and critically appraised topics	✔	✔	✔	✔	✔
Adapt learning style to incorporate 'life-long learning skills' rather than reliance on 'expert' teaching	✔	✔	✔	✔	✔

If the profession is serious about the adoption of evidence-based practice then it is essential that educational 'culture' is addressed both at undergraduate and postgraduate levels. Evidence-based practitioners are life-long learners and it is this attribute that we need to promote in our graduates.

The current separation that exists for some clinicians between treating patients and using research, needs to be closed. This begins in the university but should continue into the workplace and be promoted by professional bodies. There is strong evidence that we need to change the way we currently disseminate research information and conduct continuing education events.

In 1999 the NHS R&D Centre for Evidence Based Medicine in Oxford (www.jr2.ox.ac.uk/cebm) identified several areas requiring further development. These areas include the need to:

- understand better how clinicians seek information and the factors that influence and limit the application of knowledge, once found, to changing practice
- continue to develop innovative (going beyond paper to CD, websites, video clips, and so forth) evidence-based, patient-care guides for frontline health professionals in all disciplines
- promote ways to integrate evidence into information systems that can support the decisions of patients and practitioners
- understand better how health professionals, patients and managers understand, value and use evidence in decisions
- encourage researchers who are interested in studying these problems.

These areas remain relevant for speech pathologists. We do have some information about the knowledge and attitudes of our profession towards evidence-based practice but we need to better understand the barriers and determine if the same strategies used in medicine and nursing to overcome these will be effective in speech pathology.

The challenges that lie ahead in establishing the evidence base for the subspecialities within speech pathology are huge but not insurmountable. The challenges are exciting and will establish firmly the knowledge base upon which our profession rests. In this book we have exposed readers to the arguments for and against evidence-based practice, provided convincing arguments as to why evidence-based practice should be taken seriously, evaluated the evidence in some of the speech pathology subspecialities and outlined the future challenges for the profession. It is now the responsibility of each individual to take up these challenges.

References

Barratt A, Irwig L, Glasziou P, Cumming RG, Raffle A, Hicks N Gray JA, Guyatt GH. How to use guidelines and recommendations about screening. The Evidence-Based Medicine Working Group. JAMA 1999; 281: 2029–2034.

Brener L, Vallino-Napoli L, Reid J, Reilly S. Accessing the evidence to treat the dysphagic patient: can we get it? Is there time? Asia Pacific Journal of Speech Language and Hearing 2003; 8: 36-43.

Caine C, Kendrick M. The role of clinical directorate managers in facilitating evidence-based practice: a report of an exploratory study. Journal of Nursing Management 1997; 5: 157-65.

Closs SJ, Baum G, Bryar RM, Griffiths J, Knight S. Barriers to research implementation in two Yorkshire hospitals. Clinical Effectiveness in Nursing 2000; 4: 3-10.

Davis DA, Thomson MA, Oxman AD, Haynes RB. Changing physician performance: a systematic review of the effect of continuing medical education strategies. JAMA 1995; 274: 700-5.

Eddy DM. Clinical decision making: from theory to practice. Designing a practice policy. Standards, guidelines and options. JAMA 1990; 263: 3077, 3081, 3084.

Giacomini MK, Cook DJ. Users' guides to the medical literature: XXIII. Qualitative research in health care A. Are the results of the study valid? Evidence-Based Medicine Working Group. JAMA 2000; 284: 357-62.

Gresham GE, Duncan PW, Stason WB et al. Post-Stroke Rehabilitation, Clinical Practice Guideline No. 16. AHCPR Publication No. 95-0662. Rockville, MD: US Department of Health and Human Services. Public Health Service, Agency for Health Care Policy and Research, 1995.

Guyatt G, Rennie D (eds). The Users' Guides to the Medical Literature: A Manual for Evidence-Based Clinical Practice. Chicago, IL: American Medical Association, 2002.

Hayward RS, Wilson MC, Tunis SR, Bass EB, Guyatt G. How to use clinical practice guidelines. A. Are the recommendations valid? The Evidence-Based Medicine Working Group. JAMA 1995; 274: 570-4.

Macdonald G. Assessing systematic reviews and clinical guidelines. In: Moyer VA, Elliott EJ, Davis RL, Gilbert R, Klassen T, Logan S et al. (eds). Evidence Based Paediatrics and Child Health. London: BMJ Books, 2001.

Mead J. Developing, disseminating and implementing clinical guidelines. In: Bury T, Mead J (eds). Evidence Based Health Care: A Practical Guide for Therapists. Oxford: Butterworth Heinemann, 1998.

Metcalfe C, Lewin R, Wisher S, Perry S, Bannigan K, Moffett JK. Barriers to implementing the evidence base in four NHS therapies: dietitians, occupational therapists, physiotherapists, speech and language therapists. Physiotherapy 2001; 87: 433-41.

National Health Service Executive. Clinical Guidelines: Using Clinical Guidelines to Improve Patient Care within the NHS. Leeds: NHS Executive, 1996.

Nuffield Institute for Health (NIH). Effective Health Care Bulletins 8. Implementing Clinical Practice Guidelines: Can Guidelines be used to Improve Clinical Practice? University of Leeds, Nuffield Institute for Health, Centre for Health Economics; University of York: the NHS Centre for Reviews and Dissemination; London: Royal College of Physicians, 1994.

Rousseau I, Onslow M, Packman A, Robinson R. The Lidcombe program in Australia. In: Onslow M, Packman A, Harrison E (eds). The Lidcombe Program of Early Stuttering Interventions: A Clinicians' Guide. Austin, TX: Pro-Ed Rousseau, 2001.

Royal College of Speech and Language Therapists (RCSLT). Clinical Guidelines by Consensus for Speech and Language Therapists. London: RCSLT, 1998.

Sackett D, Scott Richardson W, Rosenberg W, Hynes R. Evidence Based Medicine. How to Practice and Teach EBM. New York, NY: Churchill Livingstone, 1997.

Thomson MA, Oxman AD, Davis D. Outreach visits to improve health care, professional practice and health care outcomes. In: Berow L, Grilli R, Grimshaw J, Oxman A (eds). Cochrane Collaboration on Effective Professional Practice module of the Co rane database of systematic reviews. The Cochrane Collaboration, Issue 1. Oxford: Update Software, 1998.

Index